H. O. Vetter, R. Hetzer, H. Schmutzler (Eds.)

Ischemic Mitral Incompetence

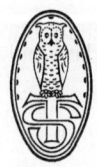 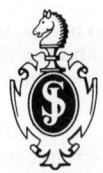

Springer-Verlag Berlin Heidelberg GmbH

Die Herausgeber:
Dr. H. O. Vetter
Ludwig-Maximilians-Universität
Klinikum Großhadern
Marchioninistraße 15
8000 München 70

Prof. Dr. R. Hetzer
Deutsches Herzzentrum Berlin
Augustenburger Platz 1
1000 Berlin 65

Prof. Dr. H. Schmutzler
Freie Universität Berlin
Universitätsklinikum Rudolf Virchow
Spanndauer Damm 130
1000 Berlin 19

CIP-Titelaufnahme der Deutschen Bibliothek

Ischemic mitral incompetence / H. O. Vetter ... (eds.). —
Darmstadt : Steinkopff ; New York : Springer, 1991

ISBN 978-3-662-08029-0   ISBN 978-3-662-08027-6 (eBook)
DOI 10.1007/978-3-662-08027-6

NE: Vetter, Herbert O. [Hrsg.]

Copyright © 1991 by Springer-Verlag Berlin Heidelberg
Originally published by Dr. Dietrich Steinkopff Verlag GmbH & Co. KG, Darmstadt in 1991.
Softcover reprint of the hardcover 1st edition 1991
Medical Editorial: Sabine Müller — English Editor: James C. Willis — Production: Heinz J. Schäfer

Preface

The International Symposium on Ischemic Mitral Incompetence was held December 2–4, 1988 at the Intercontinental Hotel, Berlin. It was organized by the German Heart Center Berlin with the primary aim to bring together experts interested in the subject of ischemic mitral regurgitation.

Our intention was to face the problems associated with diagnosis and treatment of mitral incompetence resulting from coronary artery disease. A "work-up" of the whole topic from its basic, diagnostic, and surgical aspects was initiated. In the first section we concentrate on the basic anatomical and pathophysiological knowledge, as well as on experimental work. In the second section cardiologists report on incidence of ischemic mitral incompetence, diagnostic methods that include esophageal echocardiography, follow-up studies of medical- and surgical-treated patients. This section considers interventional therapy in acute myocardial infarction, as well. The third section includes contributions by cardiac surgeons with many years' experience in operative treatment of ischemic mitral incompetence including the decision-making criteria for non-mitral valve surgery, and for valve reconstruction or replacement.

There are controversial aspects, such as indications for performing valve procedures in patients with moderate regurgitation who will undergo coronary revascularization. (Generally, our group has performed mitral valve reconstruction whenever possible.) However, with increasing numbers of operations at our Institute – from April 1986 to November 1988, we performed 3012 coronary artery bypass operations, 247 mitral valve replacements, and 111 mitral valve reconstructions – we have been increasingly confronted with the problems of ischemic mitral incompetence. It seems to us that reparative techniques, as usually used in rheumatic and degenerative mitral regurgitation, are not always applicable in ischemic mitral regurgitation. The lively discussion during the symposium revealed controversial points in this field of cardiac surgery; existing concepts thus became more clear.

The Berlin symposium brought together anatomists, physiologists, pathologists, cardiologists, experimental and cardiac surgeons from America, Belgium, Czechoslovakia, Denmark, France, Germany, Holland, Hungary, Italy, Poland, Saudi Arabia, Spain, Sweden, Switzerland, the United Kingdom, and Yugoslavia. We have included their stimulating discussions at the end of each section of this book.

A video- and poster session chaired by Drs. Frater and Fleck contained a number of excellent experimental and clinical works on ischemic mitral incompetence, but could not be included in this book. This proceedings volume includes one contribution which was not read at the symposium: Dr. R. Heuser, who has great experience in coronary angioplasty for acute mitral regurgitation due to myocardial infarction, was asked to submit a related article.

The authors thank the following persons for their help in organizing the symposium and preparing this book: Mrs. E. Kargl, Mrs. S. Müller, Miss M. Wendemuth, Mr. H. Haselbach, and Mr. M. Schwab.

This book represents the current knowledge on ischemic mitral incompetence. Our hope is that the reader will gain valuable information for the benefit of patients.

Berlin, September 1990

Roland Hetzer
Herbert O. Vetter
Horst Schmutzler

Foreword

While much progress has been made in the surgical treatment of mitral incompetence due to rheumatic valvulitis or degenerative prostheses, our understanding
and successful management of ischmemic mitral incompetence is still in an early
and primitive stage. Thus, the symposium on ischemic mitral insufficiency held in
Berlin in 1988, from which this book is derived represents an important step forward in our quest to treat this condition.

International in scope, the book assembles an up-to-date analysis on multiple
aspects of the problem from basic anatomy and physiology to diagnosis and treatment methods, and finally, to surgical indications.

A confluence of multiple development pathways lend timeliness to this analysis.
First, the availability of conventional, esophageal, and epicardial Doppler Echo to
unravel the complex interaction of muscle function in valvular performance in the
living patient; second, the growing sophistication of our surgical abilities in mitral
repair according to the concepts and techniques of Carpentier and others; third, the
greater understanding of ischemic heart disease derived from as mass experience,
both with coronary angioplasty and coronary artery bypass; and in addition the
development of information systems for the long-term tracking of such patients
over the course of decades. What emerges is an authoritative, albeit first approxi-
mation of this complex entity from reversible mitral incompetence associated with
angina or silent ischemia to end-stage, and irreversible ischemic cardiomyopathy in
which the mitral insufficiency is an associated finding.

We became interested in this problem in the early 1980s and first published on
this topic in 1984. We were, therefore, delighted to participate with the auhtors
whom we have known and admired over the past decade. A review of the text
which incorporates our own studies from Oregon provides some significant insights
into ischemic mitral incompetence, it is importance as a powerful prognostic indicator, the importance of right coronary artery occlusion common in a large portion
of these patients, and the possibility of prevention with early and aggressive revascularization. The treatment by revascularization alone in mild mitral incompetence
is now well established. The role of valve replacement versus repair in severe mitral
incompetence is discussed extensively in the text with consideration of multiple
clinical and anatomic variables.

The reader will find this volume an important landmark along the pathway to our
better understanding of ischemic mitral incompetence.

A. Starr, Portland/Oregon

Contents

I. Basic aspects

Functional anatomy of the myocardium and its interaction with the mitral valve apparatus

Anatomy of the coronary arteries with respect to chronic ischemic mitral regurgitation

Transmitral flow dynamics in the normal heart and during mitral regurgitation

Influence of papillary muscle function on the mitral valve and left ventricular mechanics

II. Diagnosis and indications for treatment

Predictors for mitral regurgitation in coronary artery disease

The influence of revascularization on ischemic mitral insufficiency

III. Surgical aspects

I. Basic aspects

Functional anatomy of the myocardium and its interaction with the mitral valve apparatus

A. Puff

Anatomical Institute, University of Freiburg, Freiburg i. Br., FRG

Introduction

The pathophysiology of "ischemic mitral incompetence" is based on a number of different factors. So far as function is concerned, the morphological structure of the valve, the papillary muscles, and also the whole myocardium — as well as the coronary system and the supporting connective tissue — must all be taken into account.

The heart as a functional unit

The heart is an organ which must be seen as a functional unit, and in health its structural elements work together to bring about a single purposeful result. The links of the functional chain influence each other, and a disturbance of one link affects the whole system. The connective tissue framework enables the myocardium to cooperate functionally with the coronary and valvular apparatus.

To understand this mechanism fully it is not only necessary to know how the ventricles themselves act, but also to have a clear picture of the morphological structures underlying the function of the heart, and to know how they develop in the embryo.

Sometimes it is difficult to analyze complicated morphological structures and to lay bare an intelligible architecture. That is why it is necessary to start by analyzing the function, and decide later what the structural elements signify. During systole the different parts of the ventricle do not contract simultaneously, but rather according to a certain temporo-spatial plan which starts with the papillary muscles and ends with the contraction of the outflow tract; in other words, the contraction of the inflow and outflow tracts must follow each other — much like a peristaltic wave moving along the main blood pathway through the ventricle — since simultaneous contraction of all the ventricular fibers would result in their individual effects cancelling each other.

It is important to realize that there are morphological differences between the spiral fiber-systems of what we call the inflow and outflow tracts (Fig. 1).

One way of verifying the mechanism outlined above was to analyze ventricular contraction with a high-speed camera [1]. The facts having been revealed by the camera, they could then be followed step-by-step by means of the most modern visualizing techniques, such as nuclear magnetic resonance and echocardiography. The idea that controlling the cups is by itself sufficient to exhaust the action of the papillary muscles is unlikely when seen from the functional point of view.

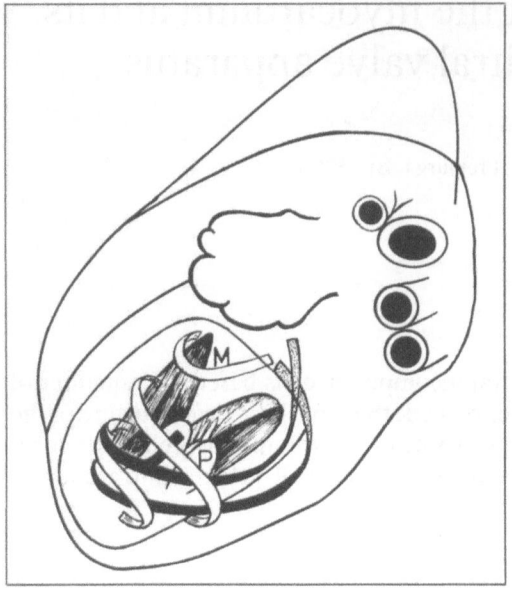

Fig. 1. Left chamber in left lateral view: muscle fiber strands in the outflow tract; muscle fiber strands in the inflow tract; M − mitral valve; p papillary muscle

The vigorous action of both papillary muscle groups − their systolic twisting which brings the lateral wall of the outflow tract into existence − can be palpated in the living ventricle (Fig. 2).

The mechanical unit of the mitral valve apparatus consists of the *valve,* the *fibrous ring,* the *tendin ous cords* and the *papillary muscles* (Fig. 3).

The size of the mitral orifice increases by 20% to 50% between systole and diastole.

This change of width of the mitral orifice during the heart-beat is the primary cause of ischemic mitral incompetence. It must be pointed out that it depends not only upon the musculature and the fibrous ring, but to a high degree on the part played by the morphology of the coronary system in this complex mechanism (Fig. 4).

During the whole of systole as far as the T-wave of the ECG, the arterial ring at the base of the heart receives the central aortic pressure. With the decrease of the T-wave − when the ventricular musculature of the inflow tract is relaxing − the ring is widened by the energy remaining in the coronary arteries. Later on (near the Q-wave) the aortic pressure also decreases, and the expanding pressure in the coronary vascular circle is diminished. The remaining diastolic tension of the ventricular musculature brings about the presystolic diminution of the orifice by its mass alone.

The fibrous skeleton of the heart

Opinions are divided as to the degree of participation of the fibrous ring. However, misunderstanding here is due solely to its false anatomical definition as a "fibrous

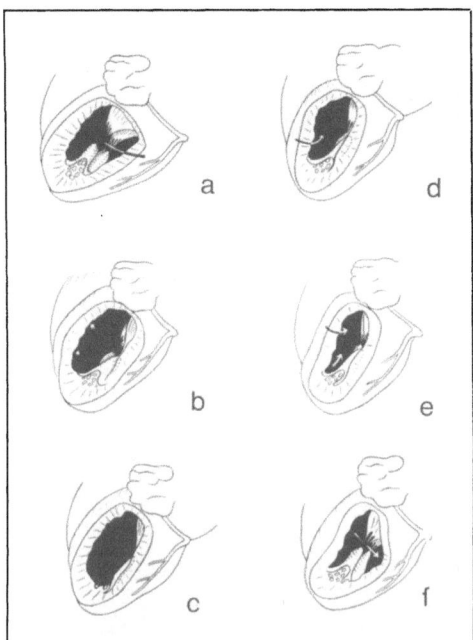

Fig. 2. Systolic phases: a) isovolumetric phase: the blood is shifted from the inflow into the outflow tract; b) distension of the outflow tract and the apex; c) the lateral wall of the outflow tract has come into existence; d) pre-ejection phase; e) ejection phase; f) relaxation of the inflow tract and its distension by the return of remaining blood (Restblut)

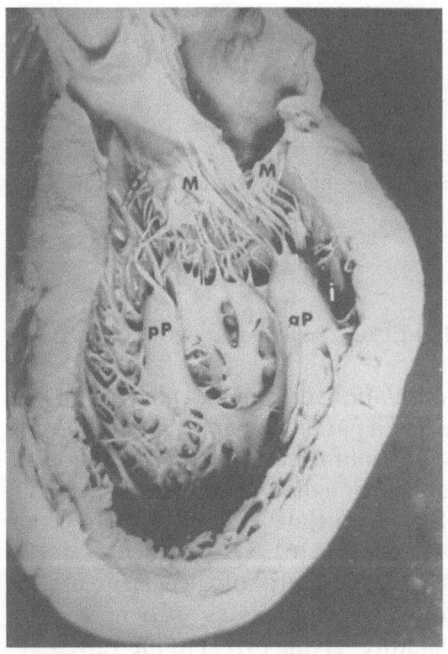

Fig. 3. Left chamber in LAO projection opened by frontal dissection. M – mitral valve; aP – anterior papillary muscle; pP – posterior papillary muscle; i – inflow tract; o – outflow tract

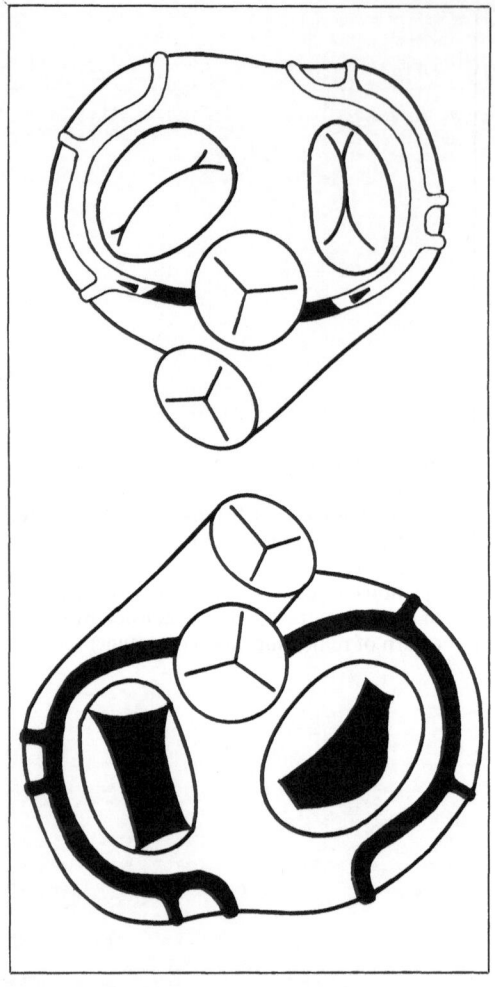

Fig. 4. Widening of the orifices in the ventricular level during the diastolic maximum of the coronary inflow (below)

collagenous ring". Consisting only of parallel fibres, such a ring would be unable either to contract or become wider.

We can now appreciate the morphological situation: only in that area of what we have called the "aortomitral septum" do we find a parallel arrangement of the collagenous fibers (Fig. 5). In the latero-dorsal or mural part of the orifice no ring exists, and the fibers here can only be seen as "intermediate tendons" between different parts of the wall musculature. They form a cruciate trellis which can widen its angles during diastole and close them in systole (Fig. 6) [3].

Such an explanation destroys our picture of these morphological structures as fibrous "rings". They can no longer be regarded as mere masses of connective tissue between the atrial and ventricular musculature, giving origin to the valves.

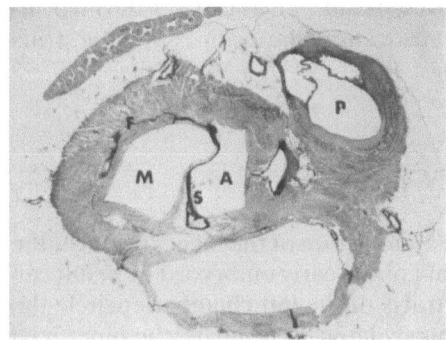

Fig. 5. Horizontal section through the ventricular level: M – mitral orifice; A – base of the aorta; P – pulmonary artery; S – aortomitral septum; F – mitral fibrous "ring"

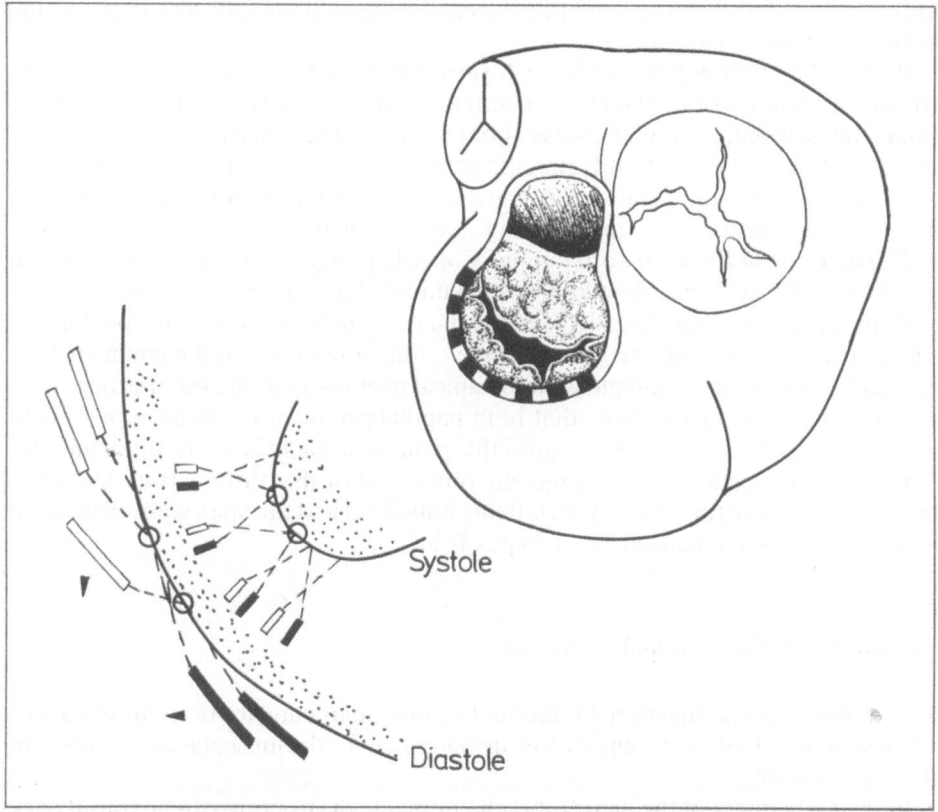

Fig. 6. How the collagenous trellis in the mitral "ring" works and brings about the shortening of the mitral orifice during systole

As ECG surface mapping has revealed, the course of activation over the myocardium is carried across the upper edge of the atrioventricular orifices as if the structure we call the "skeleton of the heart" did not exist.

The functional architecture of the myocardium

These findings impelled us to study anew the architecture of the myocardium of the left chamber in the adult heart as well as in that of the early embryo. The result can be summarized as follows. The spiral fiber tracts of the left chamber encircle the cavity. Most of them originate from the fibrous skeleton of the heart: the superficial ones from the right atrioventricular orifice and the deeper strands from the left fibrous "ring". They can be considered as the special musculature of the left chamber (Eigenmuskulatur). After their course through the wall all fibers run directly or indirectly as tendinous cords back to the fibrous heart base.

In the inflow tract, the muscle fibres form steep spirals. The papillary muscles are composed mainly from the inner, but also partly of the middle layer. The fibers of the anterior papillary muscle are continuous with the circular fiber strands of the outflow tract. This fact has a bearing during the onset of diastole on the expansion of the interpapillary space.

Within the outflow tract, which is formed by the anterior part of the interventricular septum and the neighboring anterior parts of the free wall, most muscle fibers follow a nearly circular course about this part of the cavity. Near the septum, there are some flat fiber strands running parallel to the axis of the outflow tract and anterior interventricular sulcus. They are remnants of the inner longitudinal layer, and mark the border between the inflow and outflow tracts.

The apical root fibers of both papillary muscle groups form a consistent system which, together with the fibers of the deep middle layer, gives rise to the vortex.

Connecting fibers run directly between the two papillary muscle groups (Fig. 7). The upper root fibers of one group turn over the upper edge of the chamber and, descending to the apex, mingle with the apical root fibers of the other group.

This anatomical fact ensures that both papillary muscles are twisted in the late isovolumetric phase, and it is not until this point that the twisting of these muscles during the preejection phase brings the outer wall of the outflow tract into existence. At the same time the vortex is being untwisted and the apex vigorously filled − a process long recognized as the "apex beat".

Development of myocardial structures

These structural and functional relations become clearer and more comprehensible when we take a look at the embryonic development of the muscular architecture of the myocardium.

In the early stages of the heart tube, the principle of structure can be traced back to a system of fiber spirals running in clockwise and anticlockwise directions. The inner one corresponds to the "Konturfasern" [2] in the embryo heart tube. At the

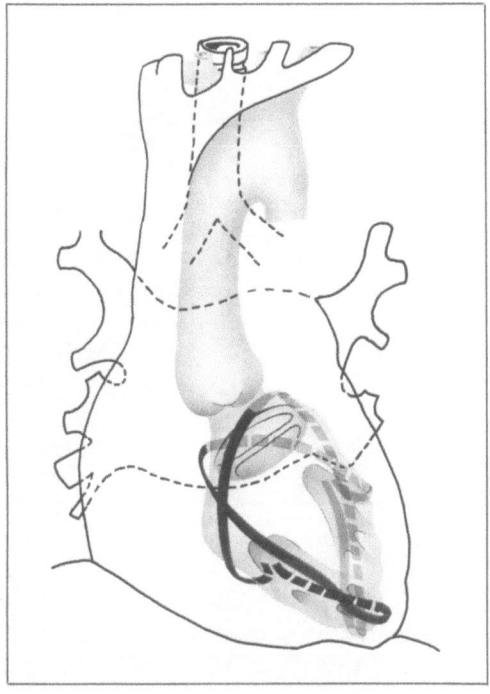

Fig. 7. Fibers connecting both papillary muscles across the heart base and the apex (vortex)

loop stage, the spirals are crowded together at the inside bend of the fold and spread apart at the convexity. The inner system of the papillary muscles and trabeculae is mostly orientated in the direction of the flow-tracts.

Mitral valve

In comparing both cusps of the mitral valve [5], one should observe the loose and almost tender structure of the mural cusp in contrast to the solid felt-like lamella within the anterior cusp. Both cusps are joined with one another by means of anterior and posterior commissures. The mural cusp originates from the posterior and lateral segments of the fibrous skeleton encircling the inflow tract, whereas the anterior cusp is fixed at the so-called "septum aortico-mitrale" – the "free part" of the fibrous ring (Fig. 5). This structure is also a part of the aortic base.

It is very important to observe that the tendinous cords of *both* papillary muscle groups insert into *both* cusps. At the mural valve (Fig. 8), two different groups of tendinous cords can be distinguished: an external group ("annuläre Chorden") travels by the shortest route to the anulus fibrosus, and at the base of the valve there is a tender, flat lamella determining its underlying structure. Another group inserts into the free edge of the valve – the "valvular cords". It includes the cords of the first and second order in the Anglo-American literature, which are connected with one another by arcades.

9

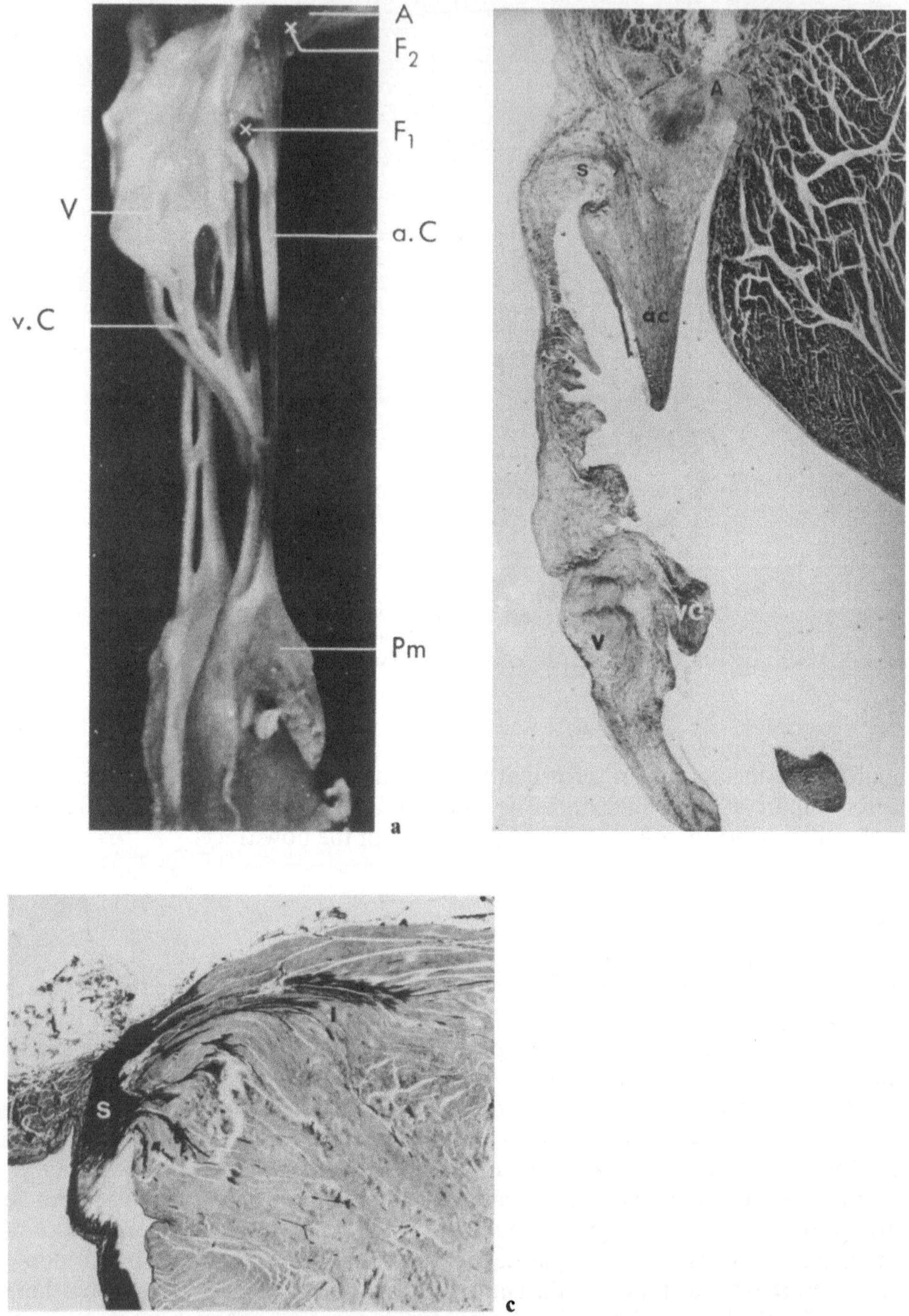

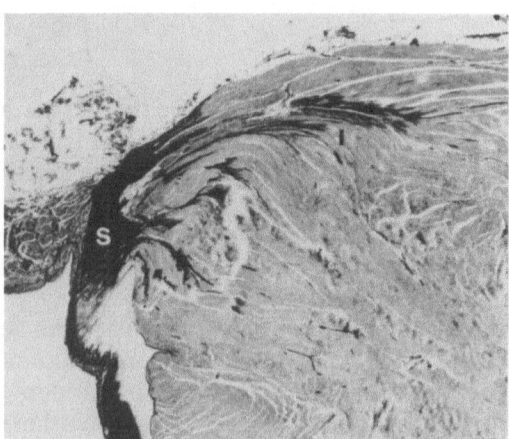

Fig. 8. The posterior (mural) cusp of the mitral valve. a) lateral view; b) longitudinal section; c) muscular insertions into the fibrous skeleton; d) the valvular "joint" (▶) elastic tissue staining. A – anulus fibrosus; F_1 – medial fornix; F_2 – lateral fornix; ac – anular cords; vc – valvular cords; V – valve; Pm – papillary muscle; S – skeleton of the valve bending down into the anular cords

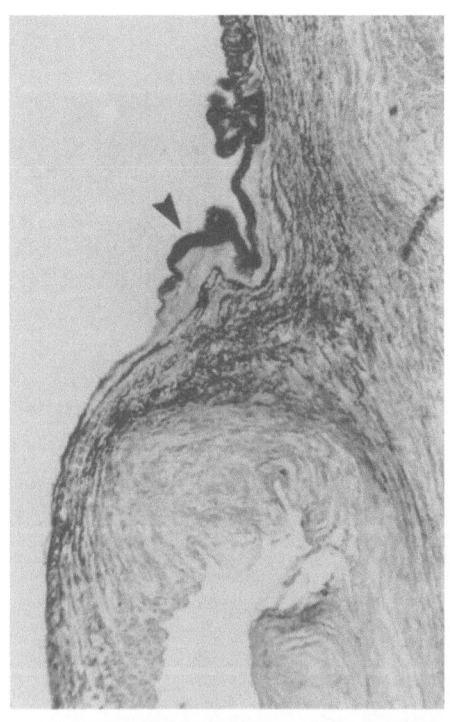

d

In the sagittal section of the *mural cusp* we can distinguish a number of structures. The mass of the connective tissue of the fibrous skeleton is the center of the whole mitral valve apparatus (Fig. 9b). In the direction of the myocardium toward the outer wall the anulus receives the ramifying muscular insertions (Fig. 8c). If one follows the main strands of these tendinous insertions (i.e., about 80% of all fibers), one can see that they bend steeply downwards into the anular cords. The most important observation in this connection is that the fibrous skeleton of the valve does not insert into the anulus directly but surrounds the inner fornix and enters the anular cords. Serial sections have shown no trace of a direct fibrous connection between the fibrous skeleton of the valve and the anulus itself. Near the endocardial surface of the origin of the valve one can see an interesting structure — "the valve joint". The endocardium is thickened here by elastic material and forms a reserve fold for the movement of the valves. Near the free edge of the valve there are regions of brawn-like tissue with little collagen.

We can see quite another scheme of distribution of the cords in the anterior or aortic cusp of the mitral valve. Most of the tendinous cords are inserted into the free edge in several layers, which overlap, one behind the other (Fig. 9).

In the *anterior valve* the valvular skeleton is directly continued into the arotic base. The subendocardial layer at the valvular base is very large, and we can imagine it to be a functional reserve for the valve as it bends during mitral opening and closure.

The *opening* of the mitral orifice is foreshadowed by the diastolic relaxation of the inflow-tract and the passive widening of the ventricular ring, the repul-

11

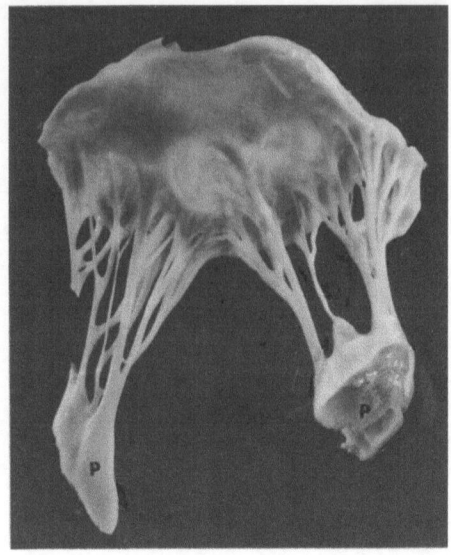

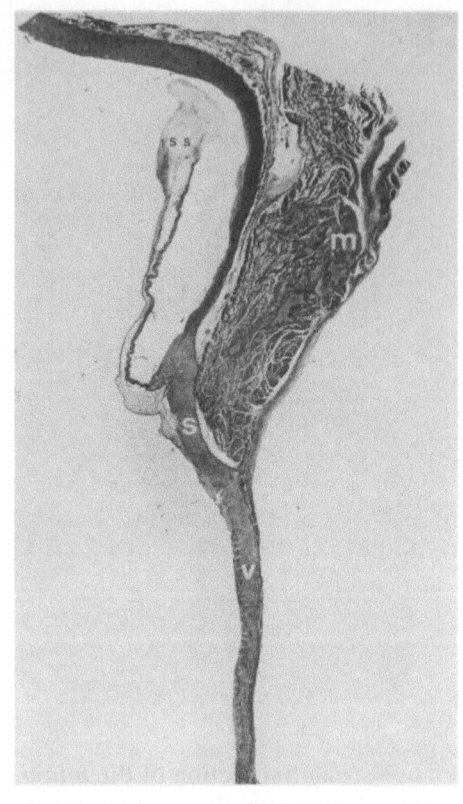

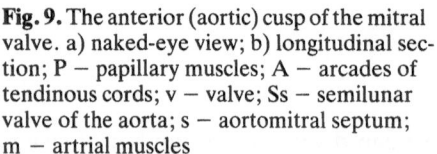

Fig. 9. The anterior (aortic) cusp of the mitral valve. a) naked-eye view; b) longitudinal section; P — papillary muscles; A — arcades of tendinous cords; v — valve; Ss — semilunar valve of the aorta; s — aortomitral septum; m — artrial muscles

sion of the remaining blood ("Restblut") from the outflow tract back into the inflow tract. This mechanism is supported by the diastolic coronary inflow. The ventricular level is elevated and the orifice pushed passively upwards over the blood already in position — much as a sock is pulled on. The opening of the valve seems to be relatively sluggish, and the free edges fall into the ventricular cavity.

In this phase the opened valve produces a funnel-shaped canal. The opening of the valves and the entry of the blood take place before the contraction of the atrium. Synchronous with the P-valve of the ECG, a sharp bend appears at the upper surface of the mural cusp (Fig. 10a) where it can be seen on x-ray; it is caused by the insertion of the atrial musculature into the valve. It somewhat resembles a wet shirt being pulled out of the washtub.

The *closure* of the valve is much more complex, as with a quick lash the free edge of the mural cusp is raised (Fig. 10). The contraction of the papillary muscle in early systole pulls on the anular cords, and simultanously the basic fibers of the skeleton of the valve are drawn in the direction of the apex (Fig. 10b). The blood beneath the valve works like a pivot around which the valve is drawn up. In this phase the interpapillary space is further distended and causes lateral systolic displacement of the wall. The musculature of the inflow tract, having previously been distended by the action, action of the anular cords, now contracts and pushed the blood from the lateral fornix under the free edge of the valve, and in this way completes closure

12

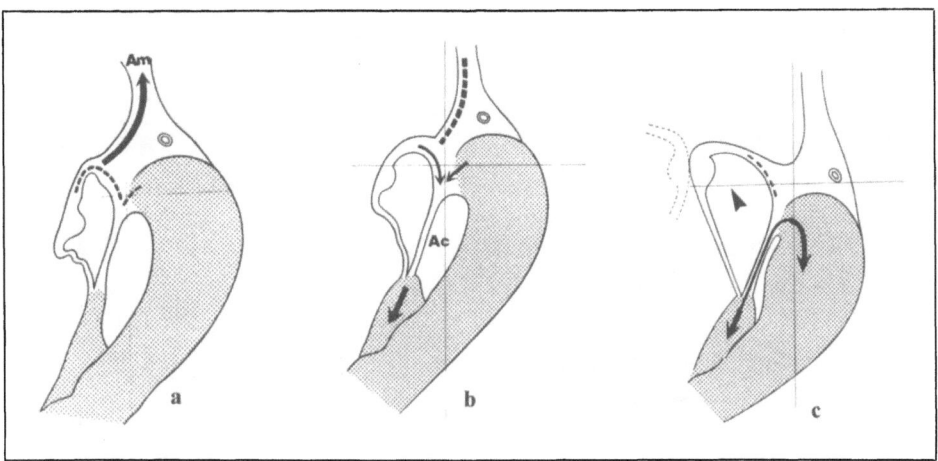

Fig. 10. The mechanism of the mural cusp. a) elevation of valvular base, brought about by the contraction of the atrial musculature Am; b) the papillary muscle pulls on the anular cords Ac and thus unrolls the cusp; c) contraction of the lateral wall

(Fig. 10c). The orifice is further shortened, and the outflow tract is in its turn distended. In the region of the apex this mechanism causes the apex beat. Only now do the valvular cords come under tension to prevent a prolapse of the cusps into the atrium, which would allow mitral regurgitation. For efficient valve function, especially that of the anterior cusp, the systolic twisting of both papillary muscle groups seems to be necessary. This cusp is therefore allowed to make contact with its mural fellow, and this may well prevent mitral regurgitation.

Conclusion

To conclude this discussion on the morphological background to mitral incompetence, let me repeat once more what we have been able to find out clinically in the levogram and with other modern techniques.

The systolic phase starts with movement of the diaphragmatic segment, brought about by the activation of the posterior papillary muscle (Fig. 11). The remaining blood between the posterior cusp and the corresponding wall works like a pivot around which this segment is distended. At the posterior lateral wall – the equator of the left chamber – it can be seen as the lateral systolic movement described by Tichonow [9]. The field around the whole posterior cusp is in its turn now contracting, the mitral orifice being in this way diminished and the apex distended during the late isovolumetric phase. The lateral wall of the outflow tract has been built, and the whole myocardium contracts in the direction of the axis of the ventricle during the ejection phase.

Tichonow demonstrated that in *ischemic hearts* the lateral systolic movement is no longer accentuated [7].

Both the increase of the deep diameter and the thinning of the posterior wall are diminished. Should too little blood be supplied by the anterior or posterior coro-

13

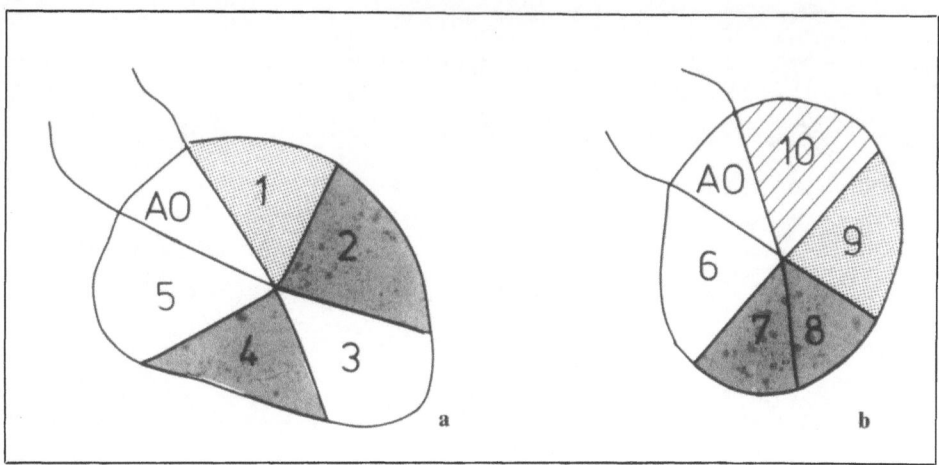

Fig. 11. Functional purpose of myocardial segments in ischemic hearts (according to [8]). a) RAO; b) LAO; (see text)

nary branches (segments 2, 4, 7, and 8), the ejection output has to be supplemented by those segments which have no share in that deficiency (segments 5, 10). This results in insufficient lifting of the basal parts of the wall needed to prepare for the ejection and construction of the lateral wall of the outflow tract (Fig. 11).

In ischemic hearts, the functional chain involving the *apical roots* of the *papillary muscles,* the *papillary muscles* themselves, the *anular cords* and the *basal loops,* does not come properly into play. This causes a functional deficiency in the "fibrous ring", which impedes closure of the angles in the collagenous cruciate trellis, and so mitral incompetence appears.

Some recently published data [6] have demonstrated that, when the posterior mitral cusp is affected, the prevalence of mitral regurgitation is significantly greater than when the anterior cusp prolapses by itself. Prolapse probably occurs in association with mitral anular dilatation, resulting in mitral regurgitation because of the greater functional impairment of the posterior cusp. When, in ischemic mitral insufficiency one or two of the links of that functional chain do not come into play correctly, this probably results in a "loosening" of the intermediate tendon — the anulus fibrosus — and that means dilatation of the orifice and mitral regurgitation owing to failure of the muscles to function properly.

There could also be some "loosening" of the collagenous material, as postulated by King and called by him "collagen dissolution" [1]. This factor makes one think about the connective tissue, and especially about the possibility of collagen being altered by hormones in women.

In ischemic mitral insufficiency and mitral regurgitation the *primary dysfunction* probably lies in the *intermediate tendons* of the anulus fibrosus.

It is possible to account for ischemic mitral incompetence on these lines: either the papillary muscles or other parts of the muscles of the outer wall are responsible for the mechanism of the trellis within the fibrous ring not working efficiently; in any case, the angles are imperfectly closed, whatever the *mechanical* reasons for this failure may be.

In this way it is possible to explain mitral incompetence, and to account for impairment of the blood-supply to the inner muscular layers and the papillary muscles themselves.

References

1. King BD, Clark MA et al. (1982) Myxomatous mitral valves: Collagen dissolution as the primary defect. Circulation 66:288
2. Benninghoff A (1929) Über die Entwicklung der Muskelarchitektur im Innern der menschlichen Herzkammern, Morph. Jb 63:208
3. Puff A (1954/55) Über die Verformung der Herzkammerbasis beim Menschen unter der Funktion. Gegenbaurs Morphol Jahrb 95:330−368
4. Puff A (1960) Der funktionelle Bau der Herzkammern. Zwanglose Abhandlungen aus dem Gebiet der normalen und pathologischen Anatomie, H 8, Thieme, Stuttgart
5. Puff A, Barrenberg M (1965) Röntgenkinematographische Untersuchungen über den Bewegungsmechanismus der Mitralklappe. Fortschr Geb Röntgenstr 102:607−618
6. Rueda B, Arvan S (1988) The relationship between clinical and echocardiographic findings in mitral valve prolapse. Herz-Kardiovasculäre Erkrankungen 13:277
   Tichonow KB (1986) Evolution of left ventricular shap through different phases of the cardiac
7. cycle in normal subjects and coronary patients. Kardiologia 11 Tom XXVI Moskau Medizina 58−63 (R)
8. Tichonow KB (1987) Left ventricular shap during ejection phase in coronary patients. Kardiologia 12:31−35 (R)
9. Tichonow KB, Puff A (1986) Funktionelle Röntgenanatomie des Herzens. Springer, Berlin Heidelberg New York Toyko

Author's address:
Prof. Dr. med. A. Puff
Anatomisches Institut
Universität Freiburg
Albertstraße 17
7800 Freiburg, FRG

Anatomy of the coronary arteries with resepct to chronic ischemic mitral regurgitation

A. E. Becker

Department of Pathology, Academic Medical Center, Amsterdam-Zuidoost, The Netherlands

Introduction

Chronic mitral regurgitation is an important complication among patients with obstructive coronary artery disease. Approximately 30% of patients considered for coronary bypass surgery show some degree of mitral valve incompetence [5]. Mitral regurgitation, moreover, has a tendency to increase steadily because of dilation of the mitral valve annulus. The left ventricular cavity dilates to accomodate the increase in diastolic volume and remodels itself by reactive hypertrophy of the non-ischemic wall segments [2]. A rise in end-diastolic pressure may develop, creating a further impediment to transmural myocardial perfusion in an already compromised myocardium because of obstructive coronary artery disease [3].

Within this setting papillary muscle dysfunction is generally accepted as the prime mechanism underlying chronic mitral regurgitation [4, 8]. The present survey will focus on some of the anatomic factors involved in this functional disorder.

Mitral valve anatomy

The mitral valve is composed of leaflets, chordae tendineae, and papillary muscles. The latter are direct continuations of ventricular myocardium and, for that reason, are dependent on coronary perfusion. The position of the papillary muscles, with respect to the overlying mitral valve leaflets, is crucial to guarantee an optimal support (Fig. 1).

Changes in left ventricular geometry may affect the position of one or both papillary muscle groups and, hence, may result in a potentially inadequate support of the leaflets. Global distension to the left ventricular cavity, for instance, due to left ventricular volume overload, may cause lateral displacement of the papillary muscle groups and mitral regurgitation. Local dilation in case of regional myocardial infarction may cause neighboring papillary muscle groups to be displaced, thus interfering with proper valve functioning. In this context it is important that considerable variations may exist in the architecture of both papillary muscle groups. The anterolateral group usually is formed by a conglommerate of papillary muscles. The posteromedial papillary muscle group, on the other hand, is tethered to the left ventricular wall over a wide area and usually contains multiple heads.

It is obvious that proper mitral valve function is jeopardized once the papillary muscles or adjacent left ventricular myocardium are affected by ischemia. From a functional point of view, therefore, the papillary muscles and left ventricular

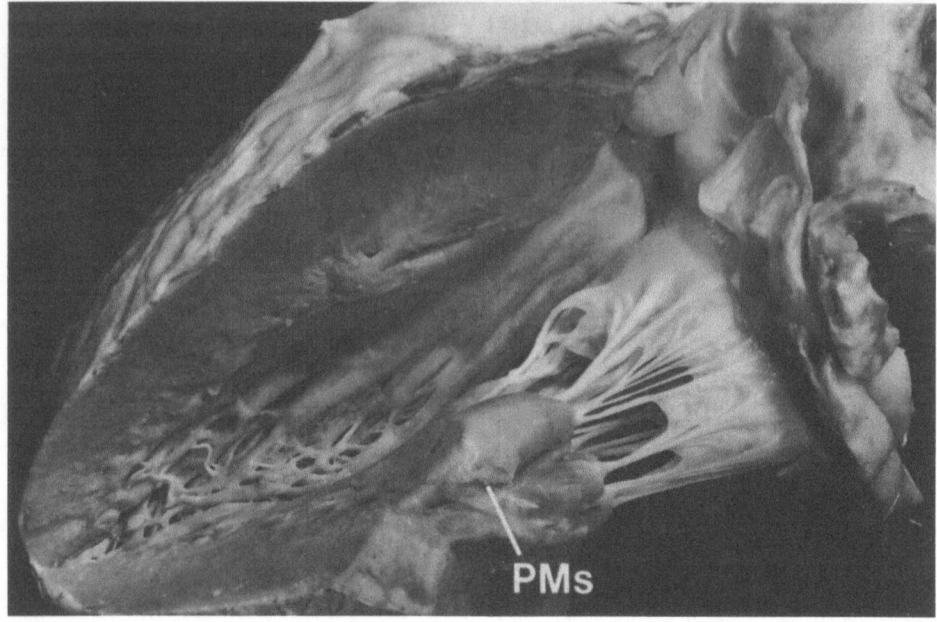

Fig. 1. Left ventricular view showing the anterolateral and the posteromedial papillary muscle groups (PMs) directly underneath the mitral valve leaflets.

myocardium are considered part of the mitral valve. The term "mitral valve apparatus" is based on this concept [7].

Mitral valve anatomy is even more complex, at least from a functional point of view, since the fibrous core of the leaflets usually is directly continuous with the fibrous annulus, while the atrial lining is a direct continuation of the left atrial endocardium. In other words, dilation of the left atrial cavity results in outward tension on the leaflets and annulus and, thus, may enhance mitral valve incompetence. The concept of mitral valve regurgitation as a self-perpetuating disease is based on these anatomic facts.

Coronary artery distribution

The right and left coronary arteries show marked variations in distribution, particularly with respect to the postero-inferior wall of the heart. In a majority of hearts the right coronary artery gives nice to the posterior descending coronary artery and then continues onto the postero-inferior wall of the left ventricle. This situation is then defined as a "dominant" right coronary artery. Once the left coronary artery gives off the posterior descending artery, the left artery is defined as the "dominant" artery. Obviously, intermediate or "balanced" forms will exist, but these are generally considered as exceptions [6]. Indeed, a right dominant pattern usually is quoted to exist in approximately 90% of hearts and a left dominant pattern in about 10% [1]. These figures differ markedly from our recent findings, based on a review

18

of 200 post-mortem angiograms followed by coronary dissection in case of doubt about the precise course or relationship. The results revealed right dominance in 76%, left dominance in 8%, and an intermediate type in 16%. The latter is characterized by a pattern in which both right and left coronary arteries contribute to the postero-inferior parts of the heart. This may consist of either two descending branches running parallel to both sides of the interventricular septum, or one artery that supplies the basal parts while the other artery courses towards the apical parts (Fig. 2). The discrepancy with literature sources most likely is due to an incorporation of intermediate types among the right dominant variety.

Be that as it may, right dominance is still by far the most common distribution pattern of the coronary arteries. The question arises what functional significance can be attributed to "right dominance". Once the artery crosses the crux of the heart how far will it reach to the postero-inferior wall of the left ventricle and, even more important, in what percentage of cases will it supply, totally or partially, the posteromedial papillary muscle group of the mitral valve apparatus? A study of 100 heart specimens, selected because of a dominant right coronary artery, showed a wide variation in this respect [9]. In this study the site of origin of the posteromedial papillary muscle group was taken as a major point of reference for categorization of right dominance (Fig. 3). In 32% of hearts the extent of the dominant right coro-

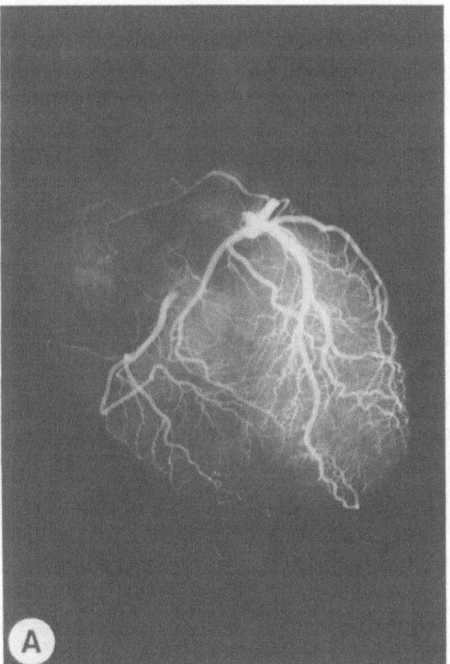 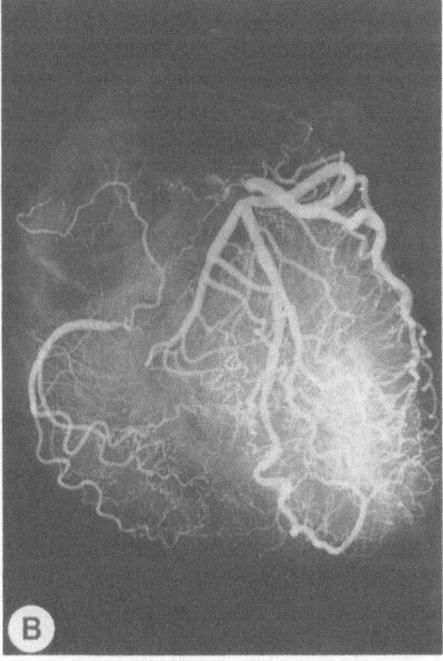

Fig. 2. Post-mortem coronary angiogram that reveals an intermediate or "balanced" coronary artery distribution pattern. Both the right and the left coronary arteries contribute to the supply of the postero-inferior wall of the heart. A) shows two descending branches running parallel to each other. B) shows the left coroncary artery contributing to the basal part and the right coronary artery to the apical part of the postero-inferior wall.

19

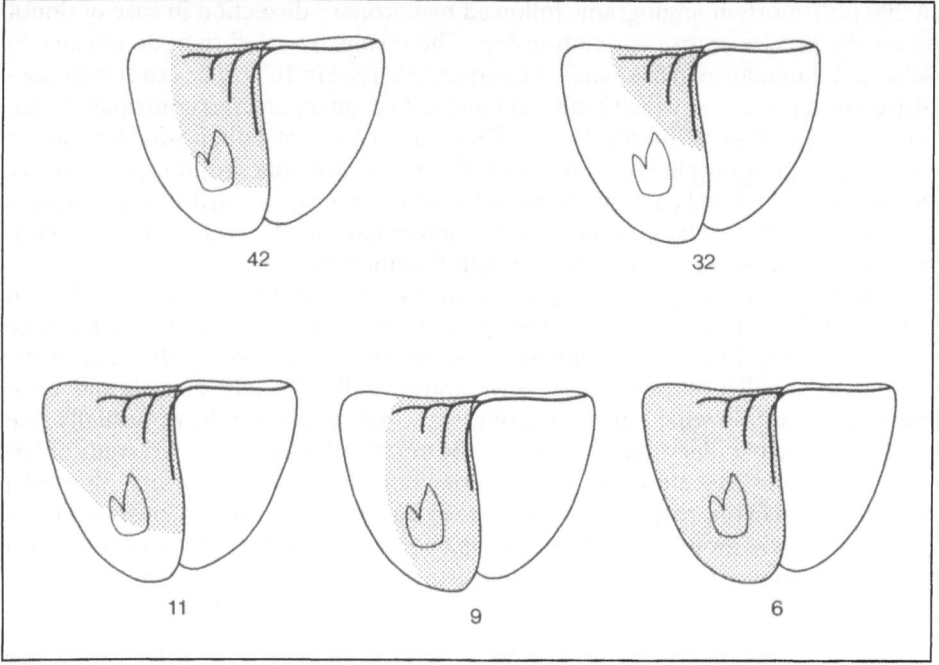

Fig. 3. Diagram of the ventricular mass and the position of the left ventricular posteromedial papillary muscle complex, viewed posteriorly, showing the incidence and variation in patterns of left ventricular extension (stippled areas) of a dominant right right coronary artery in 100 heart specimens. (Reproduced with permission from [9].)

nary artery was minimal, not reaching the level of origin of the posteromedial papillary muscle group. In 53% the artery did reach this level but the papillary muscle originated from the "watershed area" between the right and left coronary arterial systems (Fig. 4). In 15% the dominant right coronary artery reached far beyond the site of origin of the posteromedial papillary muscle group.

On the basis of these findings, one may anticipate that in approximately one-fourth of individuals a dominant right coronary artery will be of little functional significance for the left ventricular myocardium. In the majority of individuals, however, a dominant right coronary artery will contribute, partially or totally, to the vascular supply of the posteromedial papillary muscle group and the left ventricular lateral free wall. These observations appear to be of paramount significance when it comes to understanding mitral regurgitation in the setting of obstructive coronary artery disease.

Ischemic mitral regurgitation

In view of the above the question arises as to what extent the papillary muscles may be affected by obstructive coronary artery disease once myocardial infarction ensues.

20

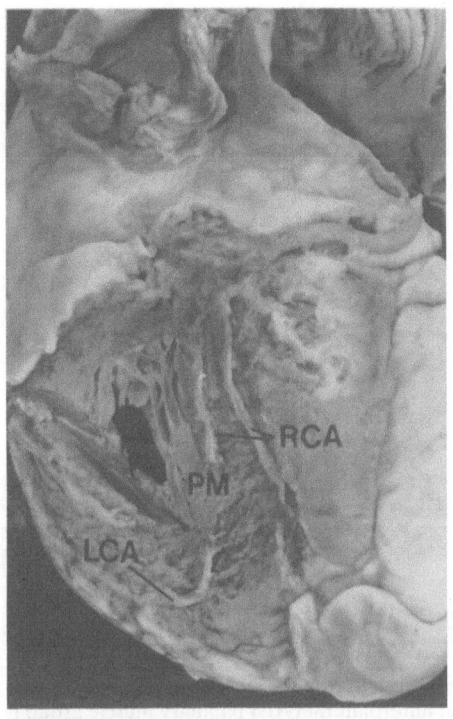

Fig. 4. Heart specimen viewed posteriorly. The "watershed area" between the dominant right coronary artery (RCA) and the left circumflex artery (LCA) has been dissected and is shown to contain the base of the posteromedial papillary muscle group (PM). (Reproduced with permission from [9].)

For this purpose 60 heart specimens have been studied, obtained from patients who died following myocardial infarction and in whom longstanding mitral regurgitation, as a consequence of the ischemic event, had been demonstrated clinically. The findings are summarized in Table 1.

An anterior wall infarction was present in 23 of the 60 hearts. An infarct in the postero-inferior wall was found in 37 hearts. Of the 23 hearts with an anterior wall infarct only 12 had the infarct extending to the anterolateral papillary muscle group (Fig. 5). Posteromedial papillary muscle involvement was not present in any of

Table 1. Evaluation of papillary muscle involvement in 60 hearts of patients with myocardial infarction and documented chronic ischemic mitral regurgitation

Anterior wall infarcts		23
Anterolateral papillary muscle	12	
Posteromedial papillary muscle	0	
Postero-inferior wall infarcts		37
Anterolateral papillary muscle	1	
Posteromdeial papillary muscle	37	

21

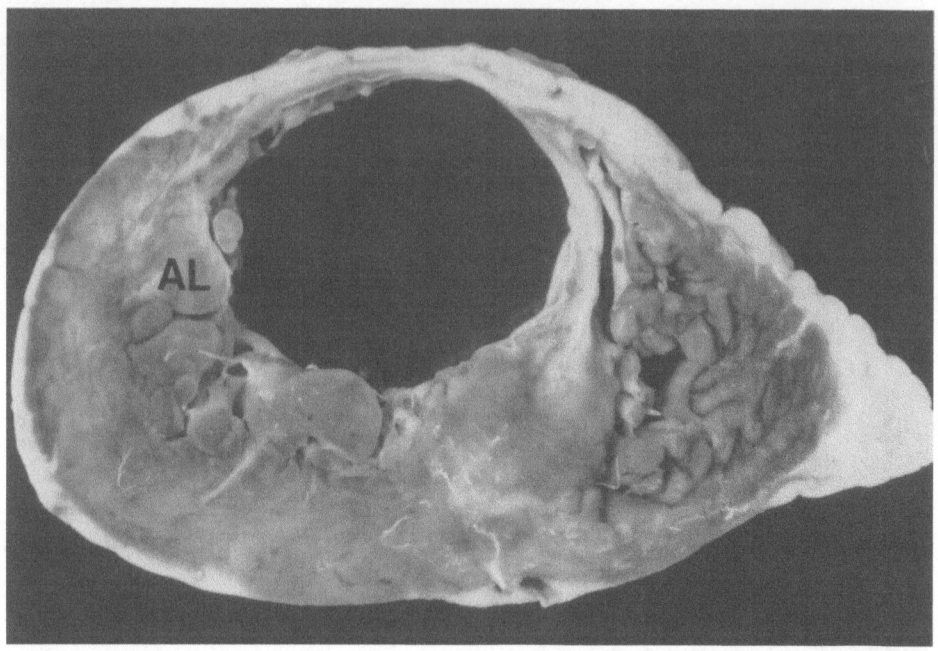

Fig. 5. Cross-section through heart of a patient with an anterior wall infarct and chronic mitral valve regurgitation. There is a large infarct, but the anterolateral (AL) papillary muscle group is not involved. A change in left ventricular geometry may have led to papillary muscle dysfunction and subsequent mitral regurgitation.

these hearts. Among the 37 hearts with a postero-inferior wall infarct, one had the infarct extending to the anterolateral papillary muscle group, but − most importantly − all 37 hearts had involvement of the posteromedial papillary muscle group (Fig. 6). Hence, there was a striking difference between anterior and postero-inferior wall infarcts, as far as involvement of the related papillary muscle groups is concerned.

The study suggests that once a postero-inferior wall infarct is complicated by longstanding mitral regurgitation the posteromedial papillary muscle group is always involved in the infarct area, be it totally or partially. In patients with an anterior wall infarct and chronic mitral regurgitation, on the other hand, the anterolateral papillary muscle is involved anatomically in approximately half of the cases. These observations lend support to clinical experiences that chronic mitral regurgitation following an anterior wall infarct is relatively rare, compared to the occurrence of this phenomenon in patients with postero-inferior wall infarcts. The present findings suggest that the difference may relate principally to direct involvement of the papillary muscles. This further underlines the significance of the papillary muscles as vital components of the mitral valve apparatus.

The 11 hearts of patients with an anterior wall infarction and chronic ischemic mitral regurgitation, but without anatomical involvement of the anterolateral papillary muscle group, all presented with large infarcts that had led to left ven-

22

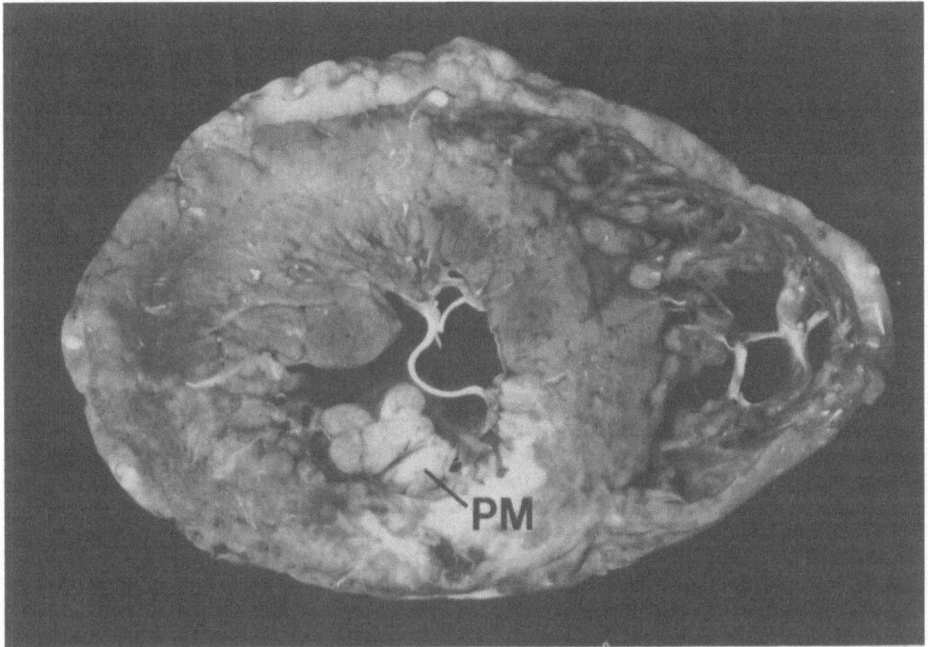

Fig. 6. Cross-section through heart of a patient with a postero-inferior wall infarct and mitral valve regurgitation. The infarct area includes the posteromedial (PM) papillary muscle group. Chronic mitral valve regurgitation is caused by direct involvement of the papillary muscle.

tricular aneurysms. Hence, a selected group of patients was definitely biased towards large-sized anterior wall infarcts. This could be an important aspect, since clinical experiences seem to indicate that an anterior wall infarction is only rarely accompanied by papillary muscle dysfunction and mitral regurgitation. An explanation could be that the usual patient with an anterior wall infarct will not present to the extent as shown in the present series. Once a left ventricular aneurysm is formed, however, the left ventricular geometry is grossly distorted and papillary muscle dysfunction may ensue.

Conclusions

Ischemic mitral incompetence is a common complication in patients with obstructive coronary artery disease, myocardial ischemia and infarction. An incompetent mitral valve apparatus is encountered both in the acute stage of the infarct and may reside as a chronic complication. The pathogenetic mechanism underlying chronic mitral regurgitation is generally considered to be due to a combination of papillary muscle dysfunction, localized or global left ventricular dilation, and myocardial dyskinesia [8]. The present study suggests a further specification of these mechanisms. In patients with chronic mitral regurgitation in the setting of a posteroinferior wall infarction, the underlying mechanism is partial or total infarction of the corresponding papillary muscle group. In patients with an anterior wall infarction, direct involvement of the anterolateral papillary muscle group is much less common. In those patients, mitral regurgitation seems to depend largely on papillary muscle dysfunction as a consequence of grossly distorted left ventricular geometry. One may also conceptualize why among patients with an anterior wall infarction is mitral regurgitation much less common than among patients with postero-inferior wall infarcts. Further studies are necessary to evaluate this concept.

References

1. Anderson RH, Becker AE (1980) Cardiac anatomy. An integrated text and colour atlas. Gower Medical Publishing, London
2. Anversa P, Ricci R, Olivetti G (1986) Quantitative structural analysis of the myocardium during physiologic growth and induced cardiac hypertrophy: a review. J Am Coll Cardiol 7:1140−1149
3. Becker AE (1988) Myocardial remodeling and its complications. In: Hurst JW, Anderson RH, Becker AE, Wilcox BR (eds) Atlas of the heart. Gower Medical Publishing, New York London, pp 2.1−2.7
4. Becker AE, Anderson RH (1975) Mitral insufficiency complicating acute myocardial infarction. Eur J Cardiol 2:351−359
5. Gahl K, Sutton R, Pearson M, Caspari P, Lairet A, McDonald L (1977) Mitral regurgitation in coronary heart disease. Br Heart J 39:13−18
6. McAlpine WA (1975) Heart and coronary arteries. An anatomical atlas for clinical diagnosis, radiological investigation and surgical treatment. Springer, Berlin Heidelberg New York
7. Perloff JD, Roberts WC (1972) The mitral apparatus. Functional anatomy of mitral regurgitation. Circulation 46:227−239
8. Rackley CE, Dear HD, Baxley WA, et al. (1970) Left ventricular chamber volume mass and function in severe coronary artery disease. Circulation 41:605−613
9. Reiss P, Becker AE (1981) Dominance of the right coronary artery: what does it mean? Anat Clin 2:369−372

Author's address:
Anton E. Becker, M.D.
Department of Pathology
Academic Medical Center
Meibergdreef 9
1105 AZ Amsterdam-Zuidoost
The Netherlands

Transmitral flow dynamics in the normal heart and during mitral regurgitation

E. L. Yellin

Departments of Cardiothoracic Surgery and Physiology and Biophysics, Albert Einstein College of Medicine, The Bronx, New York, USA

Introduction

This volume unites anatomists, pathologists, cardiologists, surgeons and physiologists, in an attempt to define the causes and to clarify the diagnosis of ischemic mitral incompetence; and then to discuss the medical and surgical approaches to solving the problem. The ability to diagnose mitral incompetence, of any origin, has been enhanced by recent developments in ultrasound technology: 2D-echocardiography, pulsed-Doppler measurement of local velocity, and color-coded flow mapping. This proceedings volume contains important applications of these methods for pre-, intra-, and post-operative examination of mitral regurgitant flow patterns. Our understanding and interpretation of the measured flow patterns is enhanced by an understanding of the physiology of flow, both antegrade and retrograde, across the mitral valve.

This paper will review the studies from our dog laboratory that have, in the course of almost two decades, defined the relations between pressure, flow, and mitral valve motion. Because this is a review paper, we will focus on the presentation and interpretation of "raw" data and on the development of applications and concepts, rather than on methodology (methods can be found in the references). We will also offer a minimum of secondary of corroborating citations; they too can be found in our original papers.

Methods

Figure 1 is a schematic of the instrumented left heart of the anesthetized open-chest dog. High fidelity micromanometers measure left atrial, left ventricular, and aortic pressures. LV dp/dt and the intracardiac phonogram are obtained from the LV catheter. Electromagnetic flow probes measure phasic blood flow across the aortic and mitral valves. In some studies the anterior and posterior mitral leaflets have been opacified [10] and in some studies mitral valve motion has been measured by M-mode echograms [11, 12, 17]. More recently we have implanted only the two intracardiac micromanometers and the mitral flow probe under sterile conditions and performed the hemodynamic studies in the conscious chronically instrumented dog [8]. In addition to studying the pressure-flow relations across the normal mitral valve we have also studied the dynamics of mitral regurgitation in the anesthetized [16, 19–21] and conscious dog [18], and in patients and models [9].

25

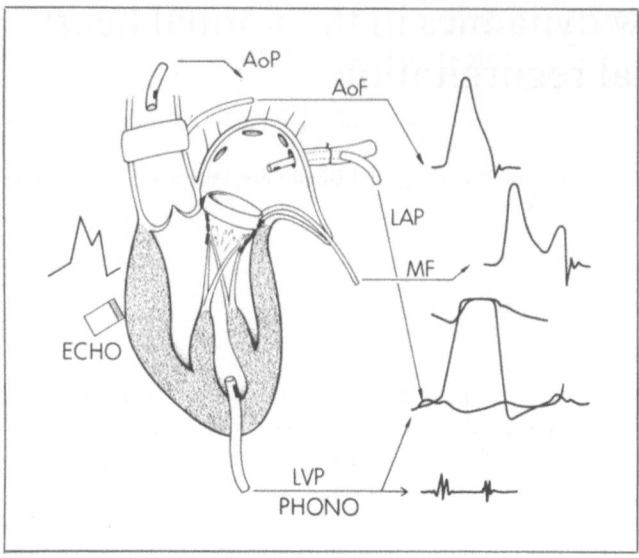

Fig. 1. Schematic of the instrumented canine heart and recorded waveforms. AoP, aortic pressure; AoF, aortic flow; LAP, left atrial pressure; MF, mitral flow; LVP, left ventricular pressure. (Redrawn from J Applied Physiol, 39:665, (1975), with permission).

Discussion of Results

Normal mitral valve
Pressure-flow relations: Figure 2 is a representative oscillographic record from a conscious chronically instrumented dog with a normal mitral valve. We restrict our description to diastolic events and note the following points. At end ejection (defined by both S2 and dp/dtmin) the left ventricular pressure falls rapidly (myocardial relaxation) until it crosses the left atrial pressure when the mitral valve opens and blood is rapidly accelerated to its maximum value (E-point on mitral flow) after which it rapidly decelerates. The driving force for this rapid filling phase is a small atrioventricular pressure gradient. Despite the fact that this AV difference quickly equilibrates at zero, forward flow continues, but at a reduced rate due to the momentum imparted to the blood by the early gradient. If diastole is sufficiently long, the flow will, of course, become zero prior to the atrial contraction (cycle 3); and very often, in the normal heart, flow rapidly decelerates to zero because the pressure gradient reverses and becomes negative (Fig. 3) [4]. Following atrial depolarization (P-wave) and mechanical contraction, flow is again reaccelerated to a new peak (A-point on mitral flow). The atrial pressure then falls due both to deactivation and emptying, the AV pressure difference becomes negative, and mitral flow decelerates. At normal PR intervals, the negative gradient is enhanced by the rapid increase in LVP due to mechanical systole. As a consequence of forward momentum of the blood, mitral flow does not become zero until c. 30 ms after the AV pressure crossover [10]. This very important result was first noted by Nolan et al. [13] and then shown in our laboratory to explain the time

26

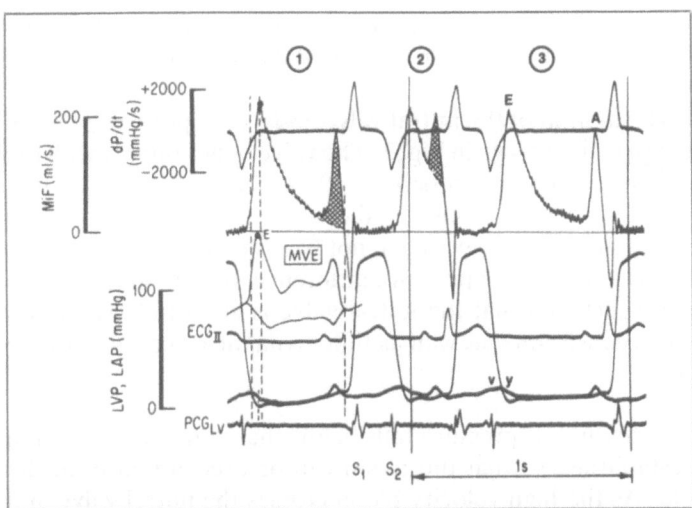

Fig. 2. Oscillographic record from a conscious chronically instrumented dog. A mitral valve echo (MVE) has been superimposed. Because of sinus respiratory variations in rhythm, the heart rate in cycle 2 is faster than in cycles 1 and 3 (127 compared to 86 and 82/min). The shaded areas in cycles 2 and 3 denote the contribution to filling of atrial systole. MVE, mitral valve echogram; S1, S2, first and second heart sounds; PCG$_{LV}$, intracardiac phonogram. The dashed vertical lines in cycle 1 denote onset of filling, peak AV pressure difference, peak flow rate, and end of filling. See text for further discussion. (Redrawn from: Recent progress in mitral valve disease, p 51, (1984), with permission.)

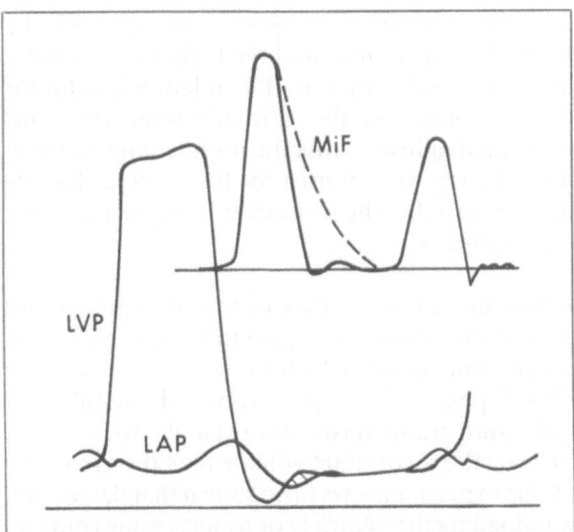

Fig. 3. Schematic pressures and mitral flow (MiF) illustrating the changes in deceleration of mitral flow during rapid filling due to a small reversal of the atrioventricular pressure difference (shaded area). The broken line represents slowed deceleration following equilibration of the AV pressure gradient in the absence of a negative gradient, as shown, for example, in Fig. 2.

delay between AV pressure crossover and the first heart sound [10]. It will be shown below that fluid momentum is also important in the interpretation of mitral regurgitant flow dynamics.

Mitral valve motion: The motion of the mitral valve and its temporal relation to the transmitral flow pattern is also shown in Fig. 2. The valve opens rapidly with the onset of flow and reaches its maximum excursion c. 20 ms before peak flow rate is reached, i.e., the mid-diastolic closing motion of the value starts while flow is still accelerating. Since large circulating vortices have not had time to form, and since accelerating flow indicates a positive AV pressure difference, both tending to keep the valve open, we have concluded that the mitral valve is almost always under chordal tension, and those constraints, as well as fluid dynamic forces, determine normal valve motion [17].

Conceptual Approach

When the ventricle relaxes and its pressure falls below that of the left atrium, a pressure difference is established so that the blood can be accelerated from the atrium into the ventricle. As the high velocity blood crosses the mitral valve and mixes with the quiescent blood in the ventricle, most of the kinetic energy is lost. The atrioventricular pressure difference is thus composed of two parts: a component required to accelerate the blood, and one required to overcome losses. This can be described by the following relation:

$$\Delta P = (L)dQ/dt + (R)Q^2$$

where ΔP is the atrioventricular pressure difference Q is the volume flow rate, and L and R are inertial and resistive coefficients. L and R together determine the impedance to flow of the mitral apparatus; both are inversely related to the area of the mitral orifice, L to the first power, and R to the area squared. As expected, the smaller the area for flow, the greater the impedance, and the higher the pressure difference necessary for maintaining the cardiac output. The relation is valid for both antegrade and retrograde flow, but note that the resistance term represents the loss of energy, and that it is very small in flow across the normal mitral configuration. But in particular, note that the regurgitant area for flow is considerably smaller than the normal mitral valve area so that the resistance across an incompetent valve is high and the loss term dominates.

Mitral regurgitation

The physical relations embodied in this equation allow us to make some useful predictions: small decreases in the effective mitral area lead to large decreases in flow; the high velocities across a regurgitant orifice make the resistive losses dominant; and because the regurgitant flow depends on the square root of the systolic AV pressure gradient, changes in the pressure gradient (due for example, to increases in afterload) have a smaller influence on the regurgitant volume than the size of the effective orifice area. In a series of dog experiments we have shown that decreasing the end diastolic volume either by unloading the ventricle or by increasing contractility, had a profound effect on decreasing the calculated mitral regurgitant area [16, 19−21]; this has recently been verified in patient studies [7, 15]. (At the anecdotal level, the cardiac surgeon frequently observes the sudden decrease in regurgitation when he "unloads" the heart during surgery.)

28

Temporal relations: Angiographic measurements in patients have led to the conclusion that almost one-half of the regurgitant volume is ejected into the left atrium *prior* to the opening of the aortic valve [6]. Although this observation has been accepted and incorporated into the best reference works [1], we have found it inconsistent with physiological principles! The pre-ejection period is only a small fraction of the total systolic period; furthermore, the time for regurgitation during the pre-ejection period is reduced by the time necessary to decelerate antegrade flow, and the duration of systolic time for regurgitation is increased during ventricular relaxation by the time necessary to decelerate retrograde flow.

These observations are illustrated in Fig. 4 showing the temporal pressure-flow relations in an anesthetized open-chest dog with a small hole (c. 5 mm diam.) in the anterior mitral leaflet instrumented as shown in Fig. 1. Time 0 is the peak of the R-wave (usually coincident with the AV pressure crossover). Note that the pre-ejection period is shortened by the time required to decelerate forward flow, t(0−1), and the actual regurgitant volume, V(1−2) is c. 10% of the total. This finding is independent of heart rate [18]. It is clear, then, that the only condition under which 50% of the regurgitant volume can occur during the pre-ejection period is a condition in which the regurgitant area is large at end diastole and becomes insignificantly small *at the onset of aortic ejection.* Although not improbable, such a condition would not lead to symptoms and would go without detection.

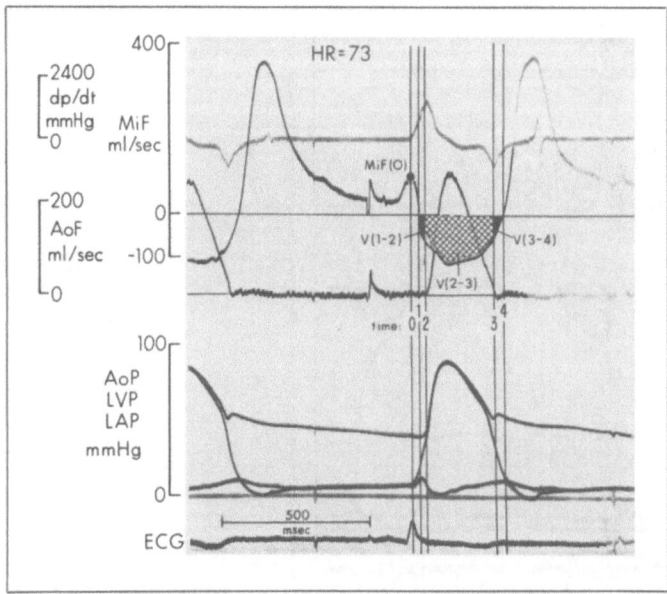

Fig. 4. Oscillographic record from an anesthetized dog with moderate, acute, mitral regurgitation (shaded area in MiF, RV = c. 35%). Time 0 is the onset of mechanical systole; note that there is some mitral flow, MiF(0), at that time, so that t(0−1) is the time necessary to decelerate the antegrade flow before regurgitation can start, at t(1). The black areas, V(1−2) and V(3−4), represent the pre- and post-ejection regurgitant volumes. Note their relativeyl small values, <10% of the regurgitant volume. (The original record has been darkened for clarity.) (From [18] with permission.)

Increased PR interval: These observations have been verified in the conscious chronically instrumented dog [18]. One condition under which significantly more than 10% of the total regurgitant volume can occur during pre-ejection is in the presence of a prolonged PR interval as illustrated in Fig. 5. Early deceleration of mitral flow following atrial contraction can reverse the pressure gradient and, when the mitral valve is incompetent, may lead to significant regurgitation during the pre-ejection period. Similarly, a slowed rate of ventricular relaxation can lead to increased regurgitation during the "isovolumic" relaxation period [18].

Role of left atrial pressure

Since it is clear from first principles that the atrioventricular pressure gradient motivates mitral flow, it must then follow that the time varying atrial pressure is a major determinant of early diastolic filling across the normal valve [8]. This conclusion from our laboratory has been verified by others in dogs [3, 5] and in patients [14]. An important application of this principle is for the understanding of the so-called "normalization" of the Doppler-derived early diastolic filling pattern by mitral regurgitation in the presence of impaired ventricular relaxation [14]. Figure 6 schematically illustrates this point. The left panel shows a normal transmitral flow pattern produced by a normal left atrial pressure and left ventricular relaxation rate. The pressure-flow relationship for impaired relaxation and high left atrial pressure due to regurgitation is shown in the right panel. Note that the elevated v-wave provides the upstream pressure to "normalize" the flow during the rapid filling phase.

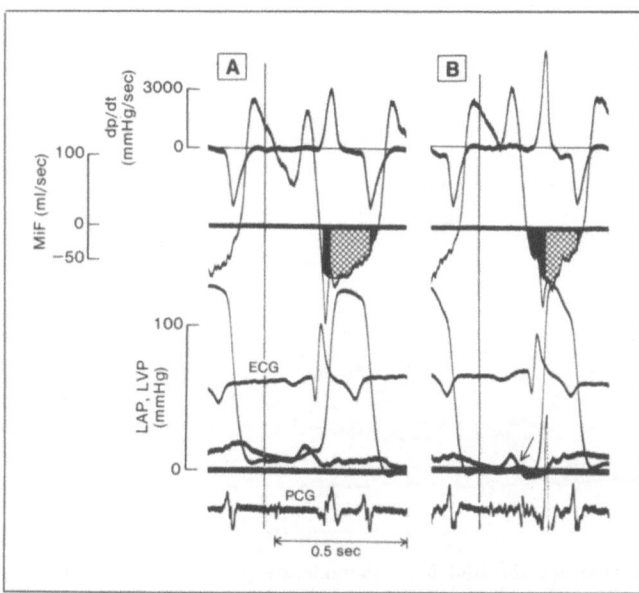

Fig. 5. Oscillographic records from a conscious dog with moderate regurgitation (RV = c. 30%), illustrating the effect on pre-ejection regurgitation of prolonged PR interval. The arrow in panel B indicates the premature atrioventricular pressure crossover that leads to increased pre-ejection regurgitation (< 30%). Further discussion in text. (From [18] with permission.)

The concept of impedance

Many, if not most, authors of papers describing the dynamics of mitral regurgitation refer to the regurgitant path from the LV to the LA as the "low impedance" path. This is physically incorrect and may become conceptually misleading. The aorta is the low impedance path because the pressure drop across the aortic valve is very small; conversely, because the pressure difference across the mitral valve in the retrograde direction is very large, the path is one of high impedance. It is, of course, true that the existence of the left atrial shunt path lowers the *total* impedance that the ventricle faces during systole, and the surgical repair of the incompetent valve therefore increases afterload. We may thus correctly refer to the phenomenon of mitral regurgitation as one that lowers the total afterload, but it is incorrect to characterize the retrograde path as one of low impedance.

Summary

The pressure-flow relations across the mitral valve, in either the antegrade or retrograde direction, can be described by a simple equation that relates the atrioventricular pressure difference to the forces of inertia and resistance. Inertia is particularly important in understanding the temporal pressure-flow relations. Forward flow is dominated by inertial forces, while backward flow is dominated by resistive forces. Because the resistive losses vary inversely with the square of the orifice area, the effective regurgitant area has a profound effect on the regurgitant volume. Maintaining a small ventricle tends to reduce the regurgitant area and volume.

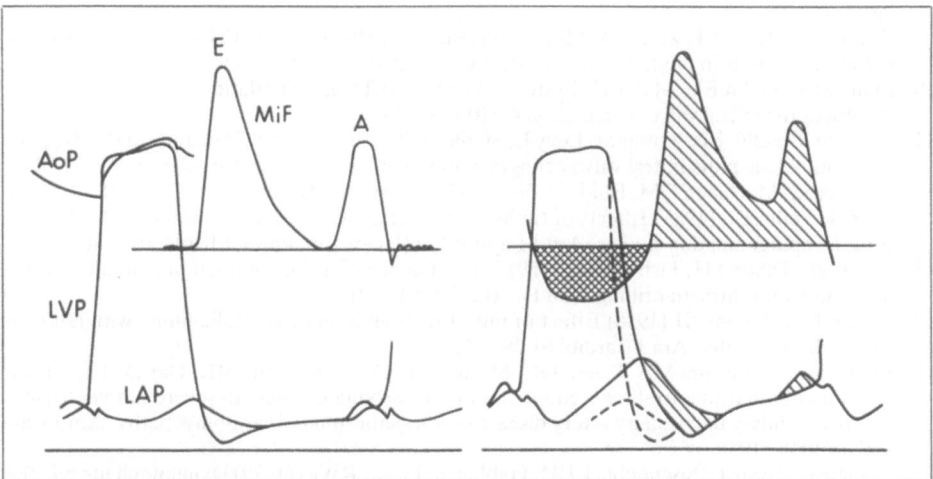

Fig. 6. Schematic pressures and flows illustrating the effect of mitral regurgitation on early filling dynamics in the presence of impaired left ventricular relaxation. The left panel shows the normal relations. The right panel shows a "normalized" early filling pattern, due to the high left atrial pressure, despite slowed LV relaxation; (compare with the broken curve that represents the normal pressures from the left panel).

31

Acknowledgements:
This review encompasses work done in collaboration with my many students, fellows, and colleagues who are listed in the References. The work could not have been done without the dedication and skills of Ms. Olivera and Messrs. Leon, Bon, and Rivera.

References

1. Braunwald E (ed) (1988) Heart disease. A textbook of cardiovascular medicine 3rd ed. Philadelphia, Saunders, p 1037
2. Choong CY, Abascal VM, Thomas JD, Guerrero JL, McGlew S, Weyman AE (1987) Combined influence of ventricular loading and relaxation on the transmitral flow velocity profile in dogs measured by Doppler echocardiography. Circulation 78:672–683
3. Choong CY, Herrmann HC, Weyman AE, Fifer MA (1988) Preload dependence of Doppler-derived indexes of left ventricular diastolic function in humans. J Am Coll Cardiol 10:800–808
4. Courtois M, Kovacs SJ, Ludbrook PA (1988) Transmitral pressure-flow velocity relation importance of regional pressure gradients in the left ventricle during diastole. Circulation 78:661–671
5. Courtois M, Vered Z, Barzilai B, Ricciotti NA, Perez JE, Ludbrook PA (1988) The transmitral pressure-flow velocity relation effect of abrupt preload reduction. Circulation 78:1459–1468
6. Eckberg DL, Gault JH, Bouchard RL, Karliner JS, Ross J (1973) Mechanics of left ventricular contraction in chronic severe mitral regurgitation. Circulation 47:1252–1259
7. Elkayam U, Roth A, Kumar A, Kuleck D, McIntosh N, McKay CR, Rahimtoola SH (1987) Hemodynamic and volumetric effects of venodilation with nitroglycerin in chronic mitral regurgitation. Am J Cardiol 60:1106–1111
8. Ishida Y, Meisner JS, Tsujioka K, Gallo JI, Yoran C, Frater RWM, Yellin EL (1986) Left ventricular filling dynamics: influence of left ventricular relaxation and left atrial pressure. Circulation 74:187–196
9. Keren G, LeJemtel T, Zelcer A, Meisner JS, Bier A, Yellin EL (1986) Time variation of mitral regurgitation flow in dilated cardiomyopathy. Circulation 74:684–692
10. Laniado S, Yellin EL, Miller H, Frater RWM (1973) Temporal relation of the first sound to closure of the mitral valve. Circulation 47:1006–1014
11. Laniado S, Yellin EL, Kotler M, Levy L, Stadler J, Terdiman R (1975) A study of the dynamic relations between the mitral valve echogram and phasic mitral flow. Circulation 51:104–113
12. Meisner JS, McQueen DM, Ishida Y, Vetter HO, Bortolotti U, Strom JA, Frater RWM, Peskin CS, Yellin EL (1985) Effects of timing of atrial systole in LV filling and mitral valve closure: computer and dog studies. Am J Physiol 249 (Heart Circ Physiol 18):H604–H619
13. Nolan SP, Dixon SH, Fisher RD (1969) The influence of atrial contraction and mitral valve mechanics on ventricular filling. Am Heart J 77:784–791
14. Shaikh MA, Lavine SJ (1988) Effect of mitral regurgitation on diastolic filling with left ventricular hypertrophy. Am J Cardiol 61:590–594
15. Weiland DS, Koustam MA, Salem DN, Marten TT, Cohen SR, Zile MR, Das D (1986) Contribution of reduced mitral regurgitant volume to vasodilator effect in severe left ventricular failure secondary to coronary artery disease or idiopathic dilated cardiomyopathy. Am J Cardiol 58:1046–1050
16. Yellin EL, Yoran C, Sonnenblick EH, Gabbay S, Frater RWM (1979) Dynamic changes in the canine mitral regurgitant orifica area during ventricular ejection. Circ Res 45:677–683
17. Yellin EL, Peskin C, Yoran C, Koenigsberg M, Matsumoto M, Laniado S, McQueen D, Shore D, Frater RWM (1981) Mechanism of mitral valve motion during diastole. Am J Physiol 241 (Heart Circ Physiol 10):H389–H400
18. Yellin EL, Yoran C, Frater RWM, Sonnenblick EH (1985) Dynamics of acute experimental mitral regurgitation: I. Changes in regurgitant orifica area. Time variation in regurgitant flow.

In: Ionescu MI, Cohn LH (eds) Mitral valve disease, diagnosis and treatment. Butterworths Scientific Ltd., London, pp 11−25
19. Yoran C, Yellin EL, Becker RM, Gabbay S, Frater RWM, Sonnenblick EH (1979) Mechanism for reduction of mitral regurgitation with vasodilator therapy. Am J Cardiol 43:773-777
20. Yoran C, Yellin EL, Becker RM, Gabbay S, Frater RWM, Sonnenblick EH (1979) Dynamic aspects of mitral regurgitation: Effects of ventricular volume, pressure and contractility on the effective regurgitant orifice area. Circulation 60:170−176
21. Yoran C, Yellin EL, Hori M, Tsujioka K, Laniado S, Sonnenblick EH, Frater RWM (1983) Effects of heart rate on experimentally produced mitral regurgitation in dogs. Am J Cardiol 52:1345−1349

Author's address:
Dr. E. L. Yellin
Department of Cardiothoracic Surgery
Albert Einstein College of Medicine
1300 Morris's Park Avenue
The Bronx, NY 10461
USA

Influence of papillary muscle function on the mitral valve and left ventricular mechanics

E. Gams, S. Hagl, W. Heimisch*, H. Meisner*, N. Mendler*, H. Schad*, F. Sebening*

Surgical University Clinic, Dept. of Cardiac Surgery, Heidelberg, and *German Heart Center Munich, Cardiovascular Surgery, Munich, FRG

Introduction

The mitral valve is not only a plain heart valve, but a very complex structure, and as such, an important part of the left ventricular chamber (Fig. 1). Valvular annulus, valve leaflets, and chordae tendineae are connected to the left ventricular wall by papillary muscles. Muscle fibers originating from the atrioventricular annulus run towards the apex, and rise from there, radiating into the papillary muscles on the inner layer of the ventricular wall [3, 16]. Consequently, the papillary muscles are not only part of the mitral valve apparatus, but also are the connecting link between the mitral valve and the left ventricular wall.

Most of our present knowledge of papillary muscle dynamics is based upon studies of isolated muscle preparations [5, 10]. Only a limited number of experimental investigations have made direct measurements of the in situ papillary muscle func-

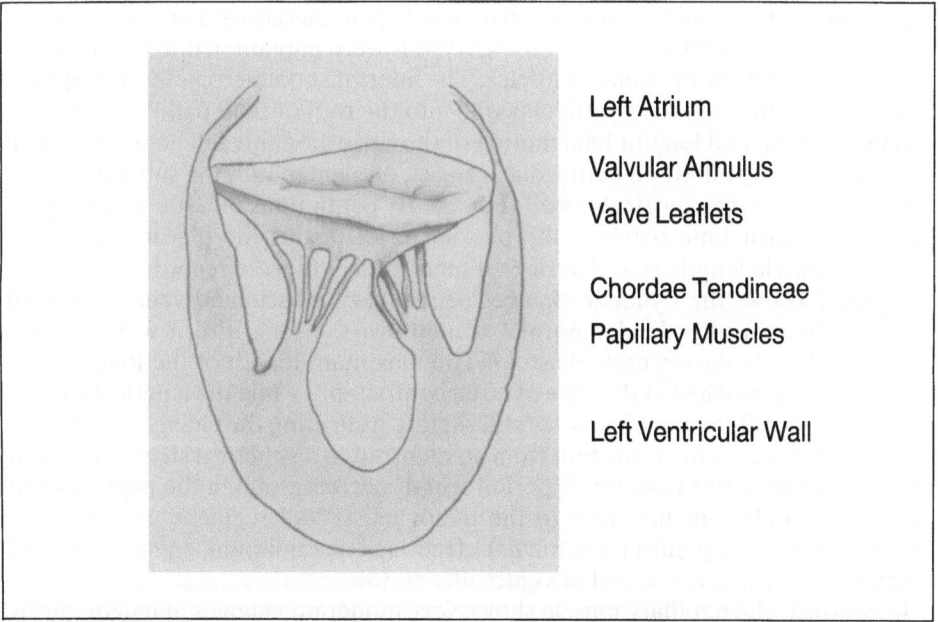

Left Atrium

Valvular Annulus

Valve Leaflets

Chordae Tendineae

Papillary Muscles

Left Ventricular Wall

Fig. 1. Components of the mitral valvular apparatus

35

tion using angiography [17], strain gauges [9], length gauges [12] or sonomicrometry [18, 19]. These studies revealed contradictory results concerning the function of the papillary muscle in the mechanics of the mitral valve: Some authors found a purely isometrie function during left ventricular contraction [6, 7, 23], others described a regular shortening of papillary muscles during systole [9, 17–19, 22]. But the question of whether the so called "dysfunction" of papillary muscles results in a significant mitral incompetence is still difficult to answer [1, 2, 4, 11, 24, 25, 27].

It is necessary to explore the function and contractile behavior of the papillary muscles in order to understand the mechanics of the mitral valve, and to analyze the significance of the close linkage of the mitral valve to the left ventricular wall in respect to ventricular performance. Both factors possibly play an important role because, on the one hand, papillary muscles are responsible for keeping the mitral valve leaflets in a competent position during cyclic changes of the left ventricular diameters [20], and on the other hand, papillary muscles are part of the contracting myocardium and belong to the left ventricular pump.

Contractile behavior of the in situ, papillary muscle

Before one studies the contractile behavior of the papillary muscle in the diseased myocardium it is necessary to know the function of the normal papillary muscle during phasic changes of the left ventricular pressure and volume. This can be demonstrated by comparing the dynamics of the left ventricular wall with those of the anterior and posterior papillary muscles.

Experiments were performed in anesthetized open-chest dogs. During cardiopulmonary bypass two miniature ultrasonic crystals were implanted into the tip of the anterior and posterior papillary muscles. The inferior sonomicrometer transducers were inserted through the ventricular wall into the root of both papillary muscles. Circumferential and longitudinal motion of the corresponding left ventricular wall were recorded by additional ultrasonic gauges, implanted into the subendocardial muscle layers of the ventricular wall (Fig. 2). By continuous measurements of the ultrasonic transit time between the piezoelectric crystals the phasic changes of papillary muscle length as well as of wall segment length were recorded.

Figure 3 shows the dynamic changes of papillary muscle and ventricular wall motion schematically. Under normal conditions, the length of a wall segment increases sharply during early diastole. The maximum length of the longitudinal wall segment is reached at the time of atrial contraction, while the length of the circumferential wall segment increases still slightly, reflecting the change in ventricular geometry due to the transition from an ellipsoid to a spherical shape of the left ventricle. During this isovolumic period length decreases along the major axis of the left ventricle, but increases in the minor axis. Wall segments shorten with almost equal velocity during ventricular ejection. The minimum length of the wall segments is reached at the end of ventricular systole.

In contrast, the papillary muscle shows very moderate changes in length during diastole. The lengthening occurs during the short isovolumic phase. During ventricular ejection the papillary muscle shortens at a velocity similar to that of the ven-

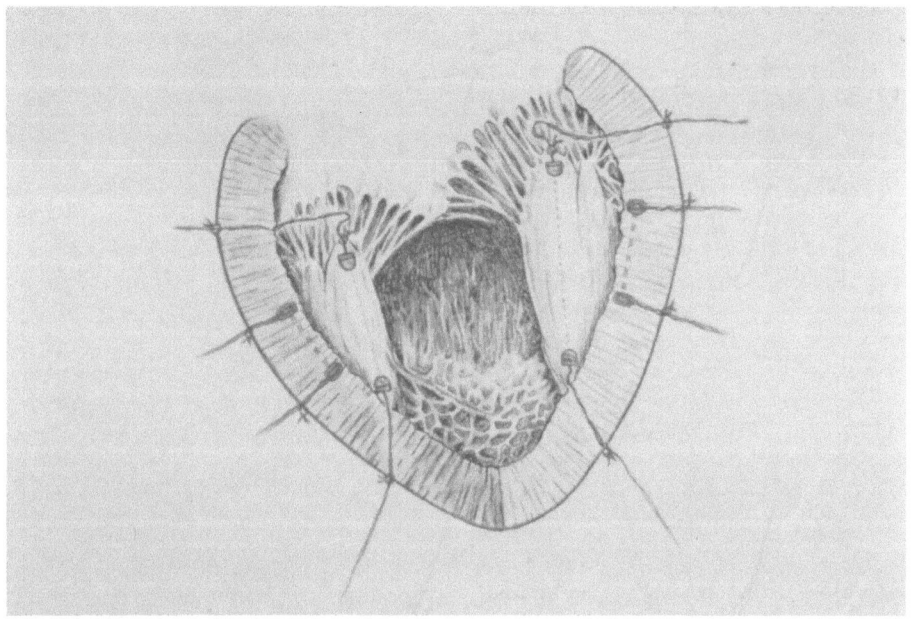

Fig. 2. Location of the ultrasonic transducers in the anterior and posterior papillary muscle and the left ventricular wall. (Used by permission of the Butterworths Company, London.)

tricular wall segments. At the end of ventricular systole minimal length of the papillary muscle is reached.

To demonstrate the contractile behavior of papillary muscles and of wall segments, left ventricular pressure was plotted against length according to the left ventricular pressure-volume-loop (Fig. 4). The shape of the pressure-length-loop of the papillary muscle differs from that of a wall segment: During isovolumic contraction papillary muscle length increases markedly, whereas only slight changes in wall-segment-length occur. This leads to a characteristic shift of the pressure-length-loop of the papillary muscle to the right. There is no difference between the function pattern of the anterior and posterior papillary muscle.

The degree of the inclination of the pressure- length-loop of the papillary muscles depends on the diastolic left ventricular pressure (Fig. 5). Increasing preload by infusion of blood results in an augmentation of enddiastolic length in the wall segment, as well as in the papillary muscle. Due to greater lengths the pressure-length-loops are shifted to the right. The increase in the area enclosed by the loop indicates an increase of the work performed by the wall segment respectively by the papillary muscle. The rise of ventricular peak pressure occurs in accordance with the Frank-Starling-mechanism.

An increase of afterload, induced by temporary occlusion of the descending aorta, leads to a marked increase in length and pressure (Fig. 6). The augmentation of afterload is followed by a similar change in dynamics of the left ventricular wall segment as well as of the papillary muscle. There is a decrease of systolic shortening

37

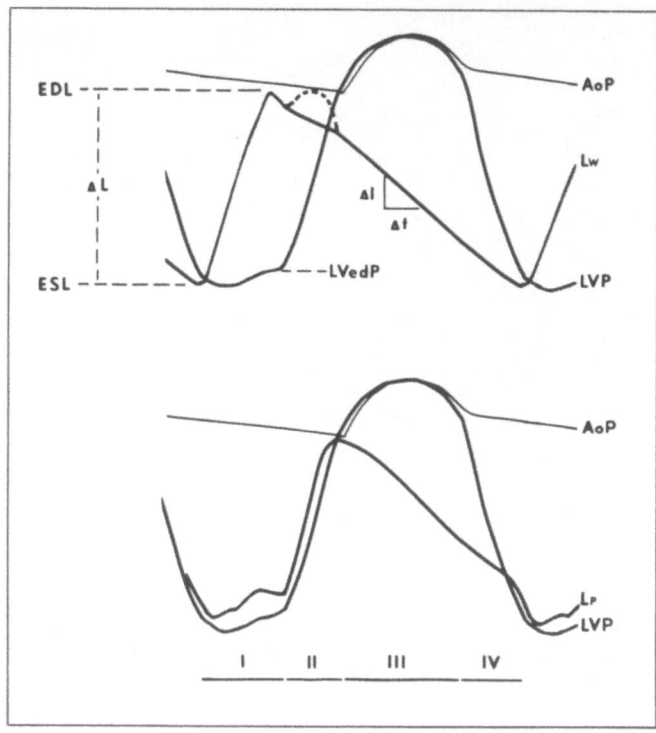

Fig. 3. Schematic drawing of the phasic changes of the left ventricular wall segments Lw (top) and the papillary muscle Lp (bottom) in relation to the left ventricular pressure LVP and aortic pressure AoP. EDL = enddiastolic length, ESL = endsystolic length, ΔL = contraction amplitude, LVedP = left ventricular enddiastolic pressure. I = diastole, II = isovolumic contraction, III = ejection phase, IV = relaxation phase

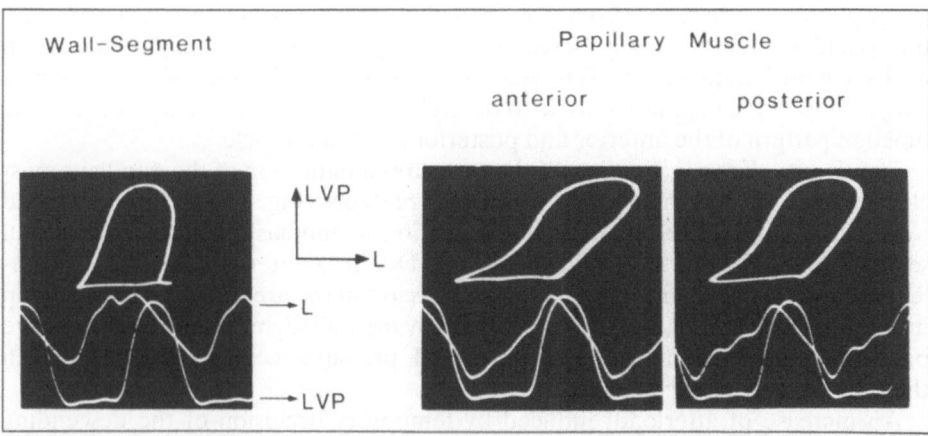

Fig. 4. Left ventricular pressure-length-loops (top) from instantaneous recordings of length L and pressure LVP (bottom) of a subendocardial wall segment (left) and the anterior and posterior papillary muscle (right). (Used by permission of the Butterworths Company, London.)

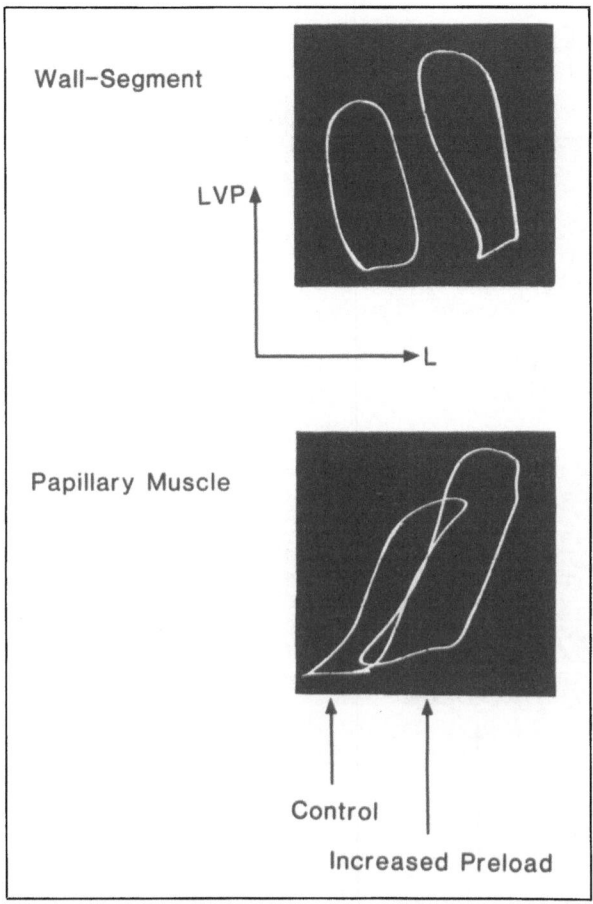

Fig. 5. Pressure-length-loops of a subendocardial wall segment and the papillary muscle during increase of preload; LVP = left ventricular pressure, L = length. (Used by permission of the Butterworths Company, London.)

in both wall segment and papillary muscle lengths, caused by the increase in ventricular outflow impedance.

In Fig. 7 the effect of changes of the contractile state is shown. Bolus injection of calcium was followed by an increase of myocardial contractility. The positive inotropic effect could be shown by an increase in total loop area and by the unchanged enddiastolic length representing unchanged preload. After calcium injection, peak systolic left ventricular pressure and the extent of shortening are augmented. Again the changes induced by calcium show a very similar shift of the pressure-length-loops of the wall segments and of the papillary muscles.

It could be demonstrated by these experiments that altering preload, afterload, and the inotropic state, the percent length changes of wall segments and papillary muscles were similar. The pressure-length-loops changed in the same direction and approximately to the same extent.

39

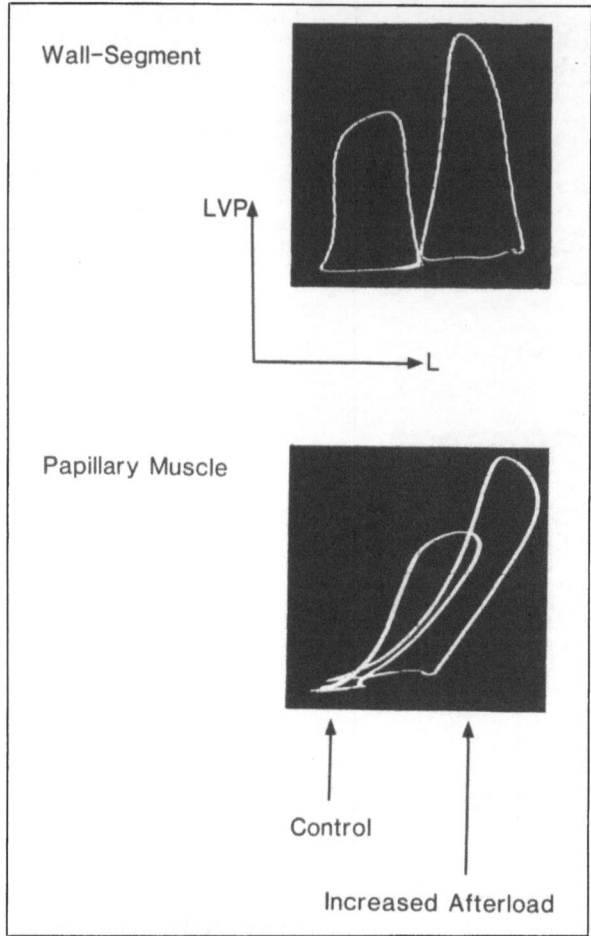

Fig. 6. Pressure-length-loops of a subendocardial wall segment and the papillary muscle during increase of afterload; LVP = left ventricular pressure, L = length. (Used by permission of the Butterworths Company, London.)

Left ventricular performance following total loss of papillary muscle function

To study the significance of papillary muscle function under pathological conditions, it is necessary to interfere with the subvalvular mitral apparatus. The most radical intervention certainly is to cut the papillary muscles, respectively, the chordae tendineae. But discontinuity of papillary muscles is followed by severe mitral incompetence. Former experiments were performed with the isovolumic heart preparation using intracavitary balloons for the left ventricle and discs for occlusion of the mitral valve orifice when the papillary muscles were disconnected from the ventricular wall [21, 26]. For this investigation we developed a new experimental model [13–15].

40

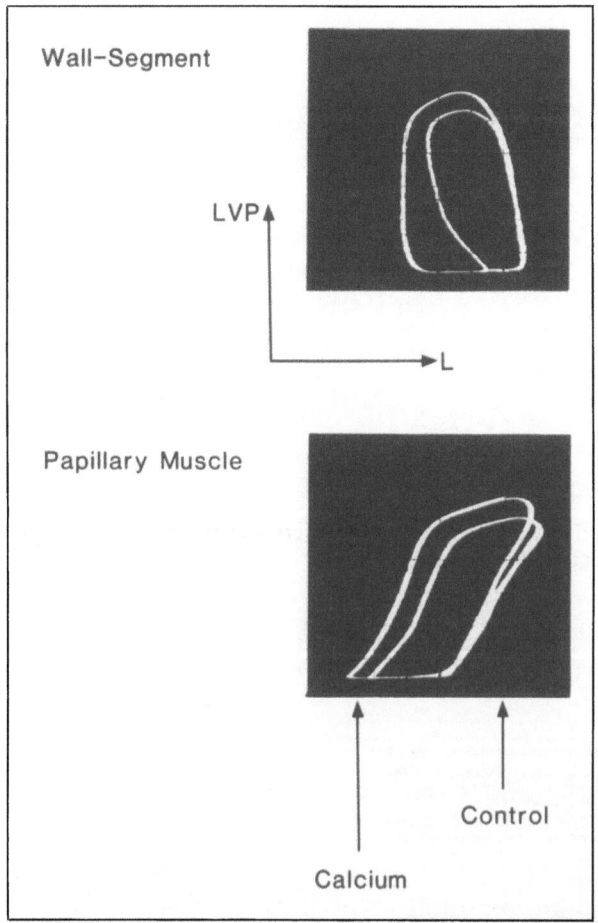

Fig. 7. Pressure-length-loops of a subendocardial wall segment and the papillary muscle during change in contractility (injection of calcium); LVP = left ventricular pressure, L = length. (Used by permission of the Butterworths Company, London.)

Mitral valve prostheses were implanted in dogs, preserving the native mitral valve apparatus, including the papillary muscles. Wires were slung around the anterior and posterior papillary muscle separately and brought through the left ventricular wall to the outside. Figure 8 shows the experimental procedure schematically. Left ventricular dimensions in the major and minor axis were measured by placing ultrasonic crystals on the inner surface of the left ventricular wall. After weaning from cardiopulmonary bypass control data were obtained during volume loading by blood transfusions. Subsequently the chordae tendineae were cut by external application of electrocautery, and volume loading was repeated.

After transsection of the chordae tendineae of the anterior and posterior papillary muscle, the left ventricular diameter in the major axis increased, whereas there was no change in the minor axis diameter (Fig. 9). The average increase of enddias-

41

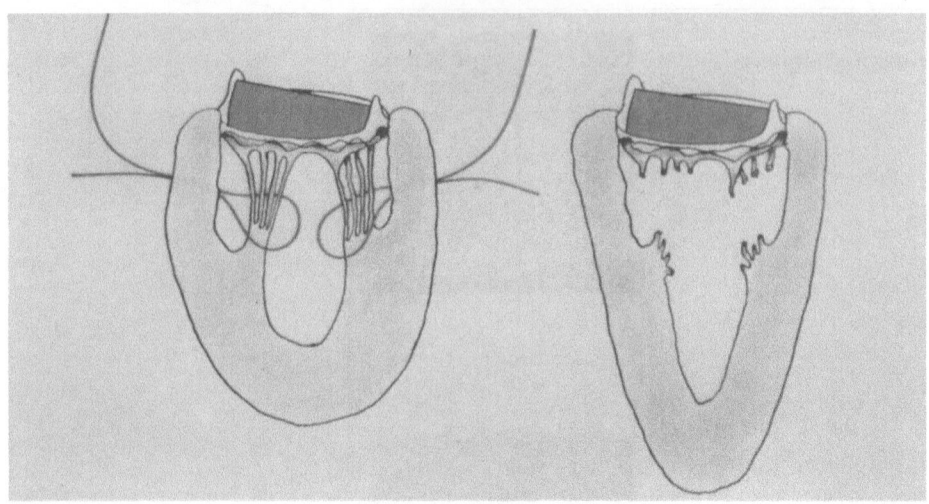

Fig. 8. Schematic drawing of the experimental arrangement for preservation (left) and loss of papillary muscle function (right) following mitral valve implantation

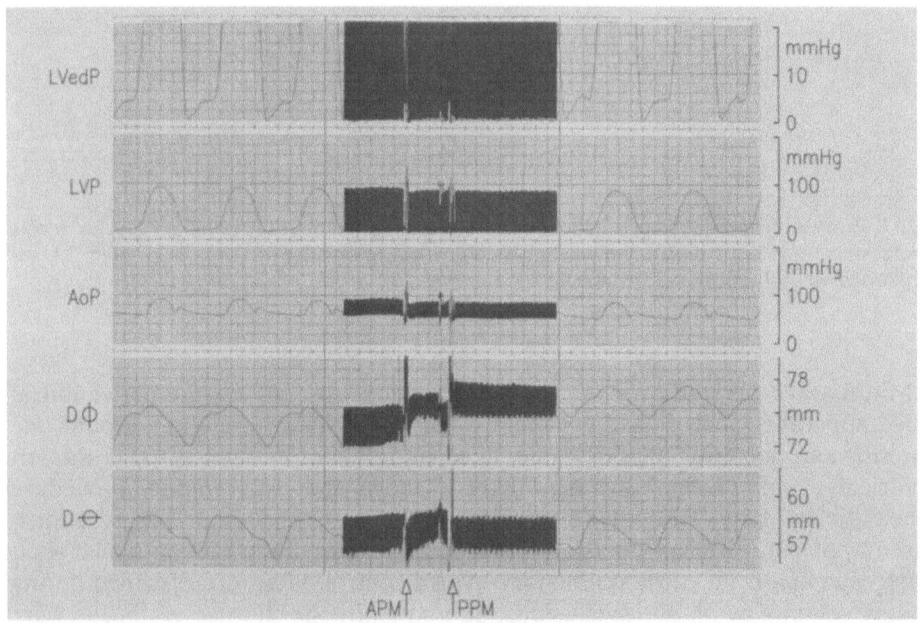

Fig. 9. Acute effects of cutting the chordae tendineae of the anterior (APM) and posterior papillary muscle (PPM) of the left ventricle following mitral valve implantation on left ventricular enddiastolic pressure (LVedP), left ventricular pressure (LVP), aortic pressure (AoP), left ventricular diameter in the major axis (DΦ), and minor axis (D$\ominus$)

tolic length in the major axis was 10 ± 1%. The increase of the enddiastolic length in the minor axis occured only at higher preload levels of 10−12 mmHg left ventricular enddiastolic pressure and ranged from 2% to 4%.

In addition to the increase of enddiastolic length there was a decay of systolic shortening, i.e., the contraction amplitude of the diameter in the major axis. The mean value of the decrease of systolic shortening in the major axis diameter was 42.8 ± 8.3% at preload levels of 12 mmHg left ventricular enddiastolic pressure, while there was no significant change of systolic shortening in the minor axis diameter.

After cutting the chordae tendineae, the left ventricular pressure-diameter-diagramm, as depicted in Fig. 10, revealed that left ventricular systolic shortening in the major axis remained decreased at the three steps of volume loading. There was a parallel shift of the pressure-length-loop to the right according to the increase of enddiastolic length not only due to volume loading, but also caused by loss of papillary muscle function.

These experiments showed that as soon as the chordae tendineae had been divided, the missing link between the mitral valve and the left ventricular wall induced changes in left ventricular geometry: The diameter in the longitudinal axis increased. At the same time deterioration of left ventricular function occured, either due to the failing active contribution of the papillary muscles to ventricular contraction, or due to the loss of passive stabilization of the left ventricular shape and size by the subvalvular apparatus. By all means, cutting the chordae tendineae

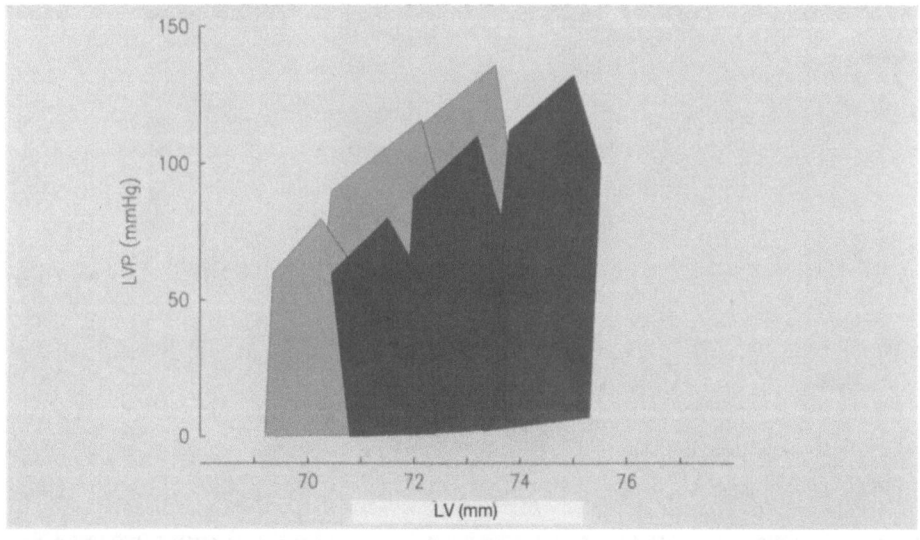

Fig. 10. Left ventricular pressure-diameter-diagram of the major axis diameter during volume loading at three steps of increasing enddiastolic lengths before (left) and after (right) cutting the chordae tendineae of both papillary muscles following mitral valve implantation; LVP = left ventricular pressure, LV = major axis diameter

of the anterior and posterior papillary muscles was followed by substantial changes of left ventricular dimensions and impaired left ventricular pump function.

Papillary muscle function and mitral valve mechanics during ischemia

Myocardial ischemia was induced by temporary occlusion of the left circumflex or left anterior descending coronary artery. Within a few beats after occlusion of the left circumflex artery, severe dysfunction of the posterior papillary muscle developed (Fig. 11). Maximal length increased, while shortening of the papillary muscle during ventricular ejection was markedly reduced. As ischemia became more pronounced, the papillary muscle continued to increase in length beyond the previous phasic maximum and a completely paradoxical motion arose. Overall pump function of the left ventricle was depressed due to the loss of regularly functioning myocardium in the left ventricle, as could be shown by the decrease of left ventricular peak pressure.

Interestingly enough, the enddiastolic length of the intact anterior wall segment and the maximal length of the normally perfused anterior papillary muscle increased at the same time, as depicted in Fig. 12. The difference in the pressure-length-loops was most impressive. The time course of contraction was completely

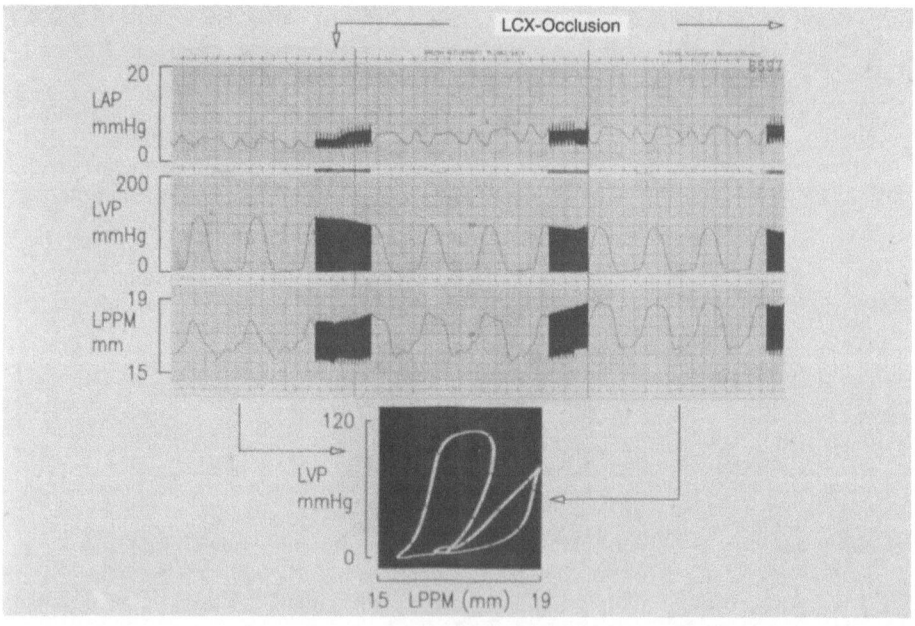

Fig. 11. Effects of acute occlusion of the left circumflex coronary artery (LCX) on left atrial pressure (LAP), left ventricular pressure (LVP), posterior papillary muscle length (LPPM) and on the pressure-length-loop of the posterior papillary muscle. Despite severe ischemic dysfunction of the papillary muscle with increase of maximal length and reduction of systolic shortening during ventricular ejection no signs of mitral incompetence can be seen in the left atrial pressure curve

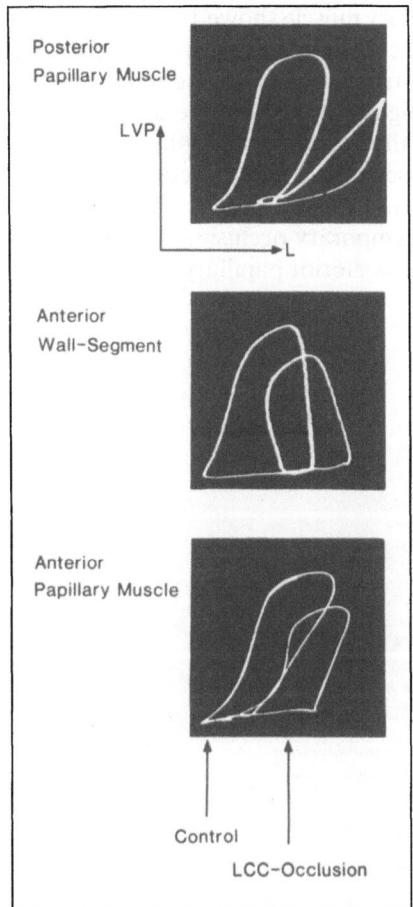

Posterior
Papillary Muscle

LVP

L

Anterior
Wall–Segment

Anterior
Papillary Muscle

Control

LCC–Occlusion

Fig. 12. Changes in the pressure-length-loops of the posterior papillary muscle, anterior wall segment and anterior papillary muscle (from top to bottom) induced by occlusion of the left circumflex coronary artery (LCC). (Used by permission of the Butterworths Company, London.)

altered during ischemia: The posterior papillary muscle was extensively stretched during isovolumic contraction and ventricular ejection, which caused the right slant of the loop. During ventricular ejection the ischemic posterior papillary muscle could not overcome the force developed by the intact ventricular wall. Under these circumstances the loop was generated paradoxically in a clockwise direction, instead of the counterclockwise direction under normal conditions. The anterior wall segment, as well as the anterior papillary muscle, also showed a shift to the right in the pressure-length-loop because of greater enddiastolic and maximal length. This indicated an overall left ventricular dilatation during myocardial ischemia.

Despite severe ischemic dysfunction of the posterior papillary muscle, none of the experimental animals developed hemodynamic signs of mitral incompetence. Mitral regurgitation could neither be seen in the left atrial pressure curves (Fig. 11) nor was it possible to detect mitral insufficiency by indicator technique. This was also true for the experiments with temporary occlusion of the left anterior descend-

45

ing coronary artery (Fig. 13). The anterior papillary muscle showed severe dysfunction with increase in maximal length and reduced shortening during ventricular ejection. The enddiastolic length of the ventricular wall segment within the ischemic zone increased as well, indicating bulging of the ventricular wall in the ischemic area, with simultaneous reduction of the contraction amplitude. In contrast, the ventricular wall segment next to the ischemic zone showed hyperkinetic reaction with augmentation of systolic shortening and increase in contraction amplitude. But similar to the findings during temporary occlusion of the left circumflex coronary artery with dysfunction of the posterior papillary muscle, mitral

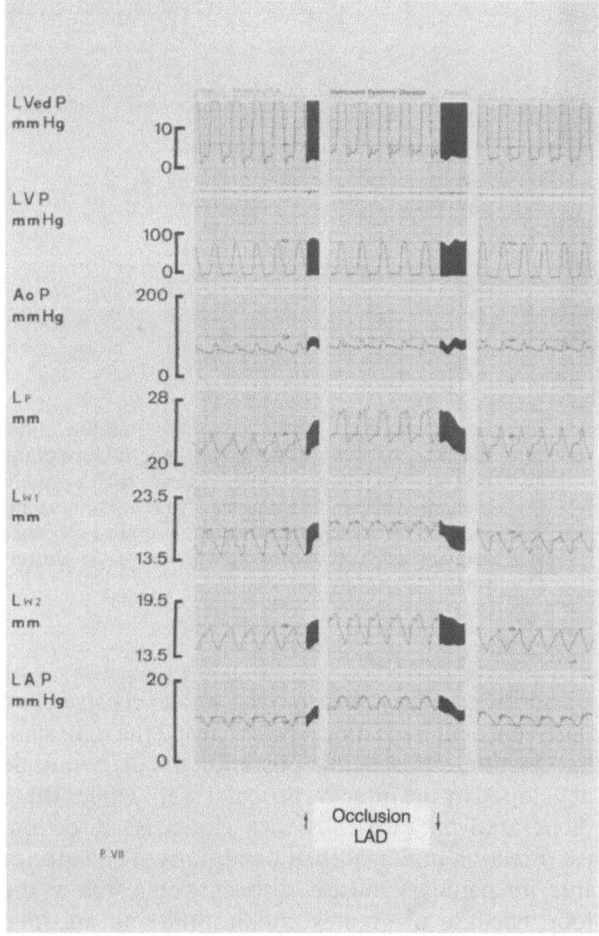

Fig. 13. Effects of acute occlusion of the left anterior descending coronary artery (LAD) on the left ventricular enddiastolic pressure (LVedP), left ventricular pressure (LVP), aortic pressure (AoP), on the anterior papillary muscle (Lp), on the left ventricular subendocardial wall segment in the ischemic zone (Lw1) and on the left ventricular subendocardial wall segment next to the ischemic zone (Lw2) and on left atrial pressure (LAP). Severe ischemic dysfunction of the anterior papillary muscle, dilatation of the left ventricular wall and reduction of systolic shortening in the ischemic myocardium can be demonstrated, but no signs of mitral incompetence can be shown.

incompetence could not be induced during severe ischemic dysfunction of the anterior papillary muscle following temporary occlusion of the left anterior descending coronary artery.

The failure to produce ischemic mitral incompetence in these experiments may be explained by several mechanism: It is possible, that the effect of systolic papillary muscle elongation is counteracted to some extent by the systolic bulging of the adjacent ventricular wall. On the other hand, it is possible that during dilatation of the ventricular wall in response to ischemia, the axis of the papillary muscle moves into a more tangential direction [20]. Both mechanisms together may reduce the net effect of the lengthening of the subvalvular apparatus on the position of the mitral valve leaflets. In addition, the presence of excessive valvular tissue of the leaflets and mitral ring contraction during systole [8] might prevent mitral incompetence. In former experimental studies with infarcted papillary muscles, mitral insufficiency could not be produced either [24, 27].

It seems that adequate papillary muscle function is only one of several factors which provide sufficient mitral valve competence. In our opinion there are three major components involved in producing ischemic mitral regurgitation:
1) the so-called papillary muscle dysfunction, in the sense of asynchronous motion of the papillary muscle and the adjacent ventricular wall;
2) the dyskinesia of the adjacent ventricular wall; and
3) the dilatation of the mitral annulus, i.e., the failing contraction during systole.

Conclusion

Papillary muscles behave like ventricular wall segments, which reflects their task in controlling the positioning of the mitral valve leaflets during cyclic changes of left ventricular pressure and diameters.

Total loss of papillary muscle function is followed by changes in shape and size of the left ventricle, and concurrently by impairment of ventricular performance.

Acute ischemic dysfunction of either the posterior or anterior papillary muscle does not result in acute mitral incompetence. In the pathogenesis of the clinical syndrom generally described as "papillary muscle dysfunction", other and associated components are necessary for induction of the ischemic mitral incompetence.

References

1. Andersen JA, Fischer-Hansen B (1973) Isolated acute myocardial infarction in papillary muscles of the heart: Clinicopathological study of 9 cases. Br Heart J 35:781
2. Aranda JM, Befeler B, Lazzara R, Embi A, Machado H (1975) Mitral valve prolaps and coronary artery disease. Clinical, hemodynamic and angiographic correlations. Circulation 52:245
3. Benninghoff A, Goerttler K (1962) Lehrbuch der Anatomie des Menschen. Urban & Schwarzenberg, München Berlin, p 424
4. Brazier JR, Maloney JV, Buckberg GD (1975) Papillary muscle ischemia with patent coronary arteries. Surgery 78:430
5. Brutsaert DL, Sonnenblick EH (1971) Early onset of maximum velocity of shortening in heart muscle of the cat. Pflugers Arch 324:91
6. Burch GE, DePasquale NP (1965) Time-course of tension in papillary muscles of the heart. JAMA 192:701

7. Burch GE, DePasquale NP, Phillips JH (1968) Syndromes of papillary muscle dysfunction. Am Heart J 75:399
8. Chiechi MA, Lees WM, Thompson R (1956) Functional anatomy of the normal mitral valve. J Thorac Surg 32:378
9. Cronin RE, Armour JA, Randall WC (1969) Function of the in situ papillary muscle in the canine left ventricle. Circ Res 25:67
10. Edman KAP, Nilsson E (1972) Relationship between force and velocity of shortening in rabbit papillary muscle. Acta Physiol Scand 85:483
11. Edwards JE (1971) Clinicopathological correlations: Mitral insufficiency resulting from "over-shooting" of leaflets. Circulation 43:606
12. Fischer VJ, Stuckey JH, Lee RF, Kavaler F (1965) Length changes of papillary muscles of the canine left ventride during the cardiac cycle. Fed Proc 24:278
13. Gams E, Heimisch W, Hagl S, Schad H, Höfter M, Muscholl M, Mendler N, Sebening F (1987) Significance of the subvalvular apparatus for left ventricular function in mitral valve replacement: A new experimental model. Thorac Cardiovasc Surg 35 (Special Issue I):89
14. Gams E, Heimisch W, Hagl S, Mendler N, Schad H, Sebening F (1987) Significance of the subvalvular apparatus following mitral valve replacement. Circulation 76 [Suppl IV]:538
15. Gams E (1989) Die Bedeutung des subvalvulären Halteapparates der Mitralklappe für die Funktion der linken Herzkammer: Untersuchungen nach experimentellem Mitralklappenersatz. Habilitationsschrift, Ludwigs-Maximilians-Universität München
16. Grant RP (1965) Notes on the muscular architecture of the left ventricle. Circulation 32:301
17. Grimm AF, Lendrum BL, Hun-Lin L (1975) Papillary muscle shortening in the intact dog: A cineangiographic study of tranquilized dogs in the upright position. Circ Res 36:49
18. Hagl S, Heimisch W, Meisner H (1976) Direkte Messung der Funktion der Papillarmuskeln des linken Ventrikels während akuter Koronarokklusion beim Hund. Thoraxchirurgie 24:303
19. Hagl S, Heimisch W, Meisner H, Braun E, Mendler N, Franklin D (1976) Function of normal and ischemic papillary muscles in the canine left ventricle. Eur Surg Res 8 [Suppl I]:129
20. Hagl S, Heimisch W, Meisner H, Mendler N, Sebening F (1984) In situ function of the papillary muscles in the intact canine left ventricle. In: Duran C, Angell WW, Johnson AD, Oury JH (eds) Recent progress in mitral valve disease. Butterworths, London Boston Durban Singapore Sydney Toronto Wellington, p 397
21. Hansen DE, Cahill PD, Decampi WM, Harrison DC, Derby GC, Mitchell RS, Miller DC (1986) Valvular-ventricular interaction: importance of the mitral apparatus in canine left ventricular systolic performance. Circulation 73:1310
22. Hirakawa S, Sasayama S, Tomoike H, Crotazier B, Franklin D, McKown D, Ross J (1977) In situ measurement of papillary msucle dynamics in the dog left ventricle. Am J Physiol 233H:383
23. Karas S, Elkins RC (1970) Mechanism of function of the mitral leaflets, chordae tendineae and left ventricular papillary muscle in dogs. Circ Res 26:689
24. Mittal AK, Langston M, Cohn EE, Selzer A, Kerth WJ (1971) Combined papillary muscle and left ventricular wall dysfunction as a cause of mitral regurgitation: An experimental study. Circulation 44:174
25. Shelburne JO, Rubinstein D, Gorlin R (1969) A reappraisal of papillary muscle dysfunction. Am J Med 46:862
26. Spence PA, Peniston CM, David TE, Mihic N, Jabr AK, Narini P, Salerno TA (1986) Towards a better understanding of the etiology of left ventricular dysfunction after mitral valve replacement: An experimental study with possible clinical implications. Ann Thorac Surg 41:363
27. Tsakiris AG, Rastelli GC, DesAmorim D, Titus JL, Wood E (1970) Effect of experimental papillary muscle damage on mitral valve closure in intact anaesthetized dogs. Mayo Clin Proc 45:275

Author's address:
Dr. med. E. Gams
Chirurgische Universitätsklinik Heidelberg,
Abteilung Herzchirurgie
(Direktor Prof. Dr. S. Hagl)
Im Neuenheimer Feld 110
6900 Heidelberg 1, FRG

Discussion

YELLIN:
Since the theme of the meeting is ischemic mitral incompetence and we have just seen some experimental work that indicates it takes more than just papillary muscle dysfunction to produce mitral regurgitation, this seems like a good time to start a discussion.

RANKIN:
I would like to address that last question by stating a hypothesis. When we looked at over 300 coronary arteriograms and left ventriculograms in our series of patients having ischemic mitral insufficiency since 1981, a certain pattern of coronary anatomy is evident. Excluding patients with complex situations, such as anterior wall left ventricular aneurysms, diffuse global infarctions, or rare patients with ruptured papillary muscles, this problem of papillary muscle dysfunction almost always occurs with posterior wall infarcts, either in the circumflex or right coronary artery distributions. Acute papillary muscle dysfunction has virtually never been seen in our experience with an isolated infarct of anterior papillary muscle. So, I would like to ask two questions of the speakers this morning: first of all, would they agree that the syndrome of acute papillary muscle dysfunctions is almost always associated with an isolated infarct of the posterior wall, and secondly, what is the mechanism of the valve incompetence? We have seen this morning, and I am glad it was emphasized, that the anterior papillary muscle anatomy is usually a single large substantial structure, whereas the posterior papillary muscle usually is comprised of multiple small heads that usually arise directly from the posterior wall. What is it that causes the syndrome to predominantly occur with posterior wall infarcts?

HUGENHOLTZ:
I suggest that Dr. Becker take on this question, as he made that point earlier during his presentation.

BECKER:
I think the point is well taken. I can agree with Dr. Rankin that anterior papillary muscle infarction is extremely rare. You made a very important point at the beginning, I think, and I would like to reemphasize that because you have introduced exclusion criteria. You have not included, in what you were saying, patients with large anterior wall infarctions, aneurysms, and by that you have probably excluded those patients who did have anterior wall infarction. You did exclude them — or did I misunderstand you there?

RANKIN:
The reason we would exclude patients with anterior aneurysms is that a very complex geometric situation may exist with diffuse annular dilation and ventricular dysfunction contributing to the regurgitation in that setting. But more relevant to the question, we have seen a large number of patients with anterior papillary muscle infarction, either in the distribution of a large first circumflex marginal or optional diagonal artery, and these patients do not seem to develop ischemic mitral regurgitation. Why does it occur as an isolated syndrome predominantly with posterior wall infarcts?

BECKER:
I don't know why. The only thing that I can say is that from my own series it also shows that the posterior area and the involvement of the posterior papillary muscle is much more frequent than the

49

infarction in the anterior wall. A reason as far as I can see, is that the variability in the posterior papillary muscle is much greater than it is anteriorly. The posterior papillary muscle almost always is in the sort of border-area, the water-shed area, if you wish, between the two major cisterns, right and left, so it is a vulnerable area; it very much will depend on the development of collaterals in the setting of progressive obstructive coronary artery disease. The second thing, which may be relevant, is that we have to realize that the posterior leaflet of the mitral valve takes up about two-thirds of the total circumference of the mitral valve annulus. Therefore, the contributions of the posterior papillary muscle to the valve may well be more "vital" than the contributions of the anterior papillary muscle.

RANKIN:

Well, I'd like to propose one possible explanation to see what you think about it, most of the incompetence in ischemic mitral regurgitation is at the posterior annulus and the posterior valve leaflet. The large number of patients we see with posterior wall infarcts do not develop ischemic mitral regurgitation; the vast majority don't. In fact, only 3% of the coronary disease population had significant ischemic mitral regurgitation in our series, and we have proposed that these patients have minor anatomic defects of the valve tissue at the posterior commissure. The posterior aspect of the posterior leaflet is a common site for persistent fetal commissure cusps and other minor anatomic defects. The specific syndrome of ischemic mitral regurgitation may occur predominantly when a posterior wall infarction and dilation of the posterior annulus is associated with previous minor anatomic defects. With the infarction, the posterior aspect of the valve opens up and produces the syndrome, so that minor preexisting abnormalities in valve anatomy may be extremely important.

BECKER:

We did an extensive study, I think way back 1976, − this was the early period of the heated debates by echocardiographers of what was the normal valve motion on the M-mode −, and when we looked into the mitral valve apparatus in normal hearts, we found such an extreme variability, minor, but still variabilities, and they could well explain all the different patterns that you could see on your tracings. Some patients have an anatomy of their mitral valve apparatus, that leaves them more prone to develop mitral valve regurgitation when something else comes to it, so one patient may have the suitable anatomy, so to speak, to develop it much more rapidly than another patient, while both of them still have a mitral valve and they have a posterior papillary muscle and the cordae are there.

RUTISHAUSER:

My question goes to Dr. Gams. I was somewhat puzzled by the slanted form of the pressure-length-loop of your papillary muscle already at rest and I would like to know how do you implant these crystals and might there be already a certain ischemia in your resting values because your slanted pressure-length-loop could eventually speak in this direction. Obviously, if you get severe ischemia you then have no energy, but even before there is a change in the form from the rectangle way to the slanted way.

GAMS:

The explanation is not the ischemia but the physiological contractile behavior of the papillary muscle. You could see this schematic drawing at the beginning that the papillary muscles reach the maximum length, not at the point where the wall segments reach the maximum. That is the reason for the right slant. So the papillary muscles reach the maximum length before the isovolumic contraction − actually at the point of isovolumic contraction − and that is the reason for the completely different shape.

HETZER:

I wanted to come back to the question that Dr. Rankin has just brought up. We have seen a few patients with ischemic mitral incompetence due to fibrosis of the anterior papillary muscle and those patients were all such who had obstruction of a large intermediate coronary artery or a large first postero-lateral branch of the circumflex coronary artery thus inflicting the basal antero-lateral surface of the left ventricle. Associated with this type of very unusual coronary distribution in some patients we found an aneurysm near the basis at the antero-lateral wall. Our explanation for the rarity of the anterior papillary muscle fibrosis or necrosis is such that, probably, in a usual coronary distribution pattern very few patients would survive an infarct inflicting both the anterior descending coronary artery and the circumflex coronary artery, which would then result in anterior papillary muscle necrosis or fibrosis. I wanted to hear your opinion about that, Dr. Becker.

BECKER:

I think that that point is well taken; I agree. I have tried to say that by indicating that if you have an anterior wall infarction with mitral regurgitation it is usually a huge infarct and even then the anterior wall, the anterior papillary muscle is not infarcted or only partially infarcted. We see patients who die with a cardiogenic shock within 24 h after onset of infarction. There we found a huge infarct, almost always accompanied by the circumferential subendocardial spreading of the infarction as part of the deterioration. In those instances it is different, because then there is infarction of the area including the antero-lateral papillary muscle. I think we have to face that because the LAD usually does not supply the blood to the base of the anterior papillary muscle, it does come from other branches. But again, it is variable.

FRATER:

I would like to suggest that it is time we drop the term "papillary muscle dysfunction" and I would like to pose a couple of questions to some of the speakers to lead into that. If we use the term papillary muscle dysfunction, it implies that we understand what the function is. If we do not know what the function is, we cannot describe dysfunction. Papillary muscles can vary from about half a centimeter in height to 3 centimeters in height, at least, and even if, according to Dr. Gams and Dr. Hagl, they can shorten by 20%. Clearly a piece of muscle that sometimes is going to change by a few millimeters and sometimes by at most 6 or 7 millimeters, is going to have such an incredible variability in its length change that it can surely not be doing very much that is consistent in the way of function. Dr. Gams's demonstration that the lengthening occurs during the ejection phase tells us precisely what the papillary muscles are doing. What the papillary muscles are doing is acting as shock absorbers, and they are, in fact, stretching in response to an increase in tension, but are not themselves actively doing anything. I think we all recognize that, in fact, it takes an infarct of some dimension to produce mitral insufficiency. The variability that has been referred to I am sure relates to the variability of infarction, as Dr. Hetzer just suggested. The anterior papillary muscle is very rarely involved except in a very large infarct. The posterior muscle is the one that is more easily involved in an infarct and more often associated with the insufficiency. But in all cases, I think, you can demonstrate that it is the ventricular wall that is the cause of the insufficiency, partly by changing annulus in some cases, partly by changing the dimension from annulus to the point of chorda-papillary attachment. If you increase the length of the posterior left ventricular wall or if you increase the dimension of the annulus in systole you will interfere with mitral valve closure. These are examples of left ventricular dysfunction not papillary muscle dysfunction. So, I would suggest that we should probably drop the term. It is an anomalous term. It does not mean anything. I grant you that there may be a very rare case of elongation of a very long papillary muscle that is ischemic that might allow prolapse, but the great majority of cases of mitral insufficiency with ischemic disease are not prolapse.

GAMS:

We used the expression of papillary muscle dysfunction because actually 20 years ago I think Burch had brought it up. It was quite clear from the experiments that papillary muscle dysfunction does not mean mitral incompetence. I think the only reason to use the expression papillary muscle dysfunction is justified when you understand it as asynchronous motion between the papillary muscle itself and the adjacent ventricular wall. Then it might be possible to get mitral incompetence.

HUGENHOLTZ:

But still, Dr. Gams and Dr. Becker, would you address yourself to the point raised by Dr. Frater, drop the term papillary muscle dysfunction. You would agree with that?

BECKER:

Yes, I would say it is spoken words right out of my heart. I think we use the term papillary muscle dysfunction on historical grounds and we really do not think very much about it and that is why we keep on using it, but as a pathologist I have been struck for years that severe ischemic mitral regurgitation may be present and the papillary muscles themselves are only partially infarcted or are not infarcted at all. And if we accept — and we have all accepted that already for a long time — that the mitral valve function relates to many aspects and they have been highlighted today so that the mitral valve apparatus heavily relates on the condition of the myocardium, then we are blaming papillary muscles for something you cannot blame them for. I agree with Dr. Frater, totally.

FEHSKE:
I just wanted to address an informative question to Dr. Becker: do you agree that even if the infarction is placed in the inferior region of the left ventricular circumference that we can see it or that we are supposed to see dysfunction of the anterior mitral leaflet, because we are looking for infarction and regurgitation in ischemic heart disease by reflected ultrasound and we cannot judge the papillary muscle dysfunction but we can look for the valve closing mechanism. We see often, or mostly, if it is not only the ring dilation or other things that have been mentioned now, we see a dysfunction of the anterior mitral leaflet in posterior or inferior infarctions in the sense of mitral prolapse, for instance, with an eccentric mitral regurgitation.

BECKER:
Yes, I agree. But you may expect that don't you, because the postero-medial papillary muscle does support part of the posterior leaflet and part of the anterior leaflet. And so the whole area the myocardium supporting that papillary muscle does. Therefore, once that is disconnected or in any other way has motion disturbance, you may see it reflected also into the anterior leaflet and particularly around the postero-medial commissure.

HUGENHOLTZ:
Could I add to that, Dr. Becker, and perhaps to ask you an answer to the question Dr. Puff has raised, namely that the AV-ring is not at all a rigid collagenous structure but a very versatile and dynamic structure. Have you studied it in this setting and found that it was, shall we say, in your pathologist's eyes "abnormal".

BECKER:
Yes, we did and I am pleased your raised the question; I was very pleased to hear Dr. Puff say this. We did look into the mitral annulus recently and we also extended that into ischemic heart disease and the point is we share this opinion that the so-called mitral annulus is highly deficient along its course. So, previously, we thought that the tricuspid fibrous annulus was deficient, or, very often absent as a fibrous cord. But we thought the mitral annulus is always well formed and is a very thick fibrous cord. We now realized that that is a mistake, that is not the case, and then we are back to your question with ischemic disease. The anatomic setting is such that you cannot expect the mitral annulus to be able to resist any dilating forces on it, and so you actually can see how it expands when the left ventricle increases its volume.

HUGENHOLTZ:
Thank you, I am sure, in the following sessions when the surgeons have a chance to talk about what they do with the ring, we will learn more.

MEYER:
Dr. Becker, I found as a clinical cardiologist that it is extremely important that you mentioned this circumferential ischemic area we often find in patients with long-standing myocardial infarctions, severe myocardial infarctions, going into pump failure. They do not always go into real cardiogenic shock, and since we do a serial echocardiogram in those patients, we always had blamed the mitral apparatus to enlarge, that means we had always the impression that the ring is going to spread since the ventricle is going up. As I have learned now, this is a combined function of the papillary muscles and also probably of the muscles Dr. Puff has demosntrated. And if those patients recover, then the ventricle shrinks and then probably also the ischemia of the interior layers improve. My question is, what do you think: is this a general disturbance of perfusion, which causes this circular ischemia, or is it going more via the endocardial layers?

BECKER:

My problem is that very few of the heart specimens that I have ssen are obtained from patients who survived, as you described it. I agree with you that it is, as far as I can see it, a combined action. I look upon it as a compromised perfusion of myocardium with dilating ventricles, with increased enddiastolic pressures, which compromises perfusion further and it gets often further complicated by the mechanisms that you described effecting the mitral valve apparatus and so then gradually you get into a condition which becomes a circulus vitiosus, it strengthens itself and you get worse perfusion in the subendocardial region, further dilation, a further compromised mitral valve and this leads to early death. We have very strong evidence for that. Looking at enzyme studies in heart specimen that have come to autopsy with this condition, you will always find this, you will always find the primary infarction, and you will see the spread being circumferential and if you correlate that with the, let's say, non-invasive studies done at the intensive care at that time, it correlates very well.

MEYER:

Sometimes in the case of following those patients we turn to the cardiac surgeons, because we can definitely demonstrate that those patients may have a degree of mitral incompetence by 40%, and this is a very badly functioning ventricle, and we then follow them serially with the echo, and if the patient then survives, this mitral incompetence goes back gradually and significantly, and if he leaves the hospital, after six months there is nearly no demonstrable mitral incompetence. This shows that this is not a total ischemia, this is a relative ischemia in many of those cases, which then normalizes, and that sometimes really is a big burden for the treatment of those patients.

RANKIN:

I would like to discuss with Dr. Frater the semantics of the term "papillary muscle dysfunction". With due respect to Dr. George Burch, we have used that term, and I think it is a good term. It very specifically describes the syndrome of mitral regurgitation occurring after infarction with an intact papillary muscle apparatus. Whenever we have used the term, however, we have defined it very clearly as actually constituting the complex of physiologic derangements including papillary muscle elongation, loss of papillary muscle shortening, posterior annular dilation, possible leaflet defects, and so on. In would certainly welcome a better term than papillary muscle dysfunction to describe this complex of physiologic derangements, but left ventricular dysfunction is not specific enough to describe it. What term would Dr. Frater propose to replace papillary muscle dysfunction? I do not believe this is a bad term, if we understand it is a complex of physiologic problems.

HUGENHOLTZ:

Dr. Frater is probably going to say mitral valve dysfunction and we are back where we were.

FRATER:

Ischemic mitral insufficiency!

RANKIN:

Yes, but there are several types of ischemic mitral insufficiency. A papillary muscle rupture is a very specific problem. Therefore, we need something to describe this syndrome of regurgitation after posterior wall infarction with an intact papillary muscle.

FRATER:

It is not even necessarily after infarction, as has been mentioned already, it can occur without infarction at all. Ischemic mitral insufficiency implies mitral insufficiency related to the consequences of reduction in coronary blood supply.

RANKIN:

So what term would you propose?

FRATER:

I am proposing precisely that term and then from there it takes more words, I grant you, it is not shorthand the way papillary muscle dysfunction is shorthand. It takes more words, but it is far more precise. Ischemic mitral incompetence due to paradoxical motion of the antero-lateral papillary muscle, due to failure of shortening in the posterior left ventricular wall, due to failure of shortening of the mural annulus, due to all three of those simultaneously, and, as a separate and completely different category is rarely — due to ischemic elongation of the papillary muscle, and, one stage beyond that, rupture of the papillary muscle. Mitral insufficiency is the common consequence, but the process may be dynamic, or may be fixed and permanent. Whatever the cases are, I think you should define it precisely.

GAMS:
I agree again. I think the problem is that it is a syndrome and not a diagnosis and that is the problem.

HUGENHOLTZ:
It is marvelous how in the medical world, the less we know, the more we like the term syndrome, and the less we like that we go to ideopathic this or that.

II. Diagnosis and indications for treatment

Predictors for mitral regurgitation in coronary artery disease

E. Frantz, F. Weininger, H. Oswald, E. Fleck

Dept. of Internal Medicine and Cardiology, German Heart Center Berlin, Berlin, FRG

Introduction

It is not yet known which factors are responsible for the occurrence of mitral regurgitation (MR) as a consequence of ischemic heart disease. The same applies to the incidence of mitral insufficiency in coronary artery disease.

Mitral valve regurgitation can be caused by ischemic heart disease in different ways. Acute myocardial infarction can cause definite rupture of a papillary muscle or of one of its heads, leading to severe mitral regurgitation with fulminant clinical deterioration. By injuring papillary muscles or ventricular myocardium to which it is inserted, infarction can also produce chronic mitral insufficiency of different grades of severity. Beside this permanent form of mitral incompetence, there may occur a transient form where ischemia leads to temporary dysfunction of parts of the mitral apparatus under conditions of stress.

The following study was designed to find criteria which make it possible to predict whether mitral regurgitation of ischemic origin will occur in a patient suffering from coronary artery disease or not. The main question was whether the incidence of ischemic mitral insufficiency depends on certain patterns of coronary artery involvement in coronary artery disease.

Reviewing the literature on this topic one finds only rare contributions reporting angiographic findings in patients with mitral regurgitation of ischemic origin. In 1963 in two publications [3, 4] the term "papillary muscle dysfunction" had been introduced, and a hypothetic model of the pathophysiology of ischemic mitral insufficiency had been created. From then on the discussion about this phenomenon [1, 5, 6, 8−10, 13] led to multiple theoretical attempts at further explanation, but did not lead to more concise results concerning its mechanisms [2].

Especially, there are no reports on the patterns of coronary vessel involvement, myocardial wall motion abnormalities of hemodynamic parameters of those patients suffering from ischemic mitral regurgitation. Only rare figures on incidence of mitral incompetence of ischemic origin and data of coronary anatomy of patients are reported; these data refer to small and selected samples only (31% in a sample of patients with three-vessel-disease pre-CABG-surgery [7]). Thus literature reveals only little information on incidence, severity, and pathophysiologic particularities of ischemic mitral incompetence.

In order to answer these questions we reviewed all patients of this clinic with angiographic proof for coronary artery disease in presence or absence of mitral regurgitation. We were especially concerned with the peculiarities which might be responsible for the occurrence of mitral regurgitation of ischemic origin.

Material and methods

Evaluated sample

In a retrospective analysis we reviewed all 2654 consecutive patients, in whom coronary angiography and ventriculography were applied between June, 1986, and November, 1988, in this clinic. This group of patients was separated according to the following procedure (Fig. 1):

In order to exclude all those patients with mitral regurgitation as part of a primarily valvular, i.e., most often rheumatic disease, we excluded all patients with angiographic evidence for (all grades of) mitral stenosis (n = 135). The remaining patients (n = 2519) were divided into a group with and a group without angiographic finding of mitral regurgitation. In each of these groups we found patients with and without evidence for coronary artery disease, for the purpose of this study defined as at least one stenosis of at least 75% reduction in diameter in one of the three major coronary arteries. By dividing the groups with and without mitral regurgitation according to this criterium, we defined the evaluated samples as 189 patients with coronary artery disease and presence of mitral regurgitation, compared to the control group (n = 1550) with coronary artery disease, but without mitral regurgitation.

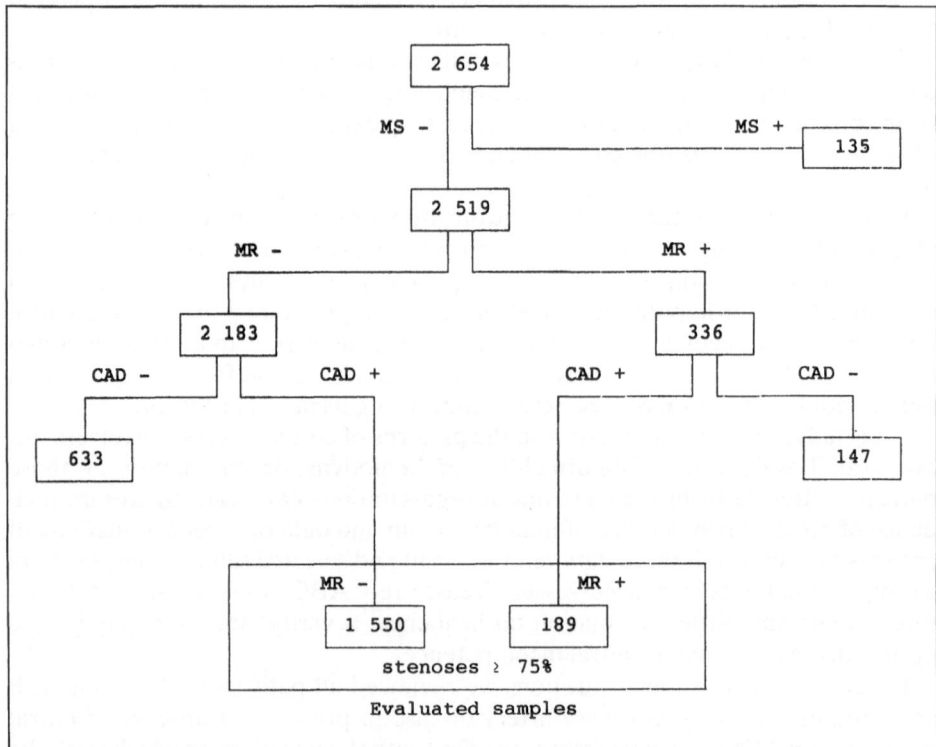

Fig. 1. Selection of Study-Group (Consecutive Patients, June, 1986 to November, 1988)

Table 1. Evaluated parameters

* age
* LV-EF
* LVEDP
* LVEDVI
* LVESVI
* PC-m
* PC-v
* PA-m

---

* wall motion
  RAO five segments,
  LAO five segments normo-,
  hypo-, a-, dys-kinetic

Methods

In order to find out predictive criteria for occurrence and severity of mitral regurgitation of ischemic origin a comparison was made. We compared possible predictive criteria in patients with and without mitral regurgitation but with identical vessel involvement patterns. Mitral regurgitation was assessed angiographically by the visualization of contrast regurgitation in the left atrium during ventricular systole; grading was based on conventionally used criteria [11]. Possible predictive criteria consisted of hemodynamic parameters, body-surface-indexed volumes of the left ventricle and wall motion abnormalities, assessed by biplane angiography (Table 1).

Patients were grouped by vessel involvement patterns, which resulted in the following seven groups: Significantly stenosed one, two or three major coronary arteries in various combinations (i.e., LAD, LCX, RCA alone, LAD and LCX, LAD and RCA, LCX and RCA, as well as involvement of all three vessels). In each of these seven groups each comparison was made between patients with and patients without mitral regurgitation.

Tables 1 and 2 show the list of evaluated parameters and the performed statistical procedures. The distribution of patients in each of the seven groups is shown in Table 3 which indicates the overall incidence of mitral regurgitation in the evaluated samples.

The comparison was performed first as an univariate analysis of the numeric data of hemodynamics, left-ventricular volume- indices, and patient age.

Wall motion abnormalities were considered by their relative frequency in the evaluated samples. Wall motion in five different ventricular regions in each of two

Table 2. Statistics

Evaluated Parameters	Procedures
Age and Hemodynamics	* Univariate analysis and *t*-Test * Discriminant analysis
Regional wall motion abnormalities	* Univariate analysis and chi-square-test

Table 3. Incidence of mitral regurgitation in coronary artery disease

Type of CAD sten. ≥ 75%	Total	Mitral regurgitation absent	Mitral regurgitation present	
	n	n	n	%
LAD	372	358	14	3.8
LCX	172	152	20	13.2
RCA	192	179	13	7.3
LAD + LCX	222	196	26	13.9
LAD + RCA	165	146	19	11.5
LCX + RCA	123	109	14	12.8
3 – VD	493	410	83	20.2
Total	1739	1550	189	10.9

Low overall incidence of mitral regurgitation; a tendency toward higher incidence of MR in groups with more than one-vessel involvement was

projections of biplane ventriculography was characterized as normal, hypokinetic, akinetic or dyskinetic. For the purpose of this study the latter three were considered as abnormal.

Relative frequency of the so defined wall motion abnormalities was compared for each group with and without mitral regurgitation, but with identical vessel involvement.

All numeric data where indicated by "±" are given as mean value with standard deviation.

A stepwise forward and backward multivariate discriminant analysis of the data was made to assess the predictive potential of the univariately analyzed numeric data.

Results

Incidence of mitral regurgitation in coronary artery disease

In the evaluated samples, i.e., 1 739 patients with coronary artery disease, the overall incidence of mitral regurgitation of all trades was 10.9% (n = 189).

Incidence varies with the extent and pattern of vessel involvement in coronary artery disease: incidence ranges from 3.8% in the group of patients with isolated LAD-stenosis to 20.2% in the group with three-vessel disease. In all groups where LCX is involved incidence of mitral regurgitation exceeds 13%.

Table 3 shows the distribution of patients with and without mitral regurgitation, according to the defined pattern of coronary artery disease-vessel-involvement.

Severity of mitral regurgitation in coronary artery disease

Nine out of 1 739 patients with coronary artery disease (= 0.52%) revealed moderately severe and severe mitral regurgitation; 1.84% (32/1 739) bore evidence of

Table 4. Angiographic grading of mitral regurgitation Patients with CAD and MR

Type of CAD sten. ≥ 75%	n	mild	Grading of MR moderate	moderately severe	severe
LAD	14	14 100%			
LCX	20	16 80%	3 15%	1 5%	
RCA	13	13 100%			
LAD + LCX	26	18 69%	5 19%	2 8%	1 1%
LAD + RCA	19	14 73.7%	5 26.3%		
LCX + RCA	14	10 71.5%	3 21.5%	1 7%	
3 – VD	83	67 81%	12 14%	4 5%	

No correlation between higher grades of MR and groups with more than one-vessel involvement was observed.

mitral regurgitation grades +2 to +4. Regarding only patients with proof for mitral regurgitation, those with grades 2+, 3+ and 4+ are a group of 16.9% (32/189), 4.76% (9/189) showing moderately severe or severe mitral regurgitation.

Incidences of mitral regurgitation not exceeding grade "1+" range between 69% (18/26) in the group of patients with combined LAD + LCX-stenosis to 100% in the group with isolated LAD- (n = 14) or RCA- (n = 13) stenoses, respectively. These incidences are noted in detail in Table 4.

Comparison of patients with and without mitral regurgitation
(Results of univariate analysis)

Comparison of patient's age: It all but one of the investigated subgroups differences in the age of patients with and without mitral regurgitation did not reach statistical significance. Only in the group of patients with isolated stenosis in LCX were patients with mitral regurgitation significantly older than those without (p < 0.01).

Comparison of hemodynamic parameters: Compared were pressures in the pulmonary artery, the pulmonary artery wedge position (peak and mean), the end-diastolic left ventricle and the left ventricular ejection fraction.

Mean pulmonary artery pressure in all subgroups with mitral regurgitation exceeds 25 mmHg (with the exception of the group with isolated RCA-stenosis – 21.7 ± 7.5 mmHg –), whereas in groups without mitral regurgitation values reach only 18 mmHg. Similarly, mean pulmonary artery wedge pressures range from 18.1 ± 6.7 mmHg (in the group with isolated LCX-stenosis) to 24.0 ± 11.2 (in the group with LAD+LCX-stenoses) in patients with mitral regurgitation, whereas in groups without mitral regurgitation, regurgitation does not exceed 12.1 mmHg.

In patients with mitral regurgitation mean left-ventricular enddiastolic pressures range from 17.3 ± 7.8 mmHg (in the group with isolated RCA-stenosis) to 24.1 ± 10.4 mmHg (in the group with LAD+LCX-stenosis), while corresponding values in patients without regurgitation do not exceed 14.1 ± 6.1 mmHg.

"V-waves" in pulmonary artery wedge pressure tracings in patients with mitral regurgitation reveal the largest value in the group with LAD+LCX-stenosis $(33.8 \pm 18.9$ mmHg), the smallest in the group with isolated LCX-stenosis $(21.6 \pm 9.8$ mmHg). In comparison, these values in groups of patients without mitral regurgitation do not exceed 15.0 ± 8.1 mmHg (in the group of patients with three-vessel disease).

The differences in these pressures between the groups of patients with and without mitral regurgitation reach a level of statistical significance in most instances: in the groups with LAD and LCX involved (either with or without RCA involvement) differences between all pressures reported reach a p-value of < 0.0005. LV-enddiastolic pressure differences are not statistically significant save in comparison of groups with isolated RCA-stenosis; the same is valid for the other pressures reported. In Table 5a–g all data are given in detail.

Table 5a. Quantitative Parameters univariate analysis, t-test. Stenosis $\geq 75\%$ isolated in LAD

Parameters	MR + n = 14	MR − n = 357	p
Age (years)	58.0 ± 11	56.0 ± 9.7	n. s.
LV-EF (%)	42.1 ± 18.4	56.0 ± 10.5	$<.05$
LVEDP (mmHg)	19.9 ± 10.9	13.1 ± 5.6	$<.05$
LVEDVI (ml/m^2)	175.4 ± 84.2	118.8 ± 36.5	$<.05$
LVESVI (ml/m^2)	113.3 ± 80.5	55.2 ± 28.7	$<.05$
PC-ṁ (mmHg)	21.2 ± 9.9	11.6 ± 4.2	$<.005$
PC-v (mmHg)	26.2 ± 12.9	14.8 ± 6.0	$<.01$
PA-ṁ (mmHg)	26.4 ± 9.6	18.3 ± 5.3	$<.01$

Significant differences in hemodynamics between subgroups with isolated LAD-stenosis with and without mitral regurgitation.

Table 5b. Quantitative Parameters univariate analysis, t-test. Stenosis $\geq 75\%$ isolated in LCX

Parameters	MR + n = 20	MR − n = 132	p
Age (years)	64.8 ± 10.3	57.6 ± 8.2	$<.01$
LV-EF (%)	42.8 ± 12.3	56.2 ± 9.1	$<.0005$
LVEDP (mmHg)	19.2 ± 8.4	13.0 ± 5.2	$<.01$
LVEDVI (ml/m^2)	152.7 ± 47.2	118.1 ± 29.9	$<.01$
LVESVI (ml/m^2)	88.2 ± 41.8	53.3 ± 23.2	$<.005$
PC-ṁ (mmHg)	18.1 ± 6.7	11.4 ± 4.0	<0.005
PC-v (mmHg)	21.6 ± 9.8	13.8 ± 6.7	$<.01$
PA-ṁ (mmHg)	25.1 ± 9.3	18.1 ± 5.5	$<.005$

Significant differences in hemodynamics between subgroups with isolated LCX-stenosis with and without mitral regurgitation.

Table 5c. Quantitative Parameters univariate analysis, *t*-test. Stenosis ≥75% isolated in RCA

Parameters	MR + n = 13	MR − n = 166	p
Age (years)	59.9 ± 8.6	55.6 ± 9.7	n.s.
LV-EF (%)	49.6 ± 12.3	55.1 ± 9.0	n.s.
LVEDP (mmHg)	17.3 ± 7.8	13.5 ± 5.8	n.s.
LVEDVI (ml/m^2)	145.6 ± 60.1	122.2 ± 32.2	n.s.
LVESVI (ml/m^2)	79.2 ± 51.8	55.6 ± 23.0	n.s.
PC-m̄ (mmHg)	16.0 ± 8.3	12.1 ± 5.0	n.s.
PC-v (mmHg)	21.5 ± 12.8	15.3 ± 6.8	n.s.
PA-m̄ (mmHg)	21.7 ± 7.5	17.8 ± 5.0	n.s.

No significant differences in hemodynamics between subgroups with isolated RCA-stenosis with and without mitral regurgitation.

Table 5d. Quantitative Parameters univariate analysis, *t*-test. Stenose ≥75% in LAD + LCX

Parameters	MR + n = 26	MR − n = 170	p
Age (years)	59.4 ± 9.3	58.4 ± 9.4	n.s.
LV-EF (%)	36.0 ± 14.9	53.1 ± 10.8	<.0005
LVEDP (mmHg)	24.1 ± 10.4	14.1 ± 6.1	<.0005
LVEDVI (ml/m^2)	191.3 ± 70.1	125.6 ± 34.8	<.0005
LVESVI (ml/m^2)	129.6 ± 69.7	60.9 ± 31.5	<.0005
PC-m̄ (mmHg)	24.0 ± 11.2	12.0 ± 4.6	<.0005
PC-v (mmHg)	33.8 ± 18.9	14.9 ± 6.6	<.0005
PA-m̄ (mmHg)	31.8 ± 12.5	18.1 ± 5.7	<.0005

Highly significant differences in hemodynamics between subgroups with combined LAD- and LCX-stenoses with and without mitral regurgitation.

Table 5e. Quantitative Parameters univariate analysis, *t*-test. Stenoses ≥75% in LAD + RCA

Parameters	MR + n = 19	MR − n = 146	p
Age (years)	58.2 ± 12.4	56.9 ± 9.0	n.s.
LV-EF (%)	41.3 ± 13.3	52.1 ± 10.4	<.005
LVEDP (mmHg)	23.5 ± 12.0	13.5 ± 6.6	<.005
LVEDVI (ml/m^2)	183.2 ± 74.8	126.1 ± 32.9	<.005
LVESVI (ml/m^2)	116.4 ± 76.3	62.3 ± 26.4	<.01
PC-m̄ (mmHg)	19.8 ± 11.1	11.6 ± 5.9	<.01
PC-v (mmHg)	26.8 ± 14.9	14.1 ± 6.6	<.005
PA-m̄ (mmHg)	28.1 ± 11.8	18.1 ± 6.1	<.05

Significant differences in hemodynamics between subgropus with combined LAD- and RCA-stenoses with and without mitral regurgitation.

Left ventricular ejection-fraction is lower in all groups of patients with mitral regurgitation compared to groups of patients with congruent vessel involvement but without mitral regurgitation. Differences are significant with p < 0.0005 in comparison to the groups of patients with isolated LCX-stenosis, combined LAD + LCX-stenosis and three-vessel involvement, with p < 0.005 in the groups with

Table 5f. Quantitative Parameters univariate analysis, *t*-test. Stenoses ≥75% in LCX + RCA

Parameters	MR + n = 14	MR − n = 95	p
Age (years)	55.4 ± 12.2	56.3 ± 8.3	n.s.
LV-EF (%)	38.1 ± 16.2	50.9 ± 9.5	<.05
LVEDP (mmHg)	21.1 ± 10.2	13.6 ± 5.5	<.05
LVEDVI (ml/m²)	164.6 ± 64.2	122.8 ± 30.7	<.05
LVESVI (ml/m²)	108.1 ± 62.4	61.5 ± 24.8	<.05
PC-ṁ (mmHg)	20.9 ± 10.4	11.7 ± 4.4	<.01
PC-v (mmHg)	24.2 ± 11.9	15.0 ± 5.7	<.05
PA-ṁ (mmHg)	27.1 ± 13.5	17.7 ± 4.8	<.05

Significant differences in hemodynamics between subgroups with combined LCX- and RCA-stenoses with and without mitral regurgitation.

Table 5g. Quantitative Parameters univariate analysis, *t*-test.
Stenoses ≥75% in LAD + LCX + RCA (3-VD)

Parameters	MR + n = 83	MR − n = 327	p
Age (years)	62.0 ± 9.5	60.0 ± 9.3	n.s.
LV-EF (%)	39.0 ± 13.1	49.3 ± 11.1	<.0005
LVEDP (mmHg)	21.0 ± 9.9	14.0 ± 6.8	<.0005
LVEDVI (ml/m²)	156.4 ± 53.9	129.6 ± 35.2	<.0005
LVESVI (ml/m²)	100.2 ± 49.7	67.6 ± 30.1	<.0005
PC-ṁ (mmHg)	19.7 ± 9.8	11.9 ± 5.5	<.0005
PC-v (mmHg)	26.5 ± 14.6	15.0 ± 8.1	<.0005
PA-ṁ (mmHg)	27.7 ± 11.1	18.2 ± 6.1	<.0005

Highly significant differences in hemodynamics between subgroups with three-vessel disease with and without mitral regurgitation.

LAD + LCX-stenosis, and $p < 0.05$ in groups with isolated LAD-stenosis being not significant in the group with isolated RCA-stenosis.

In none of the groups of patients with mitral regurgitation does LV-ejection fraction reach a mean value of 50% (range: 36.0 ± 14.9% in the group with LAD+LCX-stenosis to 49.6 ± 12.3% in the group with isolated RCA-stenosis). In comparison, in groups of patients without mitral regurgitation values range from 49.3 ± 11.1% in the group with three-vessel disease to 56.2 ± 9.1% in the group of patients with isolated LCX-stenosis. In Table 5a−g all data are given in detail.

Comparison of left ventricular volumes: Left-ventricular volumes in end-systole and end-diastole (indexed for body surface area) were compared between patients with and without mitral regurgitation but with identical coronary anatomy.

End-diastolic volume parameters were larger in all groups of patients with mitral regurgitation than in groups of patients without mitral regurgitation. The maximal volume was observed in the group of patients with stenoses in LAD+LCX (191.3 ± 70.1 ml/m²), the minimal volume in the group of patients with isolated RCA-stenosis (145.6 ± 60.1 ml/m²). The same groups revealed the extreme values for end-systolic left-ventricular volume: 129.6 ± 69.7 ml/m² in the group of patients with LAD+LCX-stenosis, 79.2 ± 51.8 ml/m² in the group of patients with isolated RCA-stenosis.

In groups without mitral regurgitation, the maximal mean value of end-diastolic volumes did not exceed 130 ml/m², the maximal mean values of end-systolic volumes reached 68 ml/m² (both values observed in the group of patients with three-vessel disease).

Univariate analysis of the differences between groups of patients with and without mitral regurgitation as to the parameter of size of the left ventricle revealed statistical significance in each comparison with the exception of patients with isolated RCA-stenosis. A level of $p < 0.0005$ was reached in the groups of patients with stenoses in LAD+LCX, with and without RCA-stenosis. In the other groups compared, p-values reached an amount of at least < 0.05. In Table 5a−g all data are given in detail.

Comparison of wall motion abnormality-incidence: The incidence and distribution of wall motion abnormalities were compared among patients with and without mitral regurgitation regarding two ventriculography projections and five different myocardial regions in each of them.

The incidence of wall motion abnormalities is higher in all but two subgroups of patients with mitral regurgitation than in corresponding subgroups of patients without mitral regurgitation but with identical pattern of coronary stenoses.

The maximal incidence of wall motion disturbance was found in the apical myocardial segment of patients with combined LAD- and LCX-stenoses (85% compared to 47% in the subgroup of patients without mitral regurgitation but identical pattern of coronary stenoses). In Table 7 all data are given in detail.

By Chi-square analysis the statistical significance of incidence-differences was determined. In four subgroups of patients such significance was reached: in the groups of patients with isolated LAD- or isolated LCX-stenoses, as well as in the group of patients with combined LAD- and LCX-stenoses, with or without additional RCA-stenosis. The p-value determined by this analysis exceeded the level of <0.0009.

The difference in incidence of wall motion disorders in two subgroups where wall motion disturbances showed a higher incidence in groups of patients without mitral

Table 6. Summary of univariate analysis (*t*-test: p-value) MR + : MR −

Parameters	LAD	LCX	RCA	LAD LCX	LAD RCA	LXC RCA	3-VD
Age	n.s.	0.01	n.s	n.s.	n.s.	n.s.	n.s.
LV-EF	0.05	0.0005	n.s.	0.0005	0.005	0.0005	
LVEDP	0.05	0.01	n.s.	0.0005	0.005	0.05	0.0005
LVEDVI	0.05	0.01	n.s.	0.0005	0.005	0.05	0.0005
LVESVI	0.05	0.005	n.s.	0.0005	0.01	0.05	0.0005
PC-m̄	0.05	0.005	n.s.	0.0005	0.01	0.01	0.0005
PC-v	0.01	0.01	n.s.	0.0005	0.005	0.05	0.0005
PA-m̄	0.01	0.005	n.s.	0.0005	0.05	0.05	0.0005

Differences in hemodynamics between subgroups with and without mitral regurgitation reach different levels of significance in univariate analysis, according to type of CAD.

Table 7. Relative frequency of involvement of left-ventricular regions in wall motion abnormalities

Type of CAD	MR	n	RAO					LAO				
			AB	AL	AP	DP	PB	SL	IL	PL	AS	BS
								%				
LAD	+	14	36	57	57	43	29	14	29	36	43	36
	−	357	4	33	34	9	4	0	4	5	28	21
LCX	+	20	15	20	55	65	55	20	45	55	40	20
	−	132	2	11	12	22	16	0	16	19	7	7
RCA	+	13	0	15	31	24	54	0	31	16	16	16
	−	166	1	9	12	35	44	0	22	26	13	7
LAD + LCX	+	26	19	77	85	70	43	8	47	58	74	70
	−	170	5	48	47	22	14	3	16	17	37	29
LAD + RCA	+	19	11	53	74	68	53	5	53	47	58	47
	−	146	4	36	45	30	25	0	18	16	49	34
LCX + RCA	+	14	14	36	43	50	43	15	43	29	36	29
	−	95	3	23	29	44	40	5	35	39	35	14
3-VD	+	83	30	75	76	63	55	22	52	53	68	47
	−	327	9	48	57	45	40	5	31	33	49	36

A higher incidence of wall motion disturbances is observed in nearly all subgroups with mitral regurgitation, compared to subgroups with identical coronary anatomy but without mitral regurgitation. For abbreviations see text.

Table 8. Differences between relative frequencies of wall motion abnormalities in groups with and without mitral regurgitation, exceeding significance level $p < 0.0009$
Univariate analysis − Chi-square-test

Type of CAD	MR+ n	MR− n	RAO					LAO				
			AB	AL	AP	DP	PB	SL	IL	PL	AS	BS
LAD	14	357	*			*	*	*	*	*		
LCX	20	132		*	*	*	*	*		*	*	
RCA	13	166										
LAD + LCX	26	170			*	*	*		*	*	*	*
LAD + RCA	19	146										
LCX + RCA	14	95										
3-VD	83	327	*	*				*	*			

* = $p < 0.0009$

regurgitation than in groups of patients with mitral regurgitation (mentioned above as exceptions) did not reach statistical significance. In Table 8 all data are given in detail.

Results of multivariate analysis

Parameter combinations: A discriminance analysis was performed to identify those of the parameters out of the univariate analysis by which the highest accuracy in

Table 9. Predictors for mitral regurgitation in CAD

Type of CAD stenoses ≥75«	Parameters	Sensitivity (%)	Sensitivity (%)
LAD	EDP, ESVI, PC-m	62	91
LCX	age, EF, PC-m	81	82
RCA	ESVI	31	92
LAD + LCX	EDP, ESVI, PC-v	74	89
LAD + RCA	EDP, EDVI, PC-m, PC-v	61	92
LCX + RCA	EF, EDVI, ESVI, PC-m	57	96
3-VD	age, EDVI, ESVI, PA-m	58	87

Results of multivariate analysis: combinations of parameters for the prediction of mitral regurgitation; different levels of sensitivity and specificity are reached, according to type of CAD.

prediction of mitral regurgitation could be reached in each group. All hemodynamic parameters and all parameters determining the size of the left ventricle were included.

Different combinations of parameters were obtained for each group of patients, defined by their coronary anatomy; the different parameters were chosen with different frequency. In Table 9 all data are given in detail.

In the result of the analysis end-systolic left ventricular volume was represented in five of the seven groups of patients: For patients with coronary stenoses in LAD alone, RCA alone, combined in LAD and LCX, LCX and RCA, and in all three major coronary vessels, a parameter combination was found that included (body-surface indexed) end-systolic left ventricular volume for the prediction of mitral regurgitation. End-systolic volume in patients with isolated LCX-stenosis is represented also by a combination of parameters including the ejection-fraction of the left ventricle.

In the only group of patients remaining (groups with isolated stenoses in LAD and RCA) prediction of mitral regurgitation can be obtained by the combination of end-diastolic left-ventricular volume and pressue, and pulmonary artery wedge pressure (mean and "v-wave"-maximum).

In all groups mentioned we find a combination of parameters containing at least one parameter of left-ventricular volume.

In five groups pulmonary artery wedge pressure is contained in the chosen combination; additionally, in the group with three- vessel disease, mean pulmonary artery pressure is contained. Thus in nearly all groups pressure in pulmonary artery is decisive for the prediction of mitral regurgitation.

Left-ventricular end-diastolic pressure is chosen for prediction of mitral regurgitation in groups with stenoses in LAD alone or combined with stenoses in LCX or RCA.

Although in univariate analysis a statistically sifnificant difference in age was not found, patient's age was obtained by the multivariate analysis for the prediction of mitral regurgitation in groups of patients with isolated LCX-stenosis and three-vessel disease.

Sensititvity and scpecificity: Multivariate analysis revealed factors of sensitivity and specificity for the predictive power of the combinations of parameters obtained:

Sensitivity exceeded 70% only in two groups (isolated LCX-stenosis, 81%, and LAD- and LCX-stenoses, 74%). For all other groups, sensitivity hardly reached 60% with a minimum of 31% in the isolated RCA-stenosis group.

In contrast to this, prediction was rather speciric in each of the investigated groups and combinations of parameters, ranging from 82% (for the group with isolated LCX-stenosis) to 96% (for the group with combined LCX- and RCA-stenosis). All combinations of parameters containing end-systolic left-ventricular volume alone reached a specificity of more than 91%, in combination with other parameters of the size of the left ventricle more than 87%. In Table 9 all data are given in detail.

Discussion

Incidence and severity of ischemic mitral regurgitation

The overall incidence of mitral regurgitation of all grades of severity in this sample was 10.9%, which demonstrates that this is — according to clinical experience — not a major problem in investigating and treating coronary artery disease. The same judgement applies to the severity of mitral regurgitation. In this sample: only 1.84% of the evaluated samples revealed mitral regurgitation-grades worse than 2+, and only in 4.76% of the group of patients with mitral regurgitation did grades 3+ or 4+ occur. Nevertheless, in each single case mitral regurgitation of ischemic origin may limit a patient's ability for physical exercise. Additionally, as it is stated in a recent review on predictors for fatal outcome after coronary surgery [11], the presence of mitral incompetence even of a moderate grade considerably worsens the perioperative risk for coronary artery disease-patients.

Only cases with ventriculographic evidence for mitral insufficiency have been included, which means that mitral regurgitation occurred under conditions of nearly complete rest. Cases in which mitral regurgitation of ischemic origin might evolve under conditions of exercise only have not been included. According to the sensitivity of possible diagnostic tools, the incidence of this disorder should exceed that of the disorder evaluated here to a considerable amount.

The occurrence of mitral insufficiency in the sample evaluated here is proved by the difference of pressures in pulmonary artery and pulmonary artery wedge position in samples with and without mitral regurgitation. The highest levels of significance ($p < 0.0005$) were mounted comparing pulmonary artery wedge pressure (mean pressure and "v-wave"-amplitude), thus proving the presence of mitral regurgitation in the subgroups, respectively. Differences in mean pulmonary artery pressure between groups of patients with and without mitral regurgitation were significant to the same extent.

Comparable figures on the incidence of mitral regurgitation and the correlation of mitral regurgitation to coronary anatomy in literature are rare. Only a few publications mention this item: One of the first papers [12] giving information about coronary anatomy in detail refers to only 14 patients with mitral regurgitation in coronary artery disease. Another paper already mentioned above [7] evaluated the data of 39 out of 127 patients (31%) in whom mitral regurgitation could be found.

All patients in this study had to undergo urgent CABG-surgery because of severe three-vessel disease.

In one later performed study [2] the data of a number of patients comparable to the number of patients in the present study were evaluated: 60 out of 1 530 coronary artery disease- cases (4%) were found with possible ischemic cause of mitral regurgitation; in contrast to the present study grades 2+ and 3+ were found in up to 75% (44/60) of patients with mitral regurgitation. As the latter paper deals with surgical or medical treatment of this disease, only little information about coronary anatomy and hemodynamic data in these cases is reported.

Thus the incidence found in this study is in accordance to the figures reported in literature; a correlation with coronary anatomy pecularities has not yet been reported in a sample of comparable extent. The 75% prevalence of more severe forms of mitral regurgitation in one previous study could not be confirmed by the present study. According to clinical experience, predominantly mild and moderate grades of mitral regurgitation could be found in the evaluated samples.

Patient's age seems to be of limited influence: With a p-value of < 0.01, the age of patients with mitral regurgitation was higher than that of the patients without mitral regurgitation only in the subgroup with isolated LCX-stenosis. Multivariate analysis resulted in combinations of parameters containing patient's age for this group of patients (with isolated LCX- stenosis) and for the group with three-vessel disease.

The influence of coronary anatomy

In analogy to the basis of the "papillary-muscle-dysfunction"- hypothesis possible correlations between certain types of coronary anatomy and the occurrence of mitral insufficiency of ischemic origin have been traced.

First, correlations between incidence of mitral regurgitation and the number of vessels involved were searched for: There can only be observed a tendency to higher incidence in samples with more vessels involved (i.e., 20.2% in the group with three-vessel disease vs 7.3% − 13.2% in the groups with one-vessel disease). These figures do not indicate striking differences of incidence so that the number of vessels involved should not be the main predicting factor for the occurrence of mitral insufficiency.

Second, certain types of vessel involvement − with high risk for papillary muscle ischemia − were observed: It is known that the posteromedial papillary muscle is involved in most of the inferior wall myocardial infarctions, whereas the antero-lateral one is not injured by most of the anterior/anterolateral infarctions [6, 13]. It should therefore be possible to observe correlations between involvement of post-erior wall supplying coronary arteries (LCX and RCA) and a higher incidence of mitral insufficiency.

Such correlations do not exist: Even in the group of patients with combined LCX- and RCA-stenoses mitral regurgitation incidence only came to 12.8%, despite the fact that in any case the posteromedial papillary muscle must be left without sufficient blood supply.

Conversely, in the group with combined LAD- and LCX-stenoses (which, in consequence, should lead to insufficient supply of the anterolateral papillary muscle) an even slightly higher incidence of mitral regurgitation was found: 13.9% of patients with this coronary anatomy revealed mitral insufficiency.

Third, there was no striking difference in severity of mitral regurgitation according to different types of coronary artery anatomy: The rare cases of mitral regurgitation with more than moderate severity did not occur predominantly in groups with more than one-vessel disease.

As a consequence, in those types of coronary artery diseases in which papillary muscles are most prone to insufficient blood supply no distinct incidence of mitral regurgitation was found. This result is contradictory to the basic assumptions of the papillary-muscle-dysfunction hypothesis in respect to manifest mitral regurgitation of ischemic origin under conditions of rest.

Wall motion disturbances and mitral incompetence

In addition to certain types of coronary anatomy certain patterns of myocardial wall motion disorders have been evaluated: hypokinesia, dyskinesia or akinesia in those areas of myocardium into which papillary muscles insert were regarded as possible predictors for the occurrence of ischemia-induced mitral regurgitation.

Such regions are the infero- and posterolateral and the diaphragmatic and posterobasal regions in respect to the posteromedial papillary muscle as well as the anterolateral, apical, superiorlateral, and posterolateral regions in respect to the anterolateral papillary muscle.

As a result, by comparing subgroups of patients with and without mitral regurgitation differences of incidence of wall motion disorders were found in all regions mentioned above. Differences were not only found in these but in nearly all myocardial regions. By limiting statistical significance to the p-value level of <0.0005 only in subgroups with involvement of LAD or LCX alone, or in subgroups with involvement of LAD and LCX combined, and in the group of patients with three-vessel disease significant differences in myocardial motion disorders were found. But even in these groups these differences were not limited to the above mentioned regions "of interest" but concerned nearly all myocardial regions.

As a consequence, neither the regions into which papillary muscles insert revealed an exceptionally high incidence of wall motion disorders, nor could wall motion disorders be observed considerably more often in those regions in case of mitral insufficiency of ischemic origin.

As a result, we cannot confirm a correlation between certain myocardial wall motion disorders and the occurrence of mitral regurgitation.

Strongest predictor: impaired left ventricular function

Impaired left-ventricular function and parameters of pathologically enlarged volumes in diastole and − most of all − in end-systole provided the strongest predictive power for the occurrence of mitral regurgitation in the evaluated samples.

As a manifestation of compromised left ventricular function end-diastolic left ventricular pressure was considerably higher in all subgroups with mitral regurgitation than in those without (with the exception of the above-mentioned group with isolated RCA-stenosis).

This corresponds to the differences in left-ventricular ejection fraction where the level of statical significance in the univariate analysis reached p-values smaller than <0.001 in most instances.

By multivariate analysis for groups of patients with LAD- stenosis alone or combined with stenoses in LCX or RCA, left ventricular enddiastolic pressure was included in the combination of parameters for the prediction of mitral regurgitation. Ejection fraction was analyzed two times as predictive (in the groups of patients with isolated LCX-stenosis or combined with RCA-stenosis).

The same result as for end-diastolic pressure in the left ventricle is reached for the left-ventricular sizes: both end-diastolic and end-systolic volumes are considerably higher in all groups of patients (with exception of the group with isolated RCA-stenosis); p-values correspond to the results of univariate analysis for the other parameters mentioned.

In all groups of patients defined by coronary anatomy the end- systolic left ventricular volume was included in the combination of parameters, which resulted out of the multivariate analysis for the prediction of mitral regurgitation either directly or indirectly by inclusion of left-ventricular ejection fraction.

Therefore, as a major result of this analysis we find end- systolic volume to be one of the most decisive circumstances of mitral regurgitation in ischemic heart disease. This not only relies on the worse-left-ventricular function found in the subgroups with mitral regurgitation – it also refers to mitral insufficiency as a systolic event. This leads to the conclusion that disturbances in left ventricular geometry, size, and function prove to be important for the occurrence of mitral regurgitation in ischemic heart disease and not special coronary anatomy pecularities.

Conclusions

This study shows a close relationship between poor left ventricular function, hemodynamic disturbances, and the occurrence of manifest mitral insufficiency of ischemic origin in coronary artery disease. A relationship between certain coronary artery blood-supply deficits and consecutive wall motion disturbances in those circumscribed myocardial regions into which papillary muscles insert, and the occurrence of mitral insufficiency could not be proved.

The strongest predictive power was gained by the impaired left-ventricular function and by enlarged left-ventricular volume. In particular, end-systolic volume enlargement correlated with the occurrence of manifest mitral insufficiency, indicating (because mitral regurgitation is a systolic event) that disturbed left-ventricular geometry allows systolic mitral regurgitation and not isolated dysfunction of papillary muscles.

This leads to the conclusion that in manifest mitral insufficiency of ischemic origin under conditions of rest the strongest predictor for mitral incompetence is the impaired left ventricular geometry and function, rather than compromised blood supply of parts of the mitral apparatus, as is the basis of the "papillary-muscle-dys-function"-hypothesis.

List of Abbreviations:

CABG   coronary artery bypass grafting
CAD   coronary artery disease
EDP   end-diastolic pressure
EDVI   end-diastolic volume index
EF   ejection fraction
ESVI   end-diastolic volume index
LAD   left anterior descending coronary artery
LCX   left circumflex coronary artery
LV   left ventricle
MR   mitral regurgitation
MS   mitral stenosis
PA-m   pulmonary artery pressure (mean)
PC-m   pulmonary artery wedge pressure (mean)
PC-v   pulmonary artery wedge pressure ("v"-wave)
RCA   right coronary artery
3-VD   three-vessel disease

Left ventricular myocardial regions:
Left anterior obliquor projection:
AB   anterobasal
AL   anterolateral
AP   apicalposterior
DP   diaphragmatic
PB   postobasal
Right anterior obliquor projection
AS   anteroseptal
BS   basalseptal
IF   inferolateral
PL   posterolateral
SL   superiorlateral

References

1. Aranda JM, Befeler B, Lazzara R, Embi A, Machado H (1975) Mitral valve prolapse and coronary artery disease. Circulation 52:245–253
2. Balu V, Hershowitz S, Zaki Maud AR, Bhayana JN, Dean DC (1982) Mitral regurgitation in coronary artery disease. Chest 81:550–555
3. Burch GE, De Pasquale NP, Phillips JH (1963) Clinical manifestations of papillary muscle dysfunction. Arch Int Med 112:112–117
4. Burch GE, De Pasquale NP, Phillips JH (1963) The syndrome of papillary muscle dysfunction. Ann Intern Med 59:508–520
5. Cheng TO (1969) Some new observations on the syndrome of papillary muscle dysfunction. Am J Med 47:924–945
6. De Busk RF, Harrison DC (1969) The clinical spectrum of papillary-muscle disease. N Engl J Med 281:1458–1467
7. Gahl K, Sutton R, Pearson M, Caspari P, Lairet A, McDonald L (1977) Mitral regurgitation in coronary artery disease. Br Heart J 39:13–18
8. Godley RW, Wann S, Rogers EW (1981) Incomplete mitral leaflet closure in patients with papillary muscle dysfunction. Circulation 63:565–571
9. Perloff JK, Roberts WC (1972) The mitral apparatus – functional anatomy of mitral regurgitation. Circulation 46:227–239

10. Ranganathan N, Burch GE (1969) Gross morphology and arterial supply of the papillary muscles of the left ventricle of man. Am Heart J 77:506−516
11. Rankin JS, Hickey MSJ et al. (1989) Ischemic mitral regurgitation. Circulation 79 [Suppl I]: 116−121
12. Sellers RD, Levy ML, Amplatz K, Lillehei CW (1964) Left retrograde cardioangiography in acquired cardiac disease. Am J Card 14:437−447
13. Shelburne JC, Rubinstein D, Gorlin R (1969) A reappraisal of papillary dysfunction. Am J Med 46:862−871

Author's address:
Dr. E. Frantz
Innere Medizin-Kardiologie
Deutsches Herzzentrum Berlin
Augustemburger Platz 1
1000 Berlin 65, FRG

The influence of revascularization on ischemic mitral insufficiency

G. Berghöfer, E. Witt, A. Desideri, M. Schartl, W. Rutsch, F. C. Dougherty, H. Schmutzler

Department of Cardiology and Pulmology, University Clinic Rudolf-Virchow, Charlottenburg, Berlin, FRG

Since Doppler echocardiography in clinical medicine we know that mitral regurgitation (MR) is a very common if not physiological phenomenon. Left ventricular angiography demonstrates regurgitation into the left atrium much less frequently – usually only if echocardiography demonstrates retrograde flow throughout systole. Left ventricular angiography has shown relatively low sensitivity [5]; furthermore, it may be associated with artifical mitral valve insufficiency caused by interference with the mitral valve apparatus or by arrhythmias.

The additional volume load, deep held inspiration, and elevated blood pressure and heart rates may all influence angiographic results. However, cineangiography is fairly suitable for detection of relevant mitral regurgitation and documents additional parameters such as ventricular volumes, ejection fraction, regional wall motion disorders and associated changes in the valve apparatus. For these reasons we performed a retrospective study on patients with left ventricular cineangiograms before revascularization procedures and at follow-up for a period of up to one year.

Table 1 presents a summary of data from literature. There is a wide range in the reported incidence of mitral regurgitation – from 4% [2] to 56% [17]. Patient selection and examination techniques are major factors in this regard. Patients with acute coronary artery disease demonstrate mitral insufficiency more often than patients with chronic coronary artery disease [7, 11, 13]. The association with anterior and inferior infarction varies widely but seems to be generally balanced.

We reviewed about 550 catheterization films from patients with left ventricular cineangiograms before and within the first year after a revascularization procedure. We defined three patient groups. Group 1 consisted of 34 patients studied between 1984 and 1987. In this group cineangiograms were performed before PTCA in acute myocardial infarction and at discharge from hospital after successful PTCA. Group 2 comprises 420 patients with successful elective PTCA and follow-up angiogram. Group 3 includes 21 patients who underwent elective coronary artery bypass surgery with follow-up studies, also within one year.

Twenty-one patients (66%) in group 1 had mitral regurgitation, compared to 8% in group 2 and 43% in group 3. The following disorders were excluded in these patients: dilated cardiomyopathy, mitral valve prolapse, history of endocarditis and calcification of the mitral valve apparatus – since these conditions may cause mitral insufficiency as well. A large proportion of the left ventricular cineangiograms at follow-up were not available or suitable for evaluation. Just 33 patients without clinical evidence of progression of coronary artery disease were compared on the basis of angiographic findings before and after revascularization (Table 2).

Table 1.

Reference	n	Presentation of CAD	Methods	Mitral-regurgita-tion (% of all pat.)	Associated with (% of al patients with MR) Anterior Infarct	Inferior Infarct	Anterior and Inferior Infarct
Breisblatt et al. 1986 [4]	150	Unstable angina	Radionuclide-ventriculography	20	45	45	
Barzilai et al. 1988 [3]	59	Acute myocardial infarction	Echo and radionuclice-ventriculography	39	46	35	
Izumi et al. 1987 [15]	81	Recent myocardial infarction	Echo and Ventriculography	53	39	56	64
Loperfido et al. 1986 [17]	72	Recent myocardial infarction	Echo and Ventriculography	56	62	37	
Servi et al. 1988 [8]	266	Recent myocardial infarction	Ventriculography	20	33	61	
Balu et al. 1982 [2]	1530	Coronary artery disease	Ventriculography	4			
Berghöfer 1988	441	Ischemic coronary artery disease	Ventriculography	10			

Table 2.

	Group I (acute PTCA)	Group II (elective PTCA)	Group III (elective CABG)	Sum
Patients with a ventriculo-graphy before and after recanalization	32	420	21	463
Patients with MR	21 (65.6%)	35 (8.3%)	9 (42.8%)	65
Remaining patients with acceptable and available follow-up ventriculography	14	15	4	33

Abbrev.: MR: mitral regurgitation; CAD = coronary artery disease; CABG: coronary artery bypass grafting

Table 3. Excluded mitral regurgitations

Dilated cardiomyopathy
Hypertrophic cardiomyopathy
Mitral valve prolapse
History of endocarditis
Calcification of the mitral valve apparatus
Catheter or arrhythmia−induced MR

Several cardiac abnormalities correlate with mitral regurgitation. These are summarized in Table 3. In addition to infarct localization and size, infarction of the papillary muscle is indisputably one cause of mitral regurgitation, as is rupture of the chordae tendineae. There is strong evidence that mitral regurgitation is more common in multi-vessel disease, especially in patients with large ventricles or with a dilated atrium. Mitral regurgitation may correlate with left ventricular enddiastolic pressure, reduced ejection fraction, the time period since myocardial infarction, and presence of refractory angina pectoris.

The schematic in Fig. 1 shows some of the possible mechanisms of mitral insufficiency [1, 6, 9, 10, 12, 18]. Normal findings of the papillary muscles and the mitral

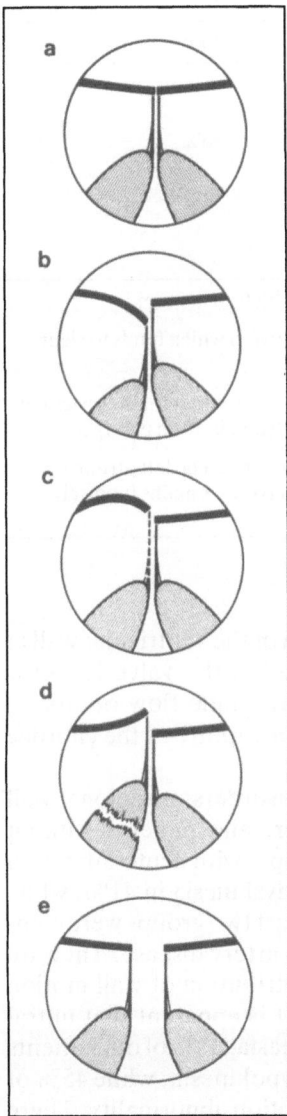

Fig. 1. Mechanisms of mitral insufficiency

77

Table 4.

	Anterior wall			Posterior wall			Both	Without wall-motion abnormalities
	hypo	akin	dys	hypo	akin	dys		
1 6%	13%	41%	16%	19%	3%	9%	–	
2 n = 420	30%	11%	2%	14%	7%	1%	16%	9%
3 n = 21	33%	14%	8%	5%	10%	–	30%	–
2 and 3	31%	10%	2%	13%	7%	1%	30%	9%
Patients of Group 2 and 3 with MR	45%	5%	5%	5%	5%	–	36%	–

Table 5. Grading of mitral regurgitation (modified from [19]):

I.   Shows a regurgitant jet with minimal staining of the left atrium, which clears rapidly.

II. There is a regurgitant jet with moderate opacification of the left atrium which tends to clear rapidly.

III. The left atrium shows distinct filling with every ventricular contraction and remains opacified for a few beats. The pulmonic veins are usually seen and the left atrium is often enlarged.

IV. The left atrium is more densely opacified than the left ventricle or aorta. The left atrium is usually markedly enlarged and the left ventricle dilated. The left atrium remains intensely opacified through the entire series of films.

valve leaflets are demonstrated in a); b) shows dyskineasia of the ventricular wall at the point of origin of the papillary muscle. In this situation the valve leaflet is retracted into the ventricle, creating a fissure where retrograde flow occurs; c) demonstrates mitral valve prolapse; d) shows distension or rupture of the chordae tendinae and in e) we see MR in a dilated left ventricle.

We divided the patients into subgroups according to disorders of regional wall motion – anterior, inferior, both anterior and inferior, and patients without regional wal motion disorders (Table 4). Patients in group 1 with acute infarction and successful balloon dilatation demonstrated anterior dyskinesia in 41%, while hypokinesia predominated in group 2 and in group 3. The last two groups were combined, since they both showed a chronic form of coronary artery disease. They are presented in the next column and compared with the distribution of wall motion abnormalities in the patients with mitral regurgitation. It is apparent that mitral regurgitation was very common in ventricles with hypokineasia. 31% of our patients with elective revascularization procedures had anterior hypokinesia, while 45% of patients with mitral valve insufficiency showed this wall motion abnormality. There

Table 6. Cardiac changes found to be correlated to mitral regurgitation

Infarct localization, and size
Dyskinesia localization, and size
Papillary muscle infarct / rupture
Chordae tendineae rupture
Multiple vessel disease
Left ventricular volume
Diameter of the mitral ring
Left ventricular enddiastolic volume
Ejection fraction
Angina refractory to medical treatment;
Time after myocardial infarct

Table 7. Therapy of mitral regurgitation

Medical:	diuretics, vasodilators, positive inotropic substances, anti-anginal drugs, [16] thrombolysis in acute myocardial infarction
Surgical:	PTCA (14), CABG, valve replacement, reconstruction

was an increased incidence of mitral regurgitation when disorders of the anterior and posterior wall were found, and in patients with anterior wall dyskinesia.

We classified mitral regurgitation using the scale proposed by Sellers in 1964 [19] (Table 5). Opacification of the left atrium was judged on a scale of 4. Faint regurgitation was detected in the majority of cases (I°). When there was a moderate opacification of the left atrium we graded II, and when this remained for some beats it was defined as III°. It should be emphasized that recognition of mitral insufficiency is closely related to the experience and attention of the observer.

Beside the number of diseased vessels the disorders of regional wall motion or left ventricular dimensions there are many other factors which may affect mitral regurgitation (Table 6). Table 7 summarizes the therapeutic possibilities; nitrates and positive inotropic agents reduce ventricular volumes and may reduce mitral regurgitation as well. Heart surgery under these principle procedures has proven to reduce MR. In our series patients were mostly treated by PTCA.

We considered the revascularization procedure successful when there was no evidence of stenoses greater than 60% in any of the three major epicardial vessels after coronary bypass grafting or PTCA. Patients with retrograde perfusion of a major artery were excluded, as were patients with progression of coronary artery disease in vessels which had not undergone revascularization. Figure 2 summarzies findings in all successfully treated patients. With the exception of one patient approximately half of the patients remained in the same grade following revascularization, while improvement was found in the remaining 54%. Some even changed from grade I to grade 0 (Fig. 2).

When these results are analyzed on the basis of subgroups it becomes apparent that nine of 14 patients with acute myocardial infarction remained unchanged in grade I or II at follow-up, while five patients demonstrated improvement (Fig. 3). There were similar findings in the group of patients with elective revascularization

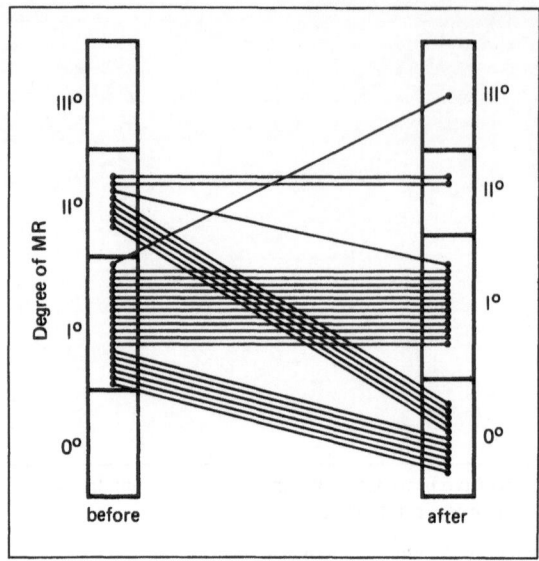

Fig. 2. Patients with coronary artery disease (CAD) (Group I, II and III). Before and after successfull revascularization (n = 27)

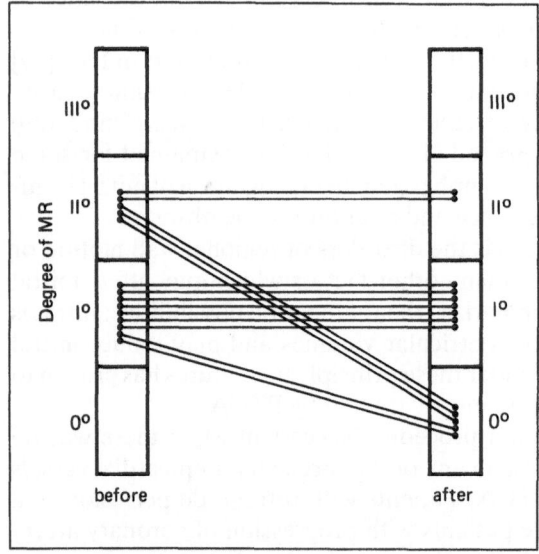

Fig. 3. Patients with acute myocardial infarct (AMI) (Group I). Before and after successfull revascularization (n = 14)

procedures (Fig. 4): six of 13 demonstrated improvement, six were unchanged, and one patient deteriorated significantly. In subgroup 2 with elective PTCA (Fig. 5) half of the patients improved and the other half remained unchanged. Six patients with significant restenosis following PTCA constitute a control group, with functional improvement in two patients and similar ventriculographic findings in the remaining four patients. The number of patients in the coronary grafting group

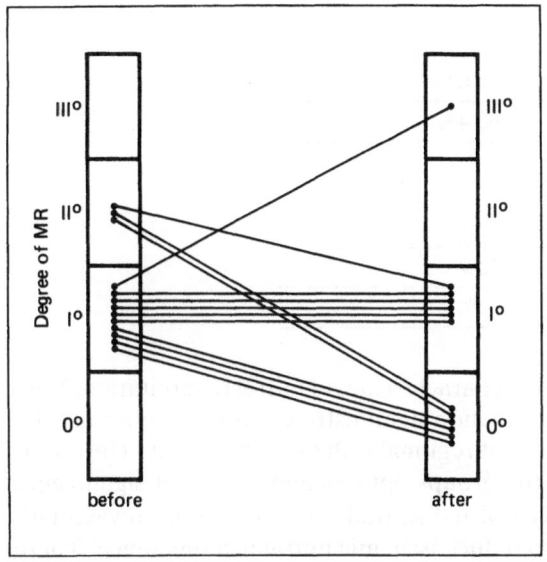

Fig. 4. Patients with CAD (Group II and III). Before and after successfull revascularization (n = 13)

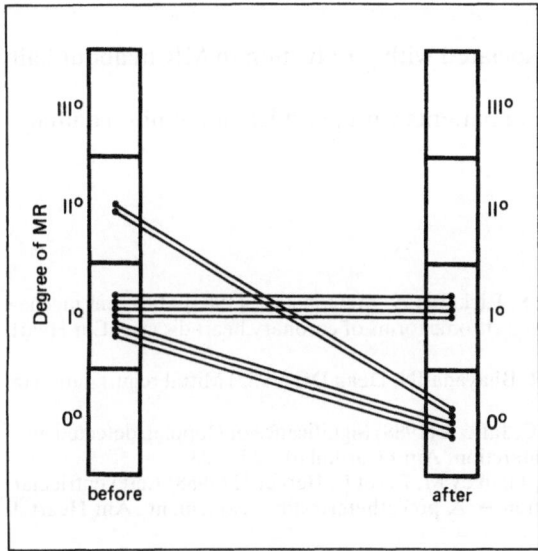

Fig. 5. Patients with elective PTCA (Group II). Before and after successfull revascularization (n = 9)

is very small so we do not comment on the effect of the bypass surgery in comparison to PTCA.

It is not clear whether the benefit from revascularization procedures was greater in patients with anterior or inferior infarction or ischemia, as the number of patients in each group was nearly the same. Analysis of the results in relation to enddiastolic volume did not reveal significant differences as well. Table 8 presents

Table 8.

	less or gone	MR after recanalisatia equal or worse
EF	67.5%	60.4%
Wall motion abnormalities		
Hypokinesia	57%	32%
Akinesia	29%	32%
Dyskinesia	14%	37%

a summary of prognostically significant characteristics of mitral regurgitation. Ventricles with relatively good residual function demonstrate improvement in mitral insufficiency, especially if the disorder of regional wall motion is slight. The difference in ejection fraction between the groups approached statistical significance ($p = 0.05$). The wall motion quality is listed as well; in hypokinesia, revascularization may especially be expected to reduce ischemic mitral incompetence. There was improvement in wall motion disorders in 10 of 14 patients with a reduction in MR.

We conclude that:
1) successful revascularization is associated with a reduction in MR in about half of all patients, and
2) the best results may be expected in patients with good EF and limited damage to the ventricle wall.

References

1. Ballester M, Tasca R, Marin L, Rees S, Rickards A, McDonald L (1983) Different mechanisms of mitral regurgitation in acute and chronic forms of coronary heart disease. Eur Heart J 4:557–565
2. Balu V, Hershowitz S, Zaki Masud AR, Bhayana JN, Dean DC (1982) Mitral regurgitation in coronary artery disease. Chest 81:550
3. Barzilai B, Gessler C, Perez J, Schaab C, Jaffe A (1988) Significance of Doppler-detected mitral regurgitation in acute myocardial infarction. Am J Cardiol 61:220–223
4. Breisblatt W, Cerqueira M, Francis C, Plankey M, Zaret B, Berger H (1988) Left ventricular function in ischemic mitral regurgitation – A precatheterization assessment. Am Heart J 115:77
5. Croft CH, Lipscomb K, Mathis K, Firth BG, Nicod P, Tilton G, Winniford M, Hillis LD (1984) Limitations of qualitative angiographic grading in aortic or mitral regurgitation. Am J Cardiol 53:1953
6. DePasquale NP, Burch GE (1971) Papillary muscle dysfunction in coronary (ischemic) heart disease. Ann Red Med 22:327–342
7. De Servi S, Vaccari L, Graziano G, Cornalba C, Codega S, Poma E, Montemartini C, Specchia G (1986) Clinical and angiographic data in early post-infarction angina. Eur Heart J 7 [Suppl C]:69–72
8. De Servi S, Vaccari L, Assandri J, Poma E, Cioffi P, Scire A, Specchia G (1988) Clinical significance of mitral regurgitation in patients with recent myocardial infarction. Eur Heart J 9 [Suppl F]:5–9

9. Donaldson M, Ballester M, Rubens M, Yacoub M (1982) Echocardiographic visualization of the anatomic causes of mitral regurgitation resulting from myocardial infarction. Postgr Med J 58:257−263
10. Estes E, Dalton F, Entmer M (1966) Anatomy and blood supply of papillary muscles of the left ventricle. Am Heart J 71:356−362
11. Gahl K, Sutton R, Pearson M, Caspari P, Lairet A, McDonald L (1977) Mitral regurgitation in coronary heart disease. Br Heart J 39:13−18
12. Godley RW, Wann LS, Roger EW, Feigenbaum H, Weymann AE (1981) Incomplete mitral leaflet closure in patients with papillary muscle dysfunction. Circulation 63:565
13. Heikkila J (1967) Mitral incompetence complicating acute myocardial infarction. Br Heart J 29:162−169
14. Heuser R, Maddoux L, Goss J, Ramo B, Raff G, Shadoff N (1987) Coronary angioplasty for acute mitral regurgitation due to myocardial infarction. Ann Int Med 107:825−855
15. Izumi S, Miyatake K, Beppu S, Park YD, Nagata S, Kinoshita N, Sakakibara H, Nimura Y (1987) Mechanism of mitral regurgitation in patients with myocardial infarction: a study using real-time two-dimensional Doppler flow imaging and echocardiography. Circulation 76:777−785
16. Keren G, Bier A, Strom JA, Laniado S, Sonnenblick EH, LeJentel TH (1986) Dynamics of mitral regurgitation during nitroglycerin therapy. A Doppler echocardiographic study. Am Heart J 112:517−525
17. Loperfido F, Biasucci L, Pennestri F, Laurenzi F, Gimigliano F, Vigna C, Rossi E, Favuzzi A, Santarelli P, Manzoli U (1986) Pulsed Doppler echocardiographic analysis of mitral regurgitation after myocardial infarction. Am J Cardiol 58:692−697
18. Ogawa S, Hubbard FE, Mardelli TJ, Dreifus LS (1979) Cross-sectional echocardiographic spectrum papillary muscle dysfunction. Am Heart J 97:312
19. Sellers RD, Levy MS, Amplatz K et al. (1964) Left retrograde cardioangiography in acquired cardiac disease. Technique, indications and interpretations in 700 cases. Am J Cardiol 14:437−445

Author's address:
Dr. med. G. Berghöfer
Abteilung für Innere Medizin
Kardiologie und Pulmologie
Universitätsklinikum Rudolf Virchow
Spandauer Damm 130
1000 Berlin 19

Intraoperative Doppler color flow mapping for assessment of ischemic mitral regurgitation

A. F. Bolger, D. C. Miller

Division of Cardiology and Department of Cardiovascular Surgery, Stanford University School of Medicine, Stanford, California, USA

Introduction

Mitral regurgitation in a common finding in patients with ischemic heart disease, accompanying more than 30% of myocardial infarctions [8, 9]. In some cases, regurgitation results solely from ischemia-related abnormalities, including annular dilatation, papillary muscle or myocardial scarring, or rupture of chordae or papillary muscle. In other cases, mitral regurgitation is the result of preexisiting mitral pathology such as myxomatous degeneration, endocarditis and congenital anomalies, with or without additional ischemic damage. Recognizing that the mitral apparatus includes many interdependent segments, from leaflets to annulus to chordae and ventricular myocardium, it can be expected that regurgitation may result from abnormalities of any one or of a combination of these. In addition, reversible dysfunction due to myocardial ischemia may contribute to the regurgitation; in the uncommon case where active ischemia but not infarction is responsible for the insufficiency, revascularization alone may be adequate to correct the regurgitation. The choice of surgical therapy for the valvular insufficiency depends upon the specific nature and extent of the abnormality as well as the accompanying ventricular function and regional wall motion.

The importance of addressing mitral regurgitation in the setting of ischemic heart disease is underscored by the increased morbidity and mortality among patients with residual mitral insufficiency after coronary artery bypass. Adler et al. at the Massachusetts General Hospital found in their series of more than 2000 consecutive revascularization procedures that residual mitral insufficiency was an independent predictor of long term mortality which more than doubled the risk of late death [3]. The high operative mortality for combined mitral valve replacement and coronary bypass [10] makes valve reconstruction an attractive alternative, with its lower perioperative mortality, good long-term durability, and fewer thromboembolic complications [3, 11]. Ultrasound imaging preoperatively and at the time of cardiac surgery offers high quality anatomic and flow information which can aid in decisions regarding the need for surgical correction of mitral insufficiency, and the choice of valve repair vs replacement in the patient with ischemic heart disease.

Doppler color flow mapping provides real-time images of intracardiac blood flow. These are generated by an autocorrelation technique which permits extremely rapid assignment of blood flow velocity on a point-by-point basis. The result is a profile of flow velocities superimposed on a morphologic black and white two-dimensional image. It provides ready visualization of abnormal intracardiac flow jets such as the turbulent systolic left atrial flow resulting from mitral insufficiency. The spatial distributions of those profiles relative to the left atrial size have been used to estimate the severity of mitral regurgitation [7]. The criteria used in our laboratory are based on the distribution of the jet within the left atrium, with mild extending into one-third or less of the left atrium, moderate involving two-thirds or less, and severe occupying more than two-thirds of the atrial cavity. These semiquantitative estimates have correlated well with angiographic grades of regurgitation in several series [5, 7]. Documentation of the systolic blood pressure, heart rate, and rhythm is performed with each study, as changes in color Doppler regurgitant grade may occur with changes in the patient's hemodynamic state [5].

Most quantitative uses of color Doppler technology are based on the assumption that the area of a flow jet depicted with color Doppler reflects the regurgitation volume. In vitro work has clearly demonstrated that color jet area is indeed a function of flow volume, but that the relationship between area and volume is not a linear one [2]. In addition, the apparent spatial distribution of a regurgitant jet is extremely sensitive to many technical and patient-related variables. The frequency of the imaging transducer and the pulse repetition, the gain setting, as well as make and model of the color Doppler system all impact jet area [2, 12]. Further, the driving pressure [13], atrial size and compliance can affect the color area. Therefore, when using color Doppler as a measure of regurgitant severity it is critical to recognize these complicating factors and control them whenever possible.

The preoperative evaluation of patients with ischemic mitral regurgitation with conventional transthoracic echocardiography yields information regarding left ventricular size and wall motion abnormalities, gross valvular structure and function, and estimates of regurgitant severity. Color Doppler studies performed in the operating suite offer higher quality morphologic and intracardiac flow detail under well-defined hemodynamic conditions. The small distances involved during epicardial imaging permit the use of higher frequency transducers which provide excellent anatomic information regarding every component of the mitral apparatus, as well as wall motion and estimates of regurgitant severity. The anatomic information is complementary to direct surgical inspection of the valve; it can demonstrate dynamic abnormalities in wall and valve motion which may be difficult to assess during cardiac standstill, and can guide and expedite surgical inspection of valve structures. Importantly, careful interrogation of all structures can be performed without increasing aortic cross clamp time. This information can be invaluable in planning complicated repair procedures and assessing their success.

We use a 5.0 MHz transducer draped with a sterile plastic sheath and placed on the exposed epicardium of the beating heart prior to cardiopulmonary bypass. Images are recorded from multiple views, including long and short axis views as well as many nonstandard views adapted to the specific anatomy at hand. Careful attention is paid to thorough interrogation of all levels of the mitral apparatus. This involves careful medial and lateral sweeps to visualize all portions of the valve leaflets, annulus and chordae. Ventricular wall motion is described, with attention to active thickening of papillary muscles and adjacent myocardium. Color Doppler is used to define the mitral insufficiency in its greatest extent, and the orientation and site of origination of the regurgitation jet is identified. In this fashion, the culprit portion of the valve may be anticipated. Finally, associated abnormalities are sought, including intracardiac thrombi, ventricular or atrial septal defects, and other valvular insufficiency. As the extent of the regurgitation is determined in part by the afterload to ventricular ejection, the patient's heart rate, rhythm, and blood pressure are noted. If the blood pressure at the time of the prepump imaging is significantly less than the patient's documented ambulatory pressure, a small quantity of phenylephrine is administered to raise the blood pressure to representative levels. Repeat color Doppler imaging following this challenge often reveals more extensive regurgitation; in some cases significant regurgitation would have been missed without this provocation [5].

Color Doppler images are recorded from the beating, ejecting heart. As a result, it is superior to other, more time-honored ways of assessing valvular competence at the time of cardiac surgery. Fluid filling of the arrested left ventricle and inspection of the atrial aspect of the mitral valve to localize leakage is not highly predictive of the amount of eventual regurgitation after reinstitution of contraction [5]. Another intraoperative indicator of mitral regurgitation is the height of v waves of the pulmonary capillary wedge pressure tracing. These are monitored from the beating heart, and can be followed sequentially. However, neither their absolute height or magnitude relative to the mean wedge pressure is highly predictive of the presence or extent of mitral insufficiency, either before ar after repair [5]. Intraoperative color Doppler imaging, therefore, offers morphologic and quantitative gitation. Several pieces of information offered by this technique are useful in predicting a valve's potential for successful reconstruction and in choosing the appropriate valve's potential for successful reconstruction and in choosing the appropriate repair procedure. Significant abnormalities of the anterior leaflet, extensive mitral annular calcification and central jets or jets with a broad origin extending over more than one-third of the valve coapture all portend a lower likelihood of adequate repair [4, 6]. In contrast, morphologically normal valves whose insufficiency results from annular dilatation, or valves with abnormalities restricted to the posterior leaflet with jets originating from the posterior commissure are more likely to be corrected by repair procedures. Both the need for surgical attention to the mitral valve at the time of coronary revascularization and the type of procedure appropriate to the patient can be better addressed intraoperatively with information from epicardial imaging.

After coronary bypass with or without mitral valve replacement or repair, epicardial color Doppler imaging is repeated after reinstitution of sinus rhythm and normal circulation. At this time, the amount of residual regurgitation is assessed and wall motion reexamined. Insufficiency may be increased early in the resuscitative period and during ventricular pacing; therefore, imaging is performed when the patient is as hemodynamically stable as possible. Challenge with phenylephrine or other pressor agent is again used in order to assess the mitral regurgitation under settings of comparable afterload. The amount of regurgutation detected during the immediate postoperative, open-chest period has been shown to be representative of the longer term course. In the series by Czer, et al. the amount of residual regurgitation seen immediately postpump did not change by more than one grade over up to 24 weeks of follow-up in any of their 49 patients with mitral valve reconstruction [4]. The use of comparable equipment and imaging settings at similar blood pressures minimizes the variability between intraoperative and follow up studies.

Doppler color flow mapping in the operating suite offers high quality anatomic and flow information which can be of great help in assessing the severity of mitral insufficiency and the potential for valve repair. Epicardial imaging allows detailed interrogation of all valvular structures from multiple views; it can identify culprit portions of the valve before aortic cross-clamping, and confirm the adequacy of the procedure postpump. This, in combination with it's ability to reliably track changes in regurgitation severity and its usefulness in long term follow up, makes it a valuable tool in indicating, predicting, and confirming successful valve repair.

References

1. Adler DS, Goldman L, O'Neil A, Cook EF, Mudge GH, Shemin RJ, DiSea V, Cohn LH, Collins JJ (1986) Long-term survival of more than 2000 patients after coronary artery bypass grafting. Am J Cardiol 58(3):195−202
2. Bolger A, Eigler N, Pfaff JM, Resser K, Maurer G (1988) Computer analysis of color Doppler images for quantitative assessment of in vitro fluid jets. J Am Col Cardiol 12(2):450−457
3. Carpentier A, Chauvaud S, Fabiani J, Deloche A, Relland J, Lessana A, d'Allaines C, Blondeau P, Piwnica A, Dubost C (1980) Reconstructive surgery of mitral valve incompetence: 10-year appraisal. J Thor Cardiovasc Surg 79:338−348
4. Czer LSC, Maurer G, Bolger AF, DeRobertis M, Gray RJ, Chaux A, Matloff JM (In Press, 1988) Valve repair versus revascularization for ischemic mitral regurgitation: evaluation by Doppler color flow mapping. Circulation (in press)
5. Czer LSC, Maurer G, Bolger AF, DeRobertis M, Resser KJ, Kass RM, Lee ME, Blanche C, Chaux A, Gray RJ, Matloff JM (1987) Intraoperative evaluation of mitral regurgitation by Doppler color flow mapping. Circulation 76:III-108−116
6. Galloway AC, Colvin SB, Baumann FG, Harty S, Spencer FC (1988) Current concepts of mitral valve reconstruction for mitral insufficiency. Circulation 78(5):1087−1098
7. Helmcke F, Nanda N, Hsiung M, Soto B, Adey C, Goyal R, Gatewood R (1987) Color Doppler assessment of mitral regurgitation with orthogonal planes. Circulation 75:175−183
8. Izumi S, Miyatake K, Beppu S, Park Y-D, Nagata S, Kinoshita N, Sakakibara H, Nimura Y (1987) Mechanisms of mitral regurgitation in patients with myocardial infarction: a study using real-time two-dimensional Doppler flow imaging and echocardiography. Circulation 76:777−785
9. Loperfido F, Biasucci L, Pennestri F, Laurenzi F, Gimigliano F, Vigna C, Rossi E, Favuzzi A, Santarelli P, Manzoli U (1986) Pulsed Doppler echocardiographic analysis of mitral regurgitation after myocardial infarction. Am J Cardiol 58:692−697
10. Miller DC, Stinson EB, Rossiter SJ, Oyer PE, Reitz BA, Shumway NE (1978) Impact of simultaneous myocardial revascularization on operative risk, functional result, and survival following mitral valve replacement. Surgery 84:848−857
11. Rankin JS, Feneley MP, Hickey M, Muhlbaier LH, Wechsler AS, Floyd RD, Reves JG, Skelton TN, Califf RM, Lowe JE, Sabiston DC (1988) A clinical comparison of mitral valve repair versus valve replacement in ischemic mitral regurgitation. J Thor Cardiovasc Surg 95:165−177
12. Stewart WJ, Schiavone WA, From JA, Castle T, Salcedo EE (1985) In vitro studies of Doppler color flow mapping: dependence of spatial distribution on instrument settings. Circulation 72:III-98 (abst)
13. Wranne B, Ask P, Lods D (1985) Quantification of heart valve regurgitation: a critical analysis from a theoretical and experimental point of view. Clin Physiol 5:81−88

Author's address:
Ann Bolger, M.D.
Division of Cardiology
Stanford University Medical Center
Stanford, California 94305−5246
U.S.A.

Diagnostic value of transesophageal echocardiography in patients with coronary artery disease and mitral insufficiency

R. Erbel, M. Drexler, S. Mohr-Kahaly, N. Wittlich, J. Meyer

II. Medical Clinic, Johannes Gutenberg-University, Mainz, FRG

Introduction

Any diagnosis of mitral regurgitation must always include the etiology. The clinical history is only rarely informative, as are chest x-ray examinations. The ECG is of value to diagnose coronary artery disease with or without previous myocardial infarction − but further differentiation is not possible. During heart catheterization mitral insufficiency can be diagnosed and quantified according to Seller's classification [1]. A differentiation of etiology is only rarely possible. Rheumatic heart disease and mitral valve prolapse can be differentiated.

The most important clinical diagnostic method is echocardiography. Using this method differentiation between mitral ring dilation, mitral valve billowing with or without prolapse, mitral aneurysm formation, mitral valve endocarditis, chordae tendineae rupture, papillary muscle rupture or dysfunction can be performed. But in patients with obesity, pulmonary emphysema, chest deformation, dyspnoe, and particularly in patients in the intensive care unit under mechanical ventilation, it is difficult to receive good, high quality images. High quality images, however, are necessary in order to be able to diagnose the etiology of mitral regurgitation.

Transesophageal echocardiography

By transesophageal echocardiography the main limitations of transthoracic echocardiography have been overcome. Using this methods, mitral valves can be scanned with high resolution (Fig. 1). Transesophageal echocardiography has been proven to be of diagnostic value in patients with valvular heart disease, endocarditis, embolism, prosthetic valves, congestive heart disease and aortic dissection [2−4]. During surgery mitral valve reconstruction can be controlled by this method [5, 6].

Transesophageal echocardiography is performed in the fasting state (< than 4 h) after detailed analysis of the patient's history with regard to disorders of swelling and disease of the esophagus. In the case of bradycardia, a venous line is put in place and 0.5 mg atropine injected. In patients with severe gastric reactions and vomiting reflexes, 10 mg diazepam for sedation and/or 0.3 mg bupremorphine for analgesia are injected. The echoscope is introduced in the left supine position and the heart scanned in standard projection [4]. By rotation of the acoustic head by 90° the descending aorta can be scanned from the level of the stomach to the aortic arch. By the transgastric approach cross-sectional images of the left ventricle and

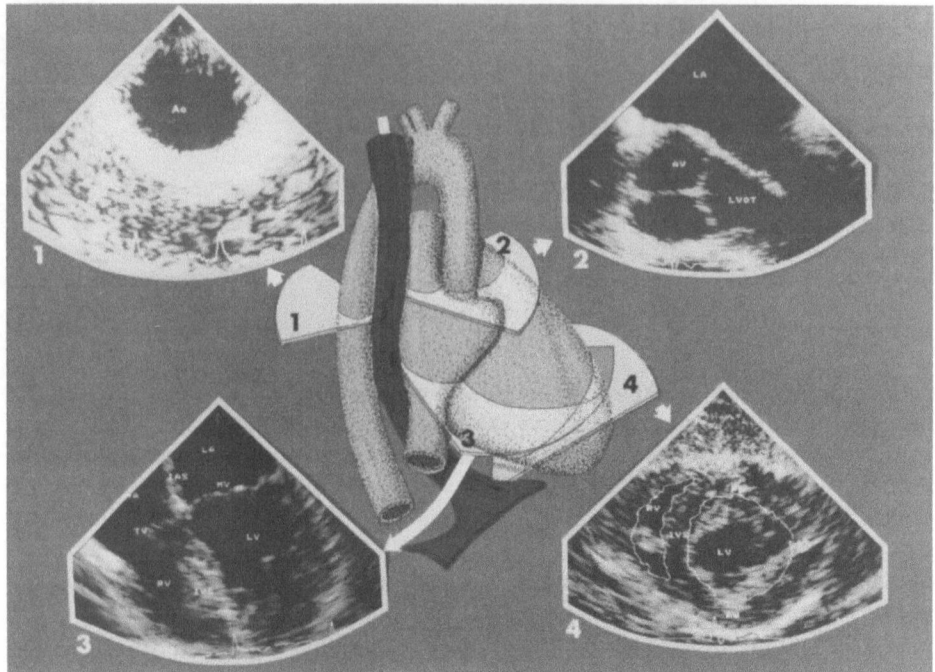

Fig. 1. Schematic of transesophageal echocardiography in the standard scan positions:
1) scanning of the descending aorta;
2) left ventricular outflow tract imaging
3) four-chamber view;
4) cross sectional imaging of the left and right ventricle;
LVILA = left ventricle/atrium, RVIRA = right ventricle/atrium, sAS/sVS = interatrial/interventricular septum, TVIUV = tricuspidal, mitral valve, AV = aortic valve

right ventricle can be received. From the transesophageal approach the four-chamber view and left ventricular outflow tract can be imaged (Fig. 1). By stepwise withdrawal of the scope the whole mitral valve can be visualized and reconstructed.

Seven different transducers from different companies are available. Usually the transducer frequency is 3.75 or 5 MHz and the transducers consist of 32 or more elements mounted to the distal end of a conventional 12 mm gastroscope. Even smaller 9 and 6 mm endoscopes are available.

Transducers with two scan planes are used for biplane imaging of the mitral valve with better spatial orientation (Fig. 2).

Using the Doppler principle, flow information can be received using the pulsed wave and color-coded Doppler imaging. A typical example of the inflow from the left atrium to the left ventricle is demonstrated in Fig. 3.

Calculation

The severity of mitral regurgitation can be judged by contrast echocardiography during heart catheterization and valve surgery. A grading of three scores seems to be useful (Fig. 4) [5, 6].

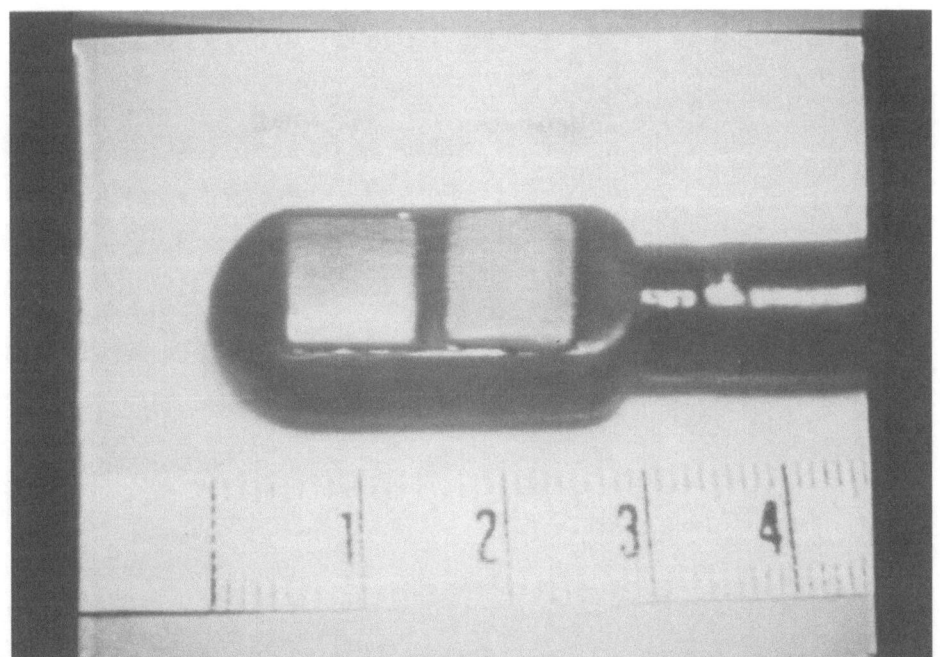

Fig. 2. Echoscope tip with two transducers for orthogonal scanning (Aloka, Hellige, Japan)

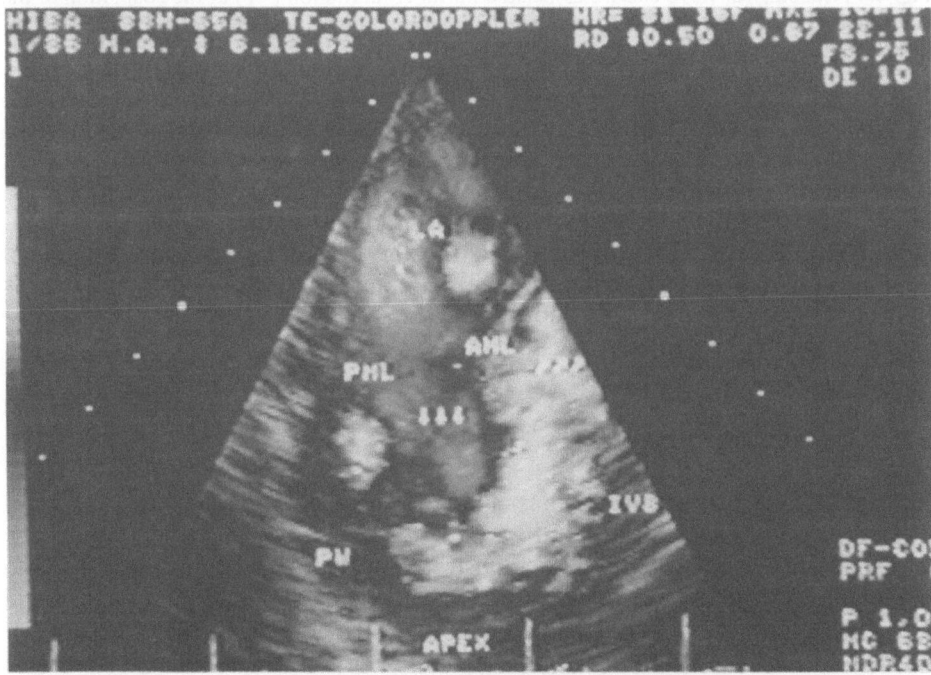

Fig. 3. Inflow during diastole into the left ventricle (LV) between the anterior (AML) and posterior (PML) mitral leaflets from the left atrium (blue) into the left ventricular outflow tract (↑↑↑) along the interventricular septum (IVS). Even the flow behind the PML can be visualized

91

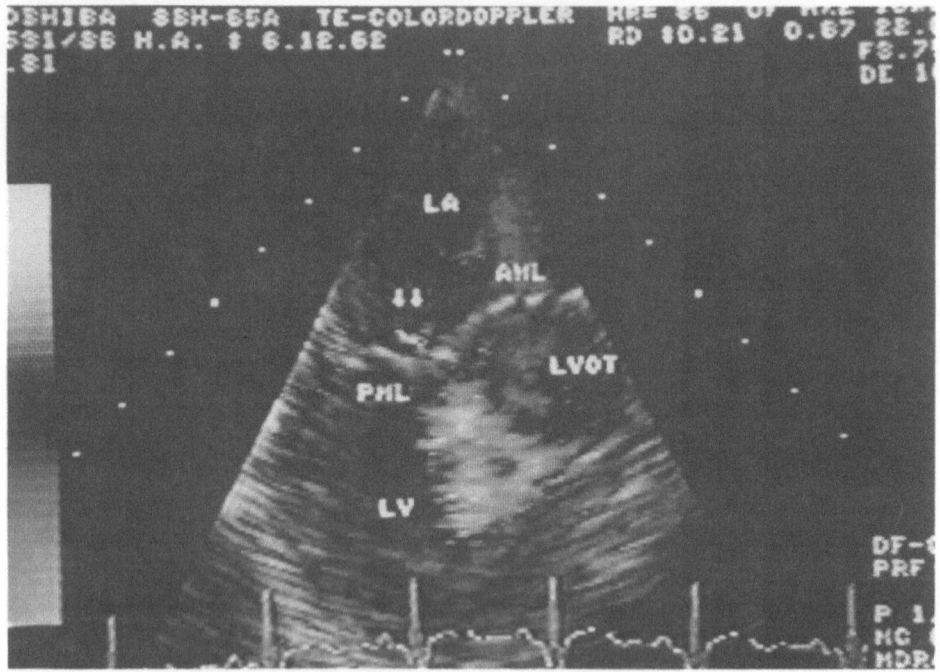

Fig. 4a. Physiological valve closure associated mitral regurgitation (↑↑) at the coaptation of the anterior and posterior (AML/PML) mitral leaflets during systole. Flow from the left ventricle (LV) into the outflow tract (LVOT) during systole.

Using color-coded Doppler imaging a semiquantitative characterization of regurgitation according to angiography (Fig. 4b) can be done, taking into account the depth and width as well as the duration of the regurgitation. Using this methodology in comparison to angiography a high grade of accuracy could be demonstrated [7]. Regarding the comparison to transthoracic echocardiography we could demonstrate that in 10% of the patients a clinical relevant discrepancy exists between both methods. Therefore, in case of preoperative analysis transesophageal echocardiography must be used.

Mitral valve regurgitation etiology

Because coronary artery disease has a high prevalence, it has to be expected that other diseases can be associated. In 307 patients the etiology of mitral insufficiency was analyzed. The distribution is demonstrated in Fig. 5. The importance of echocardiography technology is demonstrated by a patient with main stem stenosis and unstable angina with clinical and angiographically proven mitral regurgitation. Transthoracic echocardiography confirmed this finding without being able to further elucidate the etiology. Thus, transesophageal echocardiography was performed demonstrating chordae tendineae rupture and grade II–III regurgitation (Fig. 6a, b). Thus the surgical procedure changed because the previously suspected

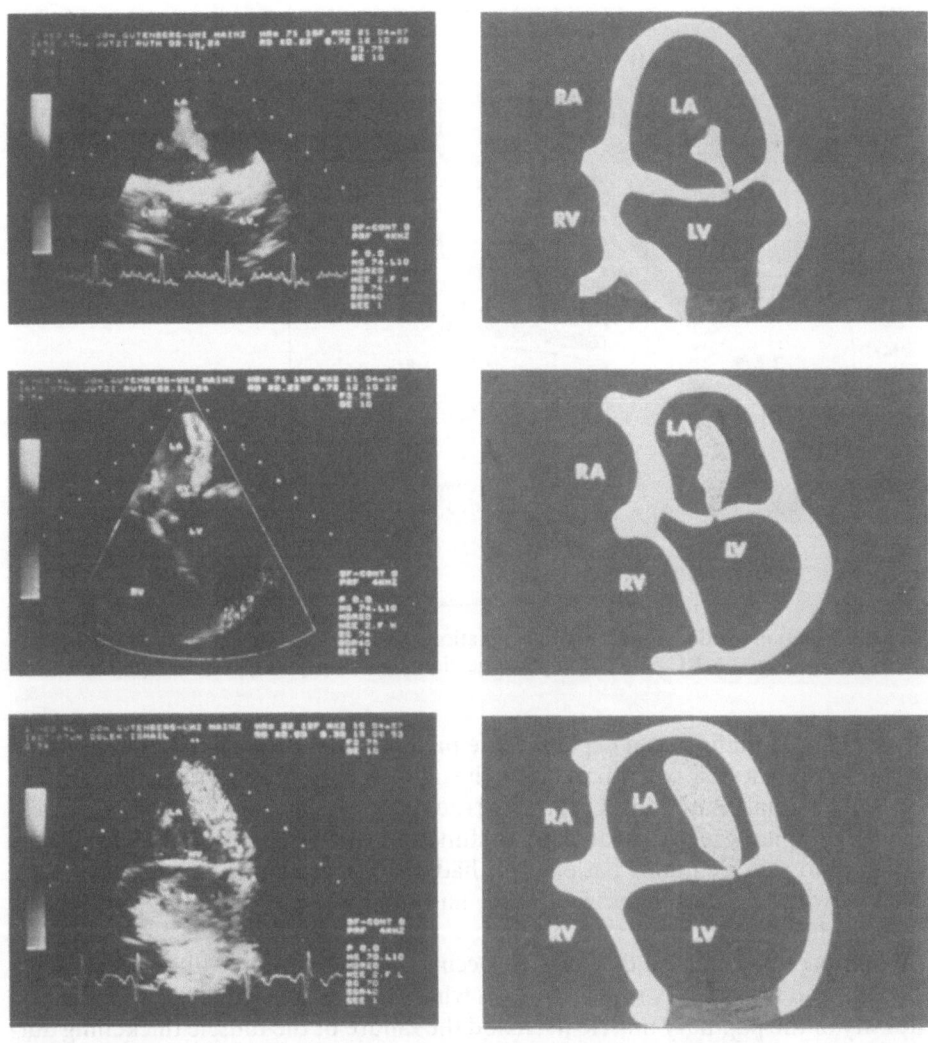

Fig. 4b. Grading of the mitral insufficiency by color Doppler echocardiography in three grades according to the degree and density of regurgitation from the left ventricle into the left atrium

ischemic mitral regurgitation could be excluded, postoperative improvement could not be expected. Mitral valve reconstruction was performed.

In patients with coronary artery disease, papillary muscle rupture is usually combined with a deterioration of the clinical situation. By transesophageal echocardiography the ruptured papillary muscle floating between the left ventricle and atrium can be demonstrated and signs of the regurgitation with volume overload of the heart be demonstrated (Fig. 7). After clarifying the coronary artery status by coronary angiography, the patient can be sent to surgery immediately without further angiography. In two patients we observed a partial rupture of the papillary muscle (Fig. 8) which could be confirmed by surgery. Diagnosis was possible prior to further deterioration of the hemodynamic situation thus avoiding emergency

93

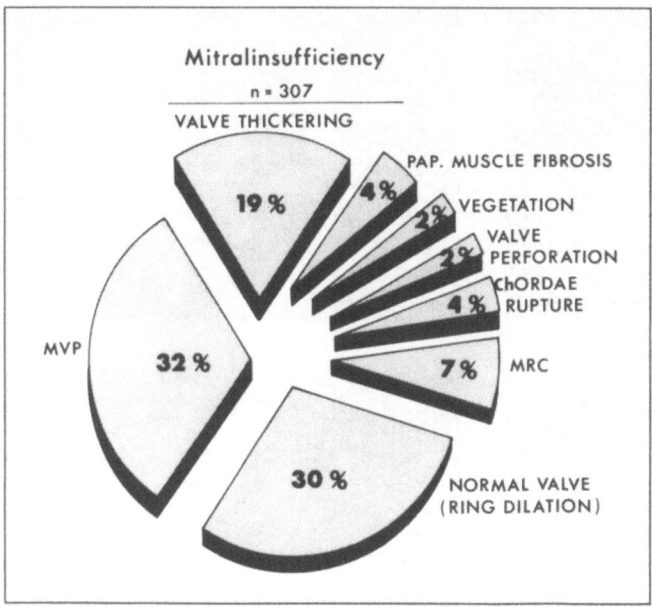

Fig. 5. Distribution of etiology of mitral regurgitation in 307 consecutive patients studied. MVP = mitral valve prolapse, MRC = mitral ring calcification, PAP = papillary muscle rupture

surgery. These findings can explain acute papillary muscle dysfunction, described by others [8]. In a series of 50 patients in the intensive and coronary care unit with 14 acute myocardial infarctions, Oh et al. [8] found 5/7 patients with cardiogenic shock. Mitral regurgitation was related to dysfunction of the papillary muscle in four patients and rupture in one patient. We had in 2/110 patients in the intensive care unit two with papillary muscle rupture, and two out of 27 patients were in cardiogenic shock [9].

When papillary muscle dysfunction occurs without rupture, fibrosis develops. This can lead to papillary muscle fibrosis which can be diagnosed by the increased intensity of the papillary muscle itself and the failure of the muscle thickening during contraction visualized by echocardiography.

In most cases with coronary artery disease only an increase of the diameter of the mitral valve ring, producing mitral insufficiency, is visible. The diameter of the mitral annulus seems to be closely related to the left ventricular enddiastolic volume [12]. The regurgitation is, as was also previously demonstrated by cineventriculogram, more often found in patients with reduced ventricular function than in those with normal ejection fraction. Thus, Barzilai et al. [11] demonstrated that patients with mitral regurgitation and myocardial infarction have volume of 112 ± 9 ml/m^2 and ejection fraction of $41 \pm 4\%$, whereas those without mitral regurgitation had an enddiastolic volume of 72 ± 4 ml/m^2 and ejection fraction of $55 \pm 3\%$. Mortality was 30% and 6%, respectively.

Mitral regurgitation was graded in 150 patients by Breisblatt et al. [12]: Grade I in 7%, grade II in 7%, grade III in 5%, and grade IV was observed in 1% of the patients. In patients with broad infarcts (n = 54) mitral insufficiency was found.

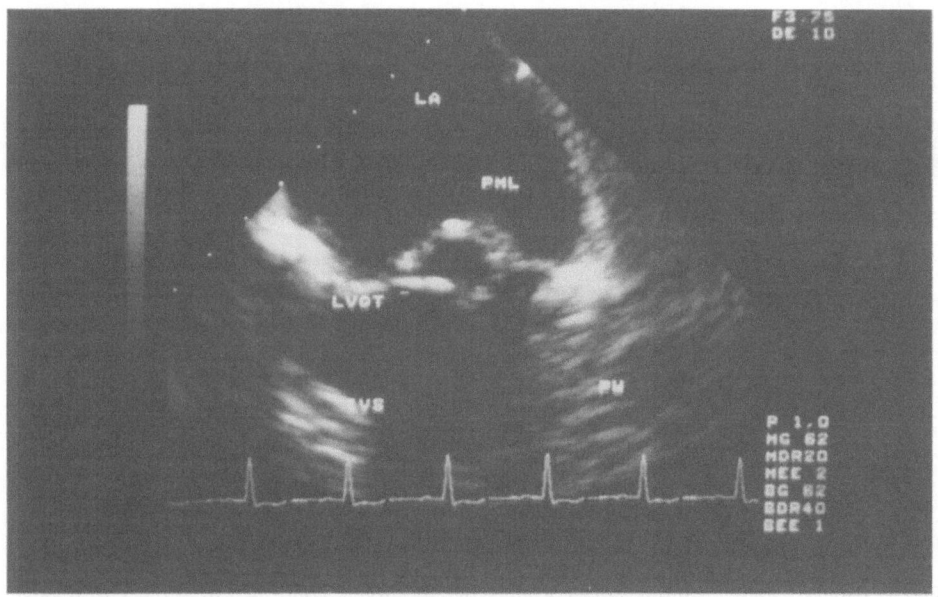

Fig. 6a. Two-dimensional transesophageal echocardiographic demonstration of ruptured chordae tendineae in a patient with mitral insufficiency and main stem stenosis. LA = left atrium, PML = posterior mitral leaflet, LVDT = left ventricular outflow tract, sVs = interventricular septum, PW = posterior wall.

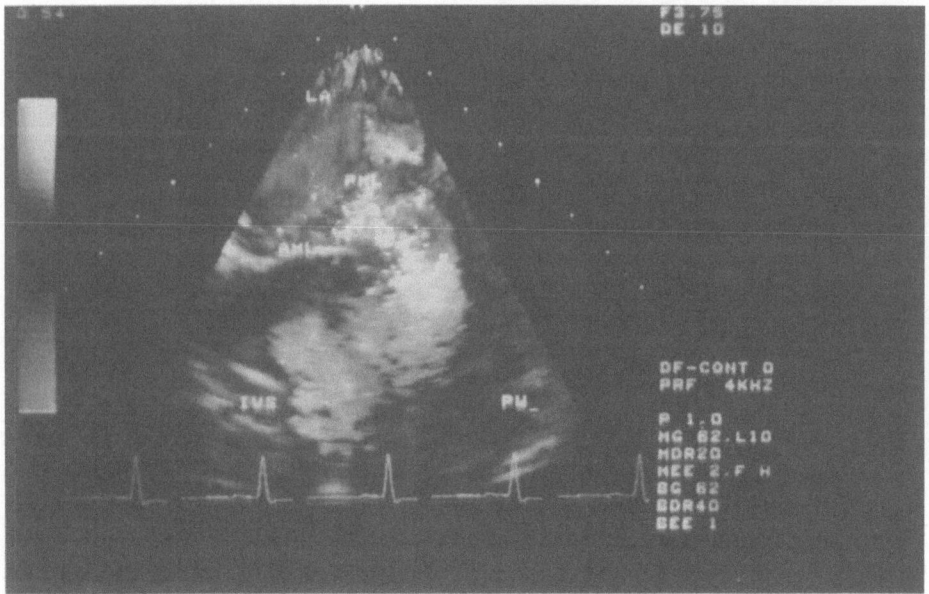

Fig. 6b. Color-coded Doppler imaging with demonstration of regurgitatin between the ruptured chordae and the anterior mitral leaflet in two scan planes during systole.

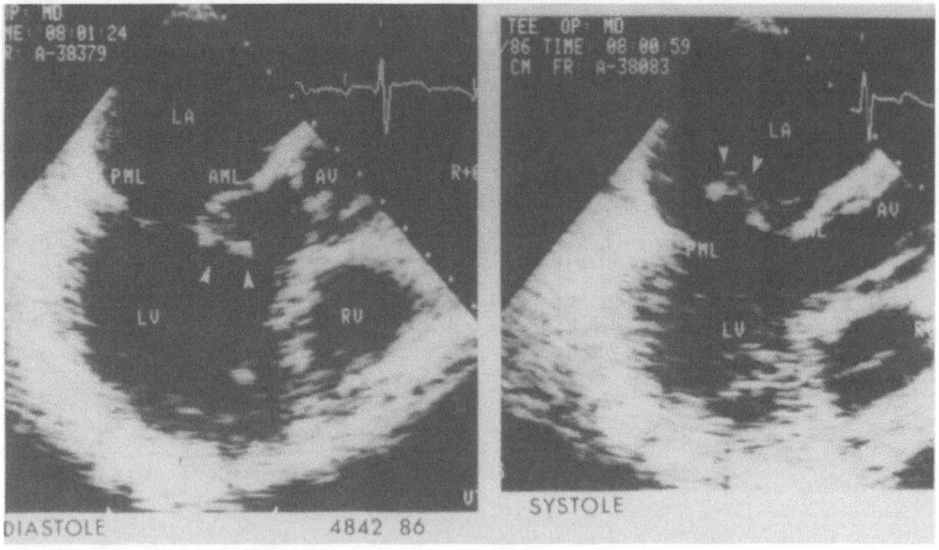

Fig. 7. Papillary muscle rupture after coronary bypass surgery confirmed by surgery with valve replacement in a patient with acute shock and severe mitral regurgitation not detected by clinical and transthoracic echocardiographic examinations, LA/LV = left atrium/ventricle, AUL/PUL = arterior/posterior mitral leaflet, AV = aortic valve.

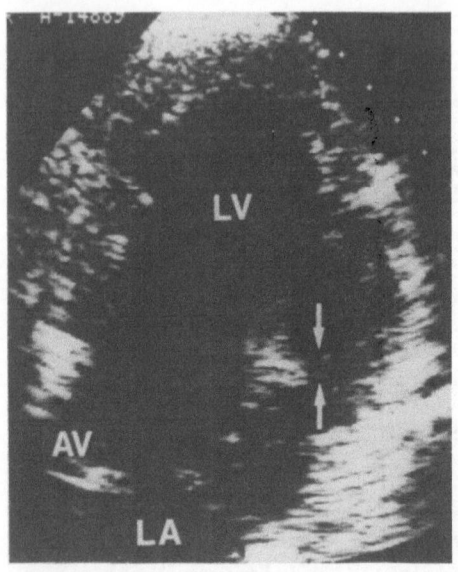

Fig. 8. Partial papillary muscle rupture after inferior myocardial infarction. LV = left ventricle, LA = left atrium, AV = aortic valve

Grade 0 in 20 patients, grade I/II in 25 patients, grade III/IV in nine patients. With small infarcts no mitral regurgitation was found in 18 patients, grade I in 27, and grade II in nine patients [10].

The degree of insufficiency seems to be dependent on the location of the infarct as depicted in the study of Izumi et al. [10]. In inferior infarcts mitral regurgitation

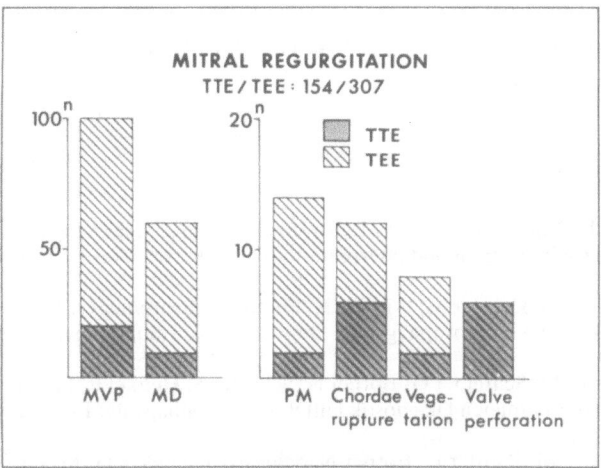

Fig. 9. Comparison of transthoracic and transesophageal demonstration of abnormalities of the mitral valve in 134/307 patients with mitral regurgitation. Demonstration of the superiority and the high accuracy of the transesophageal approach

was found in 14/25 patients (56%), in anterior infarction in 11/28 patients (39%), with bilateral infarct in 18/28 (84−60%) [10]. Arcidi et al. reported on 11/24 (46%) in anterior and 12/34 (35%) in inferior infarcts [13]. In five patients with severe mitral regurgitation a prolapse was found in 5/10 patients with jets to the anterolateral area, in 4/10 patients to the posterior area, and centrally in 3/29 patients. In anterior myocardial infarcts the jet was directed in two patients anterolaterally, in nine centrally, in inferior infarcts in six centrally and in eight posterio-medially; in bilateral infarctions in two patients anterolaterally, in 14 centrally. Thus, all patients with reinfarcts, enlarged enddiastolic volume and reduced ejection fraction, bilateral large infarcts were common in those who very often showed a mitral regurgitation and a high mortality.

Our data on 307 patients with mitral insufficiency studied by the transesophageal echocardiography approach revealed that in 32% mitral valve prolapse, in 30% mitral valve ring dilation, in 19% valve thickening, in 4% papillary muscle fibrosis, in 2% endocarditis, in 2% valve perforation, in 4% chordae tendineae rupture, and in 7% mitral calcification was present (Fig. 5).

Using the transesophageal echocardiographic approach, chordae rupture, vegetations, papillary muscle involvement or rupture were detected more often than by the transthoracic approach alone [Fig. 9].

Clinical implication

Using transesophageal echocardiography we now have the method of choice to study not only the morphology but also mitral valve function, and to estimate the degree of regurgitation. This method should be used in patients with coronary artery disease and mitral insufficiency to exlude patients with other etiologies of mitral regurgitation than ischemia, and to further elucidate the mechanism and papillary muscle function. Follow-up studies are now possible with noninvasive detailed function for cardiac surgery.

References

1. Seller RD, Levy MJ, Ampltz K, Lillehei CM (1964) Left retrograde cardioangiography in acquired cardiac disease: technical indications and interpretations in 700 cases. Am J Cardiol 14:437–447
2. Erbel R, Mohr-Kahaly S, Schuster S, Drexler M, Wittlich N, Pfeiffer C, Schreiner G, Meyer J (1987) Diagnostische Wertigkeit der transösophagealen Dopplerechokardiographie. Herz 12:177–186
3. Erbel R, Mohr-Kahaly S, Drexler M, Schreiner G, Börner N, Schuster S, Henkel B, Pfeiffer C, Meyer J (1986) Erweiterung der kardialen Diagnostik mittels transösophagealer Echokardiographie. Med Klin 81:251–257
4. Erbel R, Mohr-Kahaly S, Drexler M, Pfeiffer C, Börner N, Schuster S, Zenker G, Meyer J (1987) Diagnostischer Stellenwert der transösophagealen Echokardiographie. Dtsch Med Wochenschr 112:23–29
5. Dahm M, Iversen S, Schmidt F, Drexler M, Erbel R, Oelert H (1987) Intraoperative evaluation of reconstruction of the left ventricular valves by transesophageal echocardiography. Thorac Cardiovasc Surg 35: spez. issue, 140–142
6. Drexler M, Erbel R, Dahm M, Mohr-Kahaly S, Oelert H, Meyer J (1986) Assessment of succesful valve reconstruction by intraoperative transesophageal echocardiography (TEE). Int J Cardiol Imaging 2:21–30
7. Erbel R, Schaudig M, Mohr-Kahaly S, Wittlich N, Drexler M, Henrichs KJ, Meyer J (1987) Schweregradbeurteilung der Klappeninsuffizienz mittels transthorakaler und transösophagealer Farb-Dopplerechokardiographie. Z. f. Kardiol 76, Suppl 2:51
8. Oh J (1988) Complications of myocardial infarction. Role of TEE in diagnosis. TEE congress: A new window to the heart, Springer, Berlin Heidelberg New York Tokyo (in press)
9. Erbel R (1988) Transesophageal echocardiography in intensive care. Eur Congress Intensive Care, Stresa, Italy (in press)
10. Izumi S, Miyatake K, Beppu S, Park Y-D, Nagata S, Kinoshita N, Sakakibara H, Nimura Y (1987) Mechanism of mitral regurgitation in patients with myocardial infarction: a study using real-time two-dimensional Doppler flow imaging and echocardiography. Circulation 76:777–785
11. Barzilai B, Gessler C, Perez JE, Schaab C, Jaff AS (1988) Significance of Doppler-detected mitral regurgitation in acute myocardial infarction. Am J Cardiol 61:220–223
12. Breisblatt WM, Cergueira M, Francis CK, Plankey M, Zaret BL, Berger HJ (1987) Left ventricular function in ischemic mitral regurgitation − A precatheterization assessment. Am Heart J 115:77–82
13. Arcidi JM, Hebeler RF, Crover JM, Jones EL, Hatcher CR, Guyton RA (1988) Treatment of moderate mitral regurgitation and coronary disease by coronary bypass alone. J Thorac Cardiovasc Surg 95:951–959

Author's address:
Raimund Erbel, MD
II. Medical Clinic
Johannes Gutenberg-University
Langenbeckstr. 1
6500 Mainz, FRG

Coronary angioplasty for acute mitral regurgitation due to myocardial infarction

R. R. Heuser

Department of Interventional Cardiology, New Mexico Heart Clinic; University of New Mexico, Albfuquerque, New Mexico, USA

Introduction

When acute severe mitral regurgitation is associated with pulmonary edema in the immediate period after myocardial infarction, the patient must be treated aggressively. Because the papillary muscles are perfused by the terminal portion of the coronary vascular bed, they are particularly vulnerable to ischemia and any disturbance in coronary perfusion such as an acute occlusion of a coronary artery may result in papillary muscle dysfunction [1]. When the ischemia is severe and persistent, papillary muscle necrosis and permanent mitral regurgitation may result. The posterior papillary muscle is supplied by the posterior descending branch of the right coronary artery and is infarcted more frequently than the anterolateral papillary muscle, which is supplied by diagonal branches of the left anterior descending artery and often by the marginal branches of the circumflex coronary artery [2]. Reperfusion therapy with fibrinolytic agents or coronary angioplasty theoretically could salvage the functional integrity of the mitral valve apparatus without surgery.

We have utilized coronary angioplasty as primary therapy in 210 patients with acute transmural myocardial infarction. Of these 210 patients, three presented with severe mitral regurgitation and acute pulmonary edema. In all three patients coronary angioplasty with reperfusion resulted in reversal of the regurgitation [3]. A fourth patient presented with ongoing ischemic pain 7 days after treatment with streptokinase for inferior infarction complicated by pulmonary edema and mitral regurgitation. Subsequent angioplasty of the right coronary artery and left anterior descending artery reduced the amount of mitral regurgitation in this patient.

Patients and methods

All three patients had acute myocardial infarction defined by continuous chest pain lasting for greater than 1 h and associated with at least 2-mm ST elevation in more than one electrocardiographic lead and pain unrelieved by nitrates or morphine. Patients entered the catheterization laboratory within 4 h of the onset of chest pain with a mean of 3 h (Table 1). Patient 4 had cardiac catheterization and coronary angioplasty 7 days after treatment with streptokinase.

Treatment Protocol
All patients received intravenous morphine as required to alleviate chest pain; all procedures were done via the femoral route. After vascular sheaths were placed.

Table 1. Acute mitral regurgitation with myocardial infarction

	Patient Number 1		Patient Number 2		Patient Number 3	
Age (years)	62 (Male)		59 (Male)		62 (Male)	
Mitral murmur at time of reperfusion	III/VI		III/VI		none present	
Time of reperfusion (minutes)	180		120		240	
Myocardial infarction location	anterolateral		inferior apical		lateral	
Occluded artery	left anterior descending		circumflex graft		circumflex and left anterior descending	
Severity of mitral regurgitation	+3		+4		+4	
Blood pressure (mmHg)	78 (A)		85 (A, B)		120	
Peak creatine kinase (international units/liter)	4374		2410		3832	
Pulmonary capillary wedge (mmHg)	Pre 34	Post 10	Pre 37	Post 6	Pre 30	Post 15
V-wave (mmHg)	44	8	49	5	44	15
Ejection fraction (%)	40	55	22	67	33	NA
Doppler evidence mitral regurgitation on follow-up	0		0		+	
Follow-up Period (months)	34		33		38	
	A:	Cardiogenic Shock				
	B:	Dopamine infusion				
	NA:	Not available				

(Reprinted from [3] with permission.)

heparin (10 000 units) was administered intravenously. A Swan-Ganz catheter was placed via the femoral vein in all patients and left in place for at least 24 h. Before any intervention, left ventriculography was done in the 30° right anterior oblique projection. A total dose of 34 to 45 mL of Renografin-76 (E. R. Squibb Co., Princeton, New Jersey, USA) was administered. Selective coronary angiography was done in several views before any intervention. At the time of the intervention, surgical backup was urgently obtained so that if coronary angioplasty was unsuccessful, coronary bypass surgery plus mitral valve replacement could be done.

Coronary angioplasty was performed with USCI guiding catheters (Bard, Billerica, Massachusetts, USA) and ACS steerable balloon catheter systems (Advanced Cardiovascular System, Mountain View, California, USA). After the initial coronary angiograms were obtained either a 0.016-inch USCI steerable guidewire or a 0.018-inch ACS steerable guidewire was advanced to the coronary occlusion. If, with gentle pushing, no resistance was met the wire was advanced further. After the guidewire passed the occlusion, the balloon catheter was advanced and the balloon inflated serially until it could inflate fully. After full inflation of the catheter, coronary arteriography was done with the guidewire still present in the coronary artery to see if successful dilation had occurred. The guidewire was then removed and coronary angiography was repeated in several projections. The patients were transferred to the coronary care unit and the vascular sheaths were left in place for at least 24 h. Intravenous heparin at a dose of 1,000 units per hour was continued as a continuous drip and discontinued 24 h after the procedure and the sheaths were removed in all patients.

Angiographic Evaluation
In all patients, the coronary artery involved with the infarction was totally occluded with no flow seen distal to the occlusion. In Patient 3, at the time of initial dilation, a second coronary artery was occluded acutely; this was also dilated immediately. Coronary angioplasty was deemed successful if after the procedure the artery involved was less than 50% occluded as measured by cross-sectional area stenosis and also pain was relieved.

Grading of Mitral Regurgitation
Left ventricular cineangiograms taken in the right anterior oblique projection were reviewed for each of the four patients without previous knowledge of the diagnosis or pressures. The amount of mitral regurgitation was graded as: 0 = no systolic regurgitation of dye into the left atrium; trace = minimal amount of regurgitation, clearing entirely during each ventricular diastole; 1+ = mild regurgitation, not entirely filling the left atrium; 2+ = moderate regurgitation, entirely filling the atrium; 3+ = severe regurgitation, filling the left atrium fully such that the atrium was as opaque as the ventricle by the end of contrast injection; and 4+ = very severe regurgitation, such that the left atrium was as well opacified as the ventricle after a single systole [4]. Angiographic left ventricular ejection fraction was obtained by planimetry of the right anterior oblique ventriculograms using a standard single-plane area-length formula.

Results: Acute patients

Patient 1, a 62-year-old man, had a 6 month history of exertional chest pain. Forty-eight hours before admission, chest pain began to occur at rest with durations of several hours. On admission the electrocardiogram showed nonspecific ST- and T-wave changes. Two h before arriving at the catheterization laboratory, he had severe continuous substernal chest pain with an acute anterior wall myocardial infarction seen on an electrocardiograph. At the time of catheterization, the patient was in cardiogenic shock with a grade III/VI mitral regurgitation murmur. The systolic blood pressure was 78 mmHg and the mean capillary wedge pressure was 34 mmHg. There were V-waves of 44 mmHg on Swan-Ganz tracing. An intra-aortic balloon was placed and coronary arteriography and left ventriculography were performed. The right coronary artery was totally occluded with no collaterals seen filling the left anterior descending coronary artery. The left anterior descending was totally occluded before the origin of the first septal perforating coronary artery. The right coronary artery filled via left to right collaterals and was a large

101

dominant coronary artery. The circumflex coronary artery was totally occluded in its distal portion. The left anterior descending coronary artery was acutely dilated with a good result (Figs. 1a, b). Left ventriculography showed 3+ mitral regurgitation, (Figs. 1c, d) inferior apical hypokinesis and anterior hypokinesis with an ejection fraction of 40%.

After acute coronary angioplasty, the mean wedge dropped to 10 mmHg within 24 h and the murmur went away within 6 h. The patient left the hospital 8 days later with no heart failure or auscultative evidence of mitral regurgitation. Three months later the patient had recurrence of angina pectoris. Repeat cardiac catheterization revealed restenosis at the site of the left anterior descending coronary angioplasty. No mitral regurgitation was seen on repeat ventriculography and left ventricular function had improved to an ejection fraction of 55% (Figs. 1e, f). Because of the three-vessel coronary artery disease, uncomplicated coronary bypass surgery was done with no mitral valve replacement. Thirty-one months after surgery he is free of mitral regurgitation with no angina or heart failure.

All three patients had multiple vessel disease. All patients at the time of the coronary angioplasty had severe mitral regurgitation (two with 4+ mitral regurgitation,

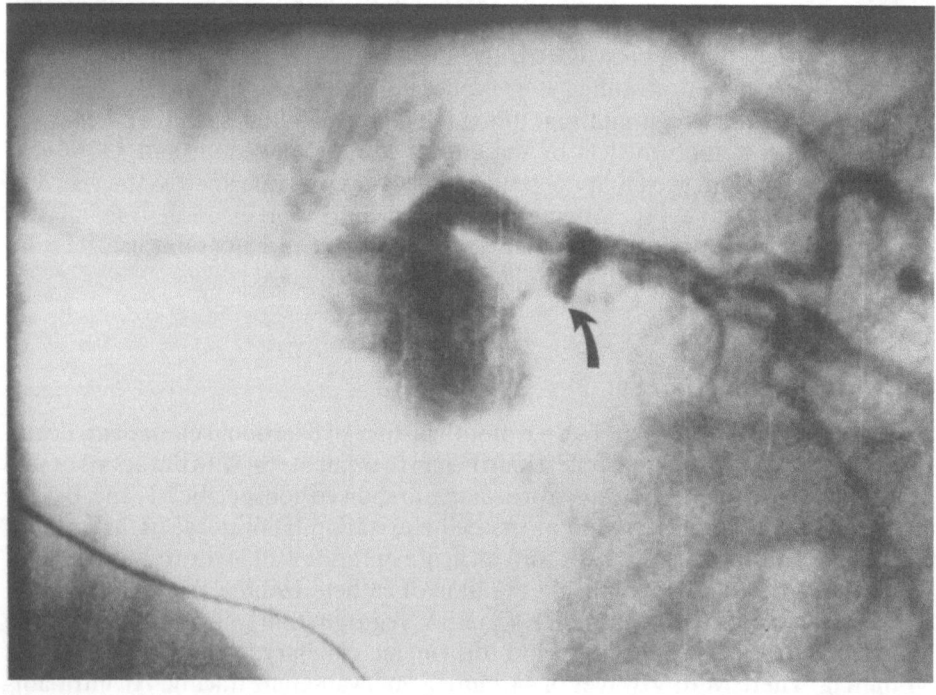

a)

Fig. 1. a) Coronary arteriography in Patient 1 before angioplasty of left anterior descending coronary artery. **b)** Coronary arteriography after successful dilatation of left anterior descending coronary artery. **c)** Left ventriculogram at time of acute infarction, at end diastole. **d)** Left ventriculogram at end systole showing 3+ mitral regurgitation. **e)** Left ventriculogram 3 months after infarction at end diastole. **f)** Left ventriculogram at end systole showing no mitral regurgitation. (Reproduced from [3] with permission.)

102

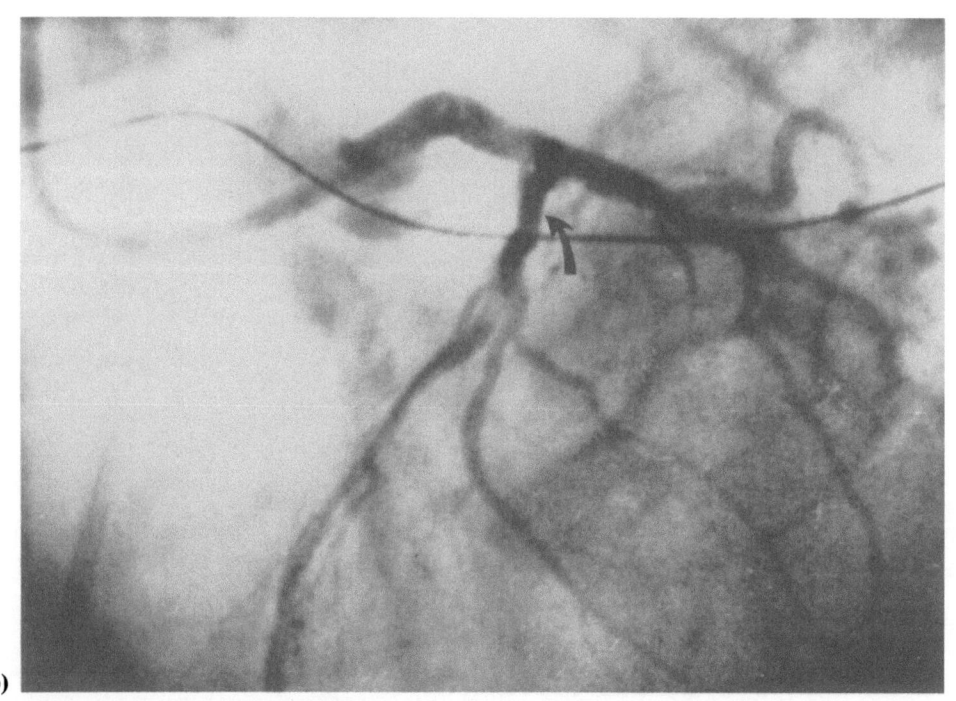

b)

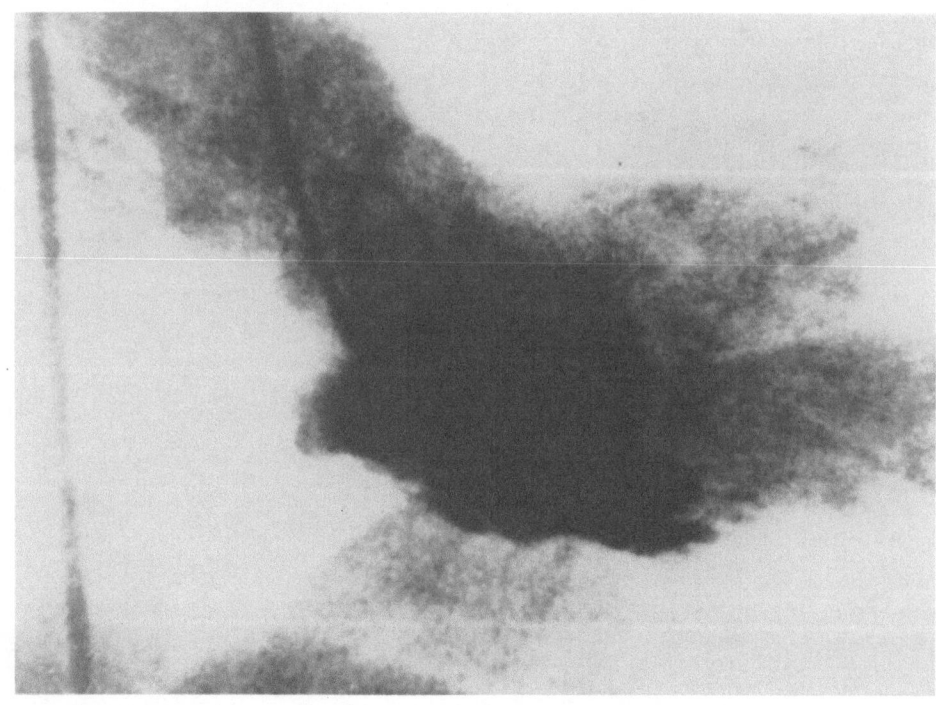

c)

103

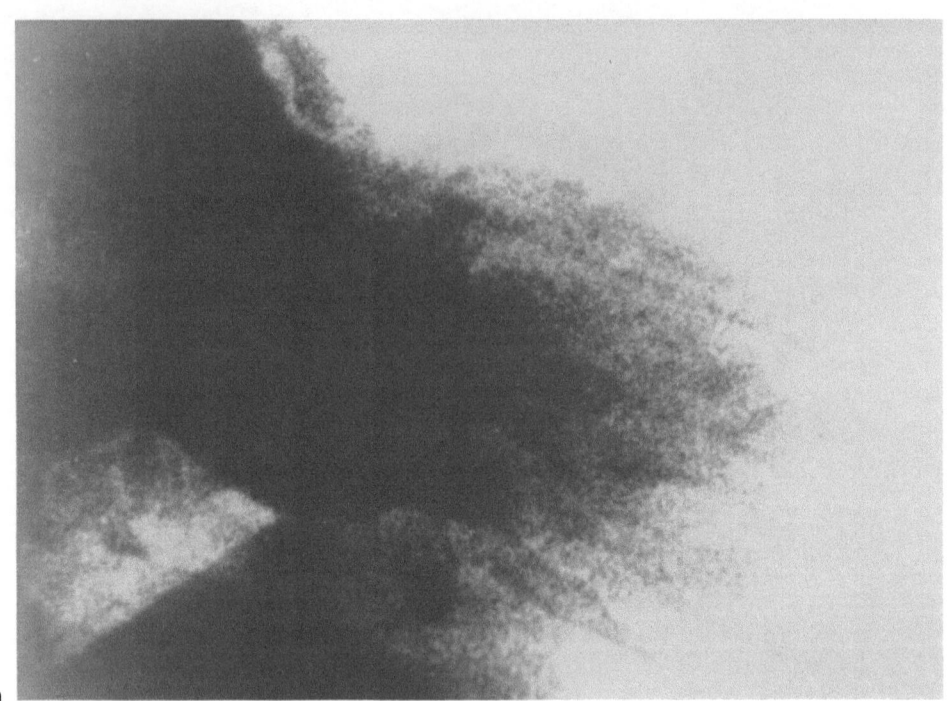

d)

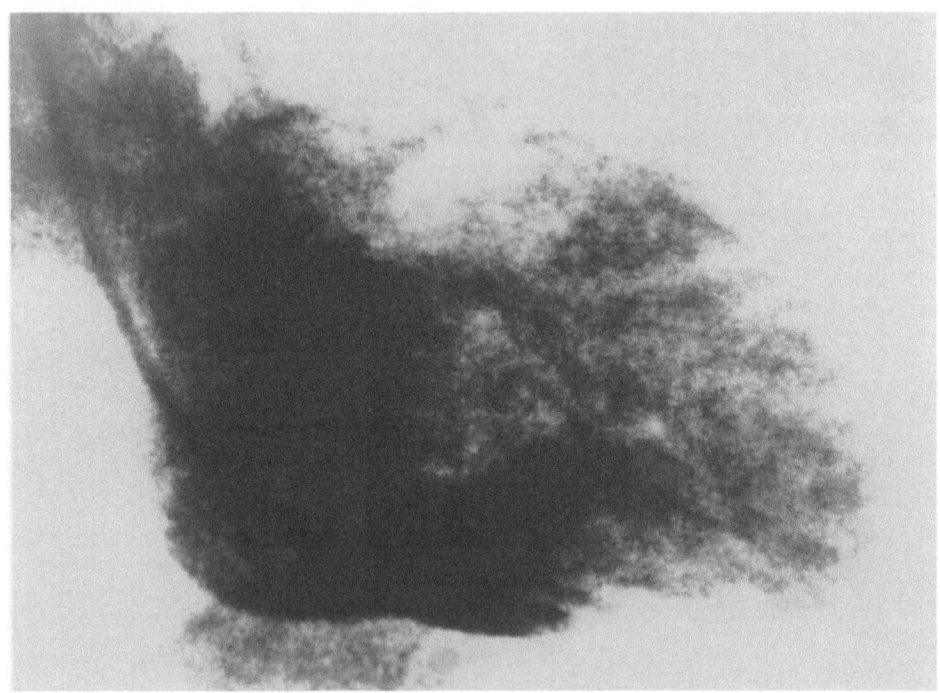

e)

104

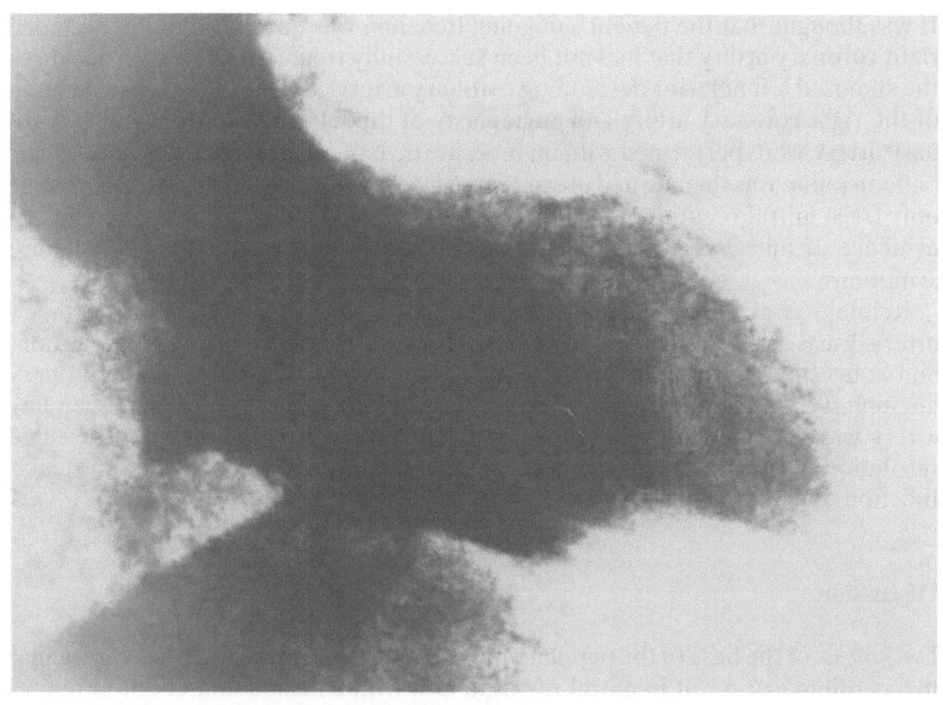

f)

one with 3+ mitral regurgitation). All patients were discharged with no mitral regurgitation murmar; the patients received calcium channel blockers, salicylates, and dipyridamole (Table 1).

Result: Subacute patient

Patient 4, a 45-year-old man, initially had cardiac symptoms in June 1985, when he suffered an acute anterior wall myocardial infarction. He was treated with intravenous streptokinase and coronary angioplasty of the left anterior descending coronary artery; he had no mitral regurgitation. In early December, 1985, he suffered an acute inferior wall myocardial infarction. Intravenous streptokinase (150000 units) was given within 3 h of the onset of chest pain. He was in acute pulmonary edema and had a murmur consistent with mitral regurgitation; 7 days later he was transferred because of recurrent chest pain. While pain-free, he had a grade II/VI murmur of mitral regurgitation. Electrocardiograph showed an old anteroseptal infarction and recent inferior infarction. Cardiac catheterization showed an occluded dominant right coronary artery, 90% stenosis of the left anterior descending artery before the septal perforator, and 30–40% stenosis of the proximal obtuse marginal branch of the circumflex coronary artery. There was poor left ventricular function (ejection fraction 22%) with mid-anterior wall hypokinesis, apical akinesis, and inferior akinesis. He had 3+ mitral regurgitation.

105

It was thought that the patient's ongoing ischemia was due either to the occluded right coronary artery that had not been successfully treated with streptokinase, or the stenosed left anterior descending coronary artery. The next day recanalization of the right coronary artery and angioplasty of the left anterior descending coronary artery were performed with an intra-aortic balloon in place. The intra-aortic balloon pump was then turned off and repeat ventriculography was done, revealing only trace mitral regurgitation. Forty-two months after the procedure, he has no evidence of mitral regurgitation; he does have Class II congestive heart failure symptoms.

Reinfeld et al. reported similar results in a patient with three-vessel coronary artery disease [5]. This patient had unstable angina, moderate mitral regurgitation, and congestive heart failure with an ejection fraction of 17% prior to coronary angioplasty. Angioplasty of a stenosed circumflex and left anterior descending artery was performed. Two months later repeat cardiac catheterization revealed resolution of the mitral regurgitation and marked improvement in left ventricular function.

Discussion

Dyskinesis of the base of the papillary muscles due to damage of the left ventricular myocardium can result in mitral regurgitation with a healed infarction. Often, as the patient recovers from the ischemia and infarction, the degree of mitral regurgitation diminishes and the patient is left without a hemodynamically significant defect. However, if ischemia to the papillary muscle continues, total rupture can occur and is usually fatal [2, 6]. Cardiogenic shock or pulmonary edema associated with severe mitral regurgitation in the setting of acute myocardial infarction is associated with a high mortality rate. Emergency coronary bypass and mitral valve replacement is complicated by technical difficulties related to repair of acutely necrotic tissue and carries a mortality as high as 60% [7, 8]. Although intra-aortic balloon counterpulsation can be used to acutely reduce afterload, the hemodynamic status often does not improve enough to defer surgical intervention. Coronary bypass surgery can result in elimination of ischemia to the papillary bed and not necessitate mitral valve replacement. Because more patients survive the initial period of acute myocardial infarction, it is thought that the incidence of papillary muscle rupture may be increasing and may be as high as 5% [9]. Unfortunately, when acute mitral regurgitation is present it is difficult to know whether acute surgical reperfusion will eliminate mitral regurgitation and therefore most surgeons replace or repair the mitral valve when severe regurgitation is present [8, 10].

These patients were treated before the GISSI and other studies [11–14] showed a decrease in short-term mortality in patients with acute myocardial infarction when treated with thrombolytic agents. Coronary angioplasty has been used effectively as sole therapy in myocardial infarction [3, 15, 16]. Coronary angioplasty has also been used as sole therapy in cardiogenic shock [15, 17, 18]. Most of the thrombolytic trials have excluded patients in cardiogenic shock [19, 20], and in trials where cardiogenic shock was included there was no difference in mortality [20]. The advantage of coronary angioplasty therapy in an evolving infarction includes the ability to quickly and fully reperfuse the vessels without the use of fibrinolytic agents.

Fibrinolytic therapy has obvious complications including bleeding (13−16%) [21]. The advantage of coronary angioplasty would be that if it were unsuccessful the patient would not be systematically fibrinolytic and acute revascularization would be done with mitral valve replacement with no increased risk in systemic bleeding. Studies of coronary angioplasty in myocardial infarction have shown the procedures to be of low risk [21]. In our institution we do not routinely have surgeons on standby for acute intervention. We were fortunate to have had surgical backup at the time when these patients arrived in the hospital. However, whether delay in obtaining surgical backup would necessarily increase the mortality associated with this procedure is unknown. Whether the use of intravenous thrombolytic agents followed by immediate coronary angioplasty in patients with acute mitral regurgitation and pulmonary edema will result in as effective an opening of the vessel and hemodynamic improvement as compared with coronary angioplasty alone is also unknown. There is a theoretical problem in the use of lytic therapy in patients who present with acute mitral regurgitation and pulmonary edema because lysis is unsuccessful 25−50% of the time depending on the agent that is used [14]. If the agent is unsuccessful and the patient does not have successful reopening of the vessel, the likelihood of mortality is quite high. In most patients who present with acute infarction who are treated with tissue plasminogen activator, immediate cardiac catheterization and coronary angioplasty are of no benefit as compared to delayed angiography [14, 22−24]. It appears in patient 4, however, that delayed cardiac catheterization and subsequent coronary angioplasty appear to be effective.

The use of coronary angioplasty in acute infarction with acute mitral regurgitation and pulmonary edema results in complete revascularization. Patients treated with intravenous lytic agents may have incomplete revascularization with only a slowly obtained small amount of flow [14, 25, 26].

References

1. Estes EH Jr, Dalton FM, Entman ML, Dixon HB, Hackel DB (1966) The anatomy and blood supply of the papillary muscles of the left ventricle. Am Heart J 1:356−362
2. Braunwald E (1984) Valvular heart disease. In: Braunwald E (ed) Heart disease: a textbook of cardiovascular medicine. 2nd ed. Saunders, Philadelphia, pp 1076−1078
3. Heuser RR, Maddoux GL, Goss JE, Ramo BW, Raff GL, Shadoff N (1987) Coronary angioplasty for acute mitral regurgitation due to myocardial infarction. Ann Int Med 107:852−855
4. Fuchs RM, Heuser RR, Yin FCP, Brinker JA (1982) Limitations of pulmonary wedge V waves in diagnosing mitral regurgitation. Am J Cardiol 49:849−854
5. Reinfeld HB, Samet P, Hildner JF (1985) Resolution of congestive failure, mitral regurgitation and angina after percutaneous transluminal coronary angioplasty of triple vessel disease. Cath CV Diag 11:273−277
6. Gahl K, Sutton R, Pearson M, Caspari P, Lairet A, McDonald L (1977) Mitral regurgitation in coronary heart disease. Br Heart J 39:13−18
7. Vlodaver Z, Edwards JE (1977) Rupture of ventricular septum or papillary muscle complicating myocardial infarction. Circulation 55:815−822
8. Tepe NA, Edmunds LH (1985) Operation for acute postinfarction mitral insufficiency and cardiogenic shock. J Thorac Cardiovasc Surg 89:525−530

9. Wei JY, Hutchins GM, Bulkley BH (1979) Papillary muscle rupture in a fatal acute myocardial infarction. A potentially treatable form of cardiogenic shock. Ann Intern Med 90:149–153

10. Pinson CW, Cobanoglu A, Metzdorff MT, Grunkemeier GL, Kay PH, Starr A (1984) Late surgical results for ischemic mitral regurgitation: role of wall motion score and severity of regurgitation. J Thorac Cardiovascular Surg 88:663–672

11. Gruppo Italiano per lo studio della streptochinasi nell' infarcto miocardico (GISSI) (1986) Effectiveness of intravenous thrombolytic treatment in acute myocardial infarction. Lancet I:397–401

12. Van de Werf F et al. (1988) Lessons from the European cooperative recombinant tissue-type plasminogen activator (rt-PA) versus placebo trial. J Am Coll Cardiol 12:14A–19A

13. Rapaport E (1989) Thrombolytic agents in acute myocardial infarction. N Engl J Med 13:861–864

14. Mark DB, Hlatky M, O'Connor CM, Pryor DB, Wall TC, Honan MB, Phillips III HR, Califf RM (1988) Administration of thrombolytic therapy in the community hospital: Established principles and unresolved issues. J Am Coll Cardiol 12:32A–43A

15. Hartzler GO, Rutherford BD, McConahay DR, et al. (1983) Coronary angioplasty with and without thrombolytic therapy for treatment of acute myocardial infarction. Am Heart J 106:965–973

16. Pepine CJ, Prida X, Hill JA, Feldman RL, Conti CR (1984) Coronary angioplasty in acute myocardial infarction. Am Heart J 107:820–822

17. Shani J, Rivera M, Greengart A, Hollander G, Kaplan P, Lichstein E (1986) Coronary angioplasty in cardiogenic shock (abstract). J Am Coll Cardiol 7:149A

18. Heuser RR, Maddoux GL, Goss JE, Ramo BW, Raff GL, Shadoff N (1986) Coronary angioplasty in the treatment of cardiogenic shock: the therapy of choice (abstract). J Am Coll Cardiol 7:219A

19. Bates ER, Califf RM, Stack RS, Aronson L, George BS, Candela RJ, Kereiakes DJ, Abbottsmith CW, Anderson L, Pitt B, O'Neill WW, Topol EJ, TIMI group (1989) Thrombolysis and angioplasty in myocardial infarction (TAMI-1) trial: Influence of infarct location on arterial patency, left ventricular function and mortality. J Am Coll Cardiol 13:12–18

20. Selzer A (1989) Does thrombolytic therapy reduce infarct size? J Am Coll Cardiol 13:1431–1434

21. Faxon DP (1988) The risk of reperfusion strategies in the treatment of patients with acute myocardial infarction. J Am Coll Cardiol 12:52A–57A

22. De Bono DP (1988) The European Cooperative Study Group trial of intravenous recombinant tissue-type plasminogen activator (rt-PA) and conservative therapy versus rt-PA and immediate coronary angioplasty. J Am Coll Cardiol. 1988; 12:20A–23A

23. Braunwald E (1988) Thrombolytic reperfusion of acute myocardial infarction: resolved and unresolved issues. J Am Coll Cardiol 12:85A–92A

24. TIMI Study Group (1989) Comparison of invasive and conservative strategies after treatment with intravenous tissue plasminogen activator in acute myocardial infarction. N Engl J Med 320:618–627

25. TIMI Study Group (1985) The thrombolysis in myocardial infarction (TIMI) trial. Phase I Findings. N Engl J Med 312:932–936

26. Topol EJ, Weiss JL, Brinker JA, et al. (1985) Regional wall motion improvement after coronary thrombolysis with recombinant tissue plasminogen activator: importance of coronary angioplasty. J Am Coll Cardiol 6:426–433

Author's address:
Richard R. Heuser, M.D.
New Mexico Heart Clinic
1001 Coal, SE
Albuquerque, NM 87106, USA

Discussion

MEYER:

I think we agreed upon that we first should discuss the first two papers, because they seem to belong together more closely. These papers include incidence, severity, and etiology.

DESIDERI:

I like to ask Dr. Fleck something about the methodology used to study his patients. You took all the mitral regurgitations and after that you selected the patients with coronary artery disease. How did you manage to select other causes of mitral regurgitation?

FLECK:

Well, we excluded, as I have shown in this scheme, every patient who had mitral valve disease out of other origin. This is easy if you look at mitral stenosis first. After that we were left with a group of patients, those with coronary disease and those without. Those without were excluded, of course, and included still in this type of analysis everybody who might have perhaps mitral valve prolapse or something in addition to coronary artery disease. Those were not excluded. But if you look in the remaining patients, which are not so many; we checked all of them only to understand what type of disease might be in those and we did not find mitral valve prolapse for one of the reasons of severe regurgitation, which I showed. We found only a few patients. These were patients with severe regurgitation who had rupturing of chordae tendineae or had additional disease. One of them had severe aortic stenosis and therefore, probably a small ventricle. But also, those patients actually had enormous endsystolic volumes. I think that this is interesting information.

SCHMUTZLER:

Dr. Berghöfer, could you explain the hemodynamic importance of these insufficiencies. You told us it is only "slight", how slight, and is there a suggestion that some of the degree of severity of the insufficiency may change within the follow-up of these cases in respect to the outcome of these patients?

BERGHÖFER:

We had a control group of six patients with restenosis after PTCA, and out of these six patients, two had less mitral regurgitation after at least 1 year. So I think mitral regurgitation will develop to a less significant stadium in most of the patients, at least in those patients with acute coronary artery disease, i.e., acute myocardial infarction. Mitral regurgitation usually is very slight, not only in angiographic findings, but in clinical findings as well.

SCHMUTZLER:

Any addition to that and also to Dr. Fleck — what do you think, what is the percentage of these patients who have to be operated on?

BERGHÖFER:

Out of 65 patients in our series there were two patients who were operated on, so it might be around 3%.

FLECK:

We have the problem that in those patients who had only bypass graft surgery without doing any surgery at the mitral valve and who had more than moderate to severe, that is grade 3 or 4 mitral incompetence, they remained in that stage and they had to be treated with large doses of ACE inhibitors together with diuretics. Finally they had to be reoperated and mitral valve repair was done.

RANKIN:
I would like to ask the first two speakers, along those same lines, what their criteria would be for approaching the mitral valve in a patient undergoing operation primarily for coronary artery disease. Secondly, what is the operative mortality rate in their series of patients with moderate to severe regurgitation that have been treated by coronary bypass alone without a valve procedure?

FLECK:
I would suggest that you should operate on the mitral valve as well in patients with large or enlarged endsystolic volumes which is the result of our study. If we did not do so the hemodynamic problems remained and therefore we had to retreat them in any form; we usually tried to have them reoperated.

BERGHÖFER:
The two patients in our series who were operated on both survived and both had repair of the mitral valve.

MEYER:
May we then turn to the echocardiographic analysis preoperatively, and also intraoperatively and postoperatively. I think the results fit very nicely into what has been shown this morning by Dr. Puff and by Dr. Becker who showed very nicely how it is related to the different coronary vessels. And I think both, Dr. Bolger and Dr. Erbel, showed how we can analyze this in the echocardiogram, also intraoperatively. So for the first time we are able not only to tell the surgeon that there is mitral incompetence but we are able to tell him which part of the valve is diseased and then during operation we are able to show whether this diseased valve is now functioning.

DREXLER:
Dr. Bolger, you nicely showed your epicardial assessment of the valve function intraoperatively. In Mainz we are using the transesophageal approach. Regardless of whether you use the epicardial or transesophageal approach, is it a problem for you to convince your surgeon that the valve is still incompetent when you perform your measurements intraoperatively or let me ask the other way around, what do you do in a case where you found still a severe mitral insufficiency on color-coded Doppler and your surgeon is quite sure that the valve is competent?

BOLGER:
Well, luckily, our surgeons have a lot of confidence in our technique at this point. We have a very good working relationship and if usually when we see severe regurgitation there was some indication that it was going to be a risky repair and this information gives them a chance to go back and modify it and they would rather know that. If there is a real question then they can look for other associated findings, but if it is still severe regurgitation you may well be able to feel the thrill.

FRATER:
If you let the surgeon be the echocardiographer then it is entirely his responsibility, and that is the way I do it. I put the thing on myself and if I see too much insufficiency, clearly I must replace the valve. I do not have to be told to replace it. But I do not want to get the reputation of being a semanticist, but I would ask the echocardiographers here if they would agree that we should use what Dr. Bolger suggested as appropriate terms for the occasions in which part of the cusp rises above the plane of the atrio-ventricular ring. I wrote a paper in 1964 in which I talked about the free edge rising above the plane of the ring and that, as far as I am concerned, is well described as prolapse. Dr. Bolger suggested that if the free edge is below the plane of the ring but the body of the cusp rises above it, this should be called billowing. To me it is fairly obvious to use those two terms: prolapse when the edge goes above the ring and billowing when only the cusp goes above. Can I ask the echocardiographers if they would agree to such terminology?

110

BOLGER:

I think that that can be a useful distinction, but part of my intraoperative experience has shown me that if you are able to angulate very carefully in many cases which would seem to be predominantly billowing, you can identify an area where the leaflet edge is acutally out of the plane. Whether or not that helps surgically to know the difference between the two then becomes a point of whether or not we should make that distinction.

FRATER:

Enormously, because if the free edges rising above the plane that explains where that particular part of the insufficiency is coming from. If it is merely billowing and you cannot demonstrate the free edge coming above, then it is a different mechanism for the insufficiency.

BOLGER:

I think that we can with color Doppler also localize the sources of regurgitation very nicely and that is also helpful.

ERBEL:

Taking into account what Roberts described as a pathologist, I think, we should talk about mitral valve prolapse when three things are detected. It is not only a billowing and that the coaptation side is upper the mitral ring, but we also look at the thickness of the mitral valve itself and we look at the mitral valve ring. Pathologists and some groups using echocardiography have demonstrated that patients with mitral valve prolapse have increased areas of the mitral valve ring.

FRATER:

That is exactly right, but you do not have to call it prolapse when the ring is large; that is ring enlargement. I have no doubt that the use of the term "mitral valve prolapse" in young ladies with billowing mitral valves is a disastrous feature of modern cardiology. These young ladies go around terribly nervous after heaving this diagnosis. They come to us, saying, "what's wrong with me, my doctor told me I had prolapse". By far it is better to say that "your valve is a little large and it is billowing, but at the moment it is not yet prolapsed".

HETZER:

I would like to add a note from the standpoint of a surgeon in respect to what Dr. Drexler brought up: we have been doing many mitral repair procedures during the last 10–12 years, it has been a routine procedure and we have been very proud about our intraoperative testing methods by just filling the left ventricle and looking at the mitral valve. With the onset of repair in ischemic mitral valve disease, this, quite obviously, has become a doubtful testing procedure. Intraoperative echocardiography certainly is much superior to any other testing procedure, as we are using it now routinely. In this respect I want to support Dr. Bolger in her results and her opinion. I would like to ask her what hemodynamic conditions you require in order to compare pre- and postoperative echocardiography in your functional tests.

BOLGER:

As I mentioned, we got to great length to match our systolic blood pressures, but we also do some other things. We try to delay our postpump imaging until the patient is hemodynamically as stable as possible, until they have been rewarmed and maintained a circulation for some time. We have seen several times that regurgitation appears much worse early on when the patient is still sightly cold. Again, it will look worse in the phase of ventricular pacing. So, if we can wait until the patient either has a sinus rhythm or atrial repaced rhythm, we will wait for that also.

VINCENT:

I have a technical question Dr. Bolger: during epicardial imaging we have got the problem to see the proper image of the mitral valve, especially because the beam is axial and if you have to make even a slight luxation of the heart, you may disturb the mitral function as well. We are still seeking for a better probe which you can slide into the pericardial back without disturbing the natural position of your heart. On your picture that was, I suppose, an axial probe too, have you got the same problems?

111

BOLGER:

Actually, we are able to usually find an acceptable view often times from the midseptum. If that is not acceptable for some reason, depending on the patient's heart, we will go apically and look up, we will go up on to the aortic root actually and look down. Some times we actually will, with the surgeon's assistance, put the transducer behind, knowing that that would distort the heart, but generally speaking even if you have to go over to the superior vena cava you can distort and use a very unorthodox view, but generally see what you need to be able to see.

RANKIN:

I would like to address the question of interactions between the surgeon and the echocardiographer intraoperatively. Now, there is no question that this interaction can be a problem. Since the early 1980s, our excellent cardiac anaesthesiology group at Duke University has pioneered trans-esophageal echocardiography through the efforts, of Norbert de Bruijn, Fiona Clemens, and Terry Reves. One of our cardiology colleagues, Dr. Shiekh, has recently completed an analysis of close to 150 valve procedures showing that residual problems with the valve were directly correlated with operative mortality. Thus, each of us is keenly aware of the dangers of residual regurgitation. However, if at the conclusion of a mitral valve repair, mild to moderate regurgitation is observed, the question arises about resuming cardiopulmonary bypass for additional valve procedures. In that setting, there is the potential for bad interaction between echocardiographer and the surgeon. Under those conditions, it is important for the echocardiographer and surgeon to trust and support eacht other. Additional concepts also have to be considered, such as the potential risk of further cardiopulmonary bypass. The ultimate decision about additional surgery has to rest with the surgeon, and if the surgeon decides to accept moderate risidual regurgitation, he has to be supported both in the operating room and in the echocardiographic note. Because of the excellent relationship that exists between our cardiac anesthesiology and surgery groups, we have largely avoided problems, but the potential is very real.

MEYER:

I think we fully agree that both sides have to learn. The echocardiographers have to learn how to interpret these echos and also keeping in mind the patient comes off cardiopulmonary bypass and it takes some time until the heart is functioning normally; that is the problem. On the other hand, we have the unique chance to give some information at the end of operation before closing the chest. I think this is mostly taken by the cardiac surgeons as a real chance to control their results as early as possible. We are both aware of the fact that on both sides there may be false positives.

ERBEL:

I want to add further comments. We found that in 10% of these patients a second repair or even valve replacement was necessary. What is your experience, Dr. Bolger?

BOLGER:

I think that we are probably in the range of 5−8% also, we have had several cases recently.

DURAN:

I feel a bit disappointed. I was hoping that by the end of the session I would understand why we have mitral regurgitation and what can we do as surgeons to repair it and I still do not know. The first paper, I think, was fascinating because of the many figures and a tremendous amount of work, and at the end all I could conclude is that the patients have mitral regurgitation. Then in the echo papers, straight away there was a division between those where there was an anatomical defect, i.e., ruptured chordae or papillary muscle, or something like that, or elongated, and those that we did not know − which were the majority; they were euphemistically called papillary muscle dysfunction. I think we could call them, those that we know, and those what we do not know. That is the best semantics I can think of, because as surgeons, the difficult cases are those in which there are no anatomical abnormalities to pinpoint. It was very interesting that there was muscle wall dysfunction but not a particular one, so it could be anywhere, the dysfunction, and either there are lots of dysfunctioning areas, or there was more regurgitation. It well justifies this meeting probably, to realize that we are still very green on this subject, for the surgeon at least, about what to do with the patient who has this unknown cause for mitral regurgitation.

112

MEYER:

Dr. Bolger, you reported on a patient in which – because of the time of the anesthesia – the surgeons did not repair the mitral insufficiency and they did only coronary bypass grafting. What was the follow-up of this patient? Did his mitral incompetence improve after being only revascularized?

BOLGER:

That particular patient you are referring to actually was very elderly and expired in the perioperative period; for the other patients I reported on the follow-up finding has generally been that the degree of regurgitation has stayed the same unless they have had an additional infarction or were imaged in a different rhythm or at a dramatically different blood pressures.

DESIDERI:

Dr. Erbel, transesophageal echocardiography is such a sensible method. So what is, for you, a normal mitral valve incompetence; what are the criteria you use for that?

ERBEL:

To define a normal valve, we have done studies in normal persons, where we think we have no mitral valve billowing or mitral valve prolapse. We have published this control group in "Stroke" and in that group we measured the mitral valve thickness. It was always below 2.5 mm, and we did not have billowing of more than 3 mm over the mitral valve ring. In these patients in the control group we have a significant difference to those where we had prolapse, where there has not only been the billowing, we had cooptation up to the left anterior atrium and thickening of the mitral valve is increased, that is the diameter of the mitral valve ring. But I want to point out that we now can, with additional transducers, carefully analyze the structure and the morphology of the mitral valve much better than we could before, and we will come to a close answer to this question in the future.

MEYER:

I would like to comment on Dr. Duran's statements. I think we have to separate between the morphology and the anatomy of the mitral valve. Dr. Erbel has pointed out that it is, up to now, very difficult to really analyze the papillary muscles in their shape, and really in their geometry. We can quite nicely show the anterior and the posterior wall leaflets and show the movement. But I think the most important thing in that special question intraoperatively is the flow, the color-coded flow, and you can rely on the flow when the heart ist beating and how much regurgitation is to be seen. If this is only a slight one you can forget it. But there are some cases where you have a complete filling of the left atrium by regurgitant flow and this is never an artefact. We are not discussing these very tiny insufficiencies. If you then combine this quantitative flow – or semi-quantitative flow – to the geometry, then you are quite one step ahead.

DESIDERI:

Thank you Dr. Meyer and Dr. Erbel, but my question was not that. I know the anatomy; I wanted to know what is the normal mitral regurgitant flow.

ERBEL:

We have looked for this and we have found that in nearly all patients we have a mitral valve regurgitant flow. But in contrast to the pathology of patients with regurgitant jets we had a decrease during systole of the extent of this regurgitant signal and that was a very striking finding.

MEYER:

The term "normal regurgitant flow" is a little bit difficult. We know that in each closing movement of the ventricle some blood is moved from the ventricle to the atrium, to the left atrium; this is not really regurgitation. This is just moving of the blood in this movement and this is not regurgitation, this is just in the closing area. In this closing phase – in the first areas – this has been called regurgitation, but this is not regurgitation in the pathological sense.

FRATER:
Yes, it is displacement of the blood in closing. In the studies that we have done over many years of the normal valve this volume is just 2 or 3% of the volume that went forward; 2 or 3% comes back as the cusps come more towards each other and then after the free edges meet a further position a small volume is displaced from between their surfaces. But it is very small and I suspect it is no more than a puff on the echo color flow immage.

MEYER:
This is what Dr. Erbel has shown. It is a very small movement with the red color going to the apex. But this is not of any relevance.

VETTER:
Dr. Bolger and Dr. Erbel, is there any difference between mitral regurgitation from rheumatic heart disease or any other cause of heart disease and ischemic mitral incompetence? From the prognosis, from the therapeutic consequences, from diagnostic tools etc.?

ERBEL:
According to my knowledge and what we observed, for me the most striking point is regarding severity; I was surprised, also on our coronary care unit, to see that the severity of the mitral regurgitation in these patients with acute myocardial infarction is severe in only a small percentage; in most patients, more than 90%, it is in a mild or moderate degree. I expected in the first setting to have more severe regurgitation than we and others have found.

III. Surgical aspects

Mechanisms of ischemic mitral insufficiency and their surgical correction

R. W. M. Frater, P. Cornelissen, D. Sisto

Division of Cardiothoracic Surgery, the Albert Einstein College of Medicine of Yeshiva University, The Bronx, NY, USA

The function of the mitral valve is dependent on the precise interaction of cusps, chordae, ventricular base, and the posterior ventricular wall. For closure to take place with or without atrial contraction, a vortex forms behind the anterior cusp and moves it posteriorly, and the ventricular muscle starts to develop tension. With this the ventricular pressure rises, reversing the diastolic forward flow of blood through the orifice. Closure occurs after systole has started, just before the aortic valve opens. The normal annulus narrows, bringing the posterior cusp nearer to the anterior cusp and the posterior left ventricular wall shortens allowing the cusps to rise to the plane of the atrioventricular ring. A small puff of regurgitation occurs as the cusps close. Most of this is blood displaced by the cusps as their contact progresses from a touching of the free edges to contact over a substantial area [2, 3].

The competent closed mitral valve has the following features:
1) The area of the cusps exceeds the systolic area of the mitral annulus. In general, the length of the anterior cusp through its center equals or exceeds the systolic diameter of the annulus from the base of the anterior cusp to the base of the central scallop of the posterior mitral cusp (at junction of ventricle, cusp, and atrium).
2) The free edges of anterior and posterior cusps in systole are a) at the same level as each other and b) on the ventricular side of the plane of the atrioventricular orifice.
3) The combination of 1) and 2) results in the body of the cusps being parallel to the plane of the orifice while appositional areas (⅓ of the anterior cusp and ½ of the posterior cusp) are in contact with each other in a plane more or less at right angles to the plane of the orifice (Fig. 1a, b) [1, 2].

The effect of coronary artery disease on the mechanisms of normal mitral valve competence

Mitral insufficiency results from the failure of cusp coaption. Coronary artery disease may affect mitral valve coaption in three basic ways:
1) It may alter left ventricular systolic funciton of a) the mural annulus (Fig. 2a); b) the posterior left ventricular wall between the annulus and the origin of one or both of the papillary muscles; (Fig. 1c, d, Fig. 2c), c) a segment of the posterior left ventricular muscle surrounding the origin of a papillary muscle (Fig. 2a, Fig. 3a, b); d) combinations of a) b) and c) (Fig. 2b, d, Fig. 3c, d), and e) the whole left ventricle producing a dilated cardiomyopathy.

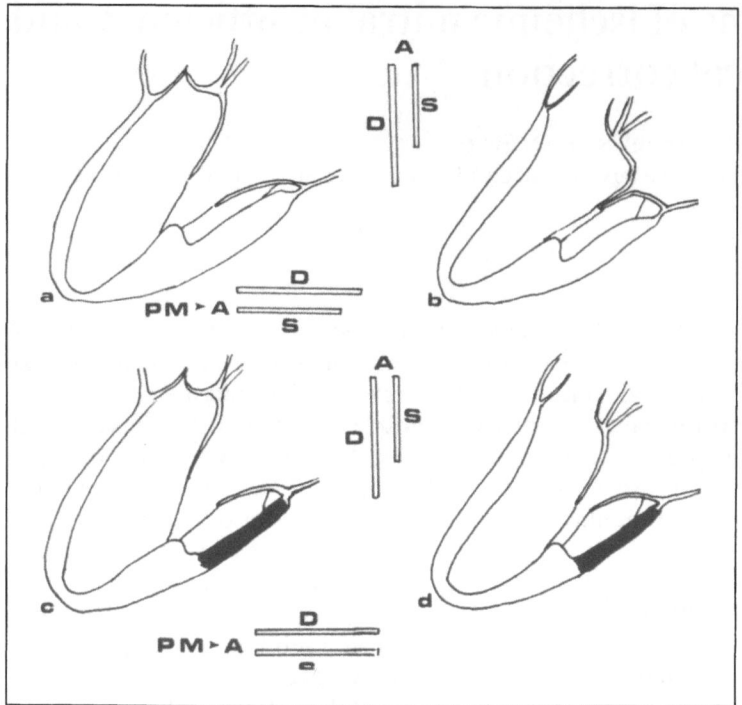

Fig. 1. In this and in all other long axis cross-sectional drawings of the left ventricle the lengths of anterior and posterior cusps and chordae are kept the same. The left ventricular dimensions change: if failure of coaption occurs it is entirely due to ventricular mechanisms. a) and b) Normal ventricle; a) Diastole, and b) Systole. The vertical bars labelled A show the annular diameter change between diastole (d) and systole (s). The bars labelled PM-A refer to the distance from the apex of the papillary muscle to the plane of the atrio-ventricular orifice in systole and diastole. Normal closure occurs as a result of combined systolic shortening of both A and PM-A

2) It may result in necrosis and full rupture of a part or all of a papillary muscle (Fig. 4a).
3) It may cause partial rupture of an infarcted papillary muscle or elongation of an infarcted or ischemic papillary muscle of the "finger"-type leading to prolapse of cusp free edges (Fig, 4b, c).

By far, the commonest of these is the first: alteration of left ventricular systolic function. This may be changed in several ways. Two are fundamental to the subject of ischemic mitral insufficiency: 1) alteration of myocardial blood supply – demand ratios; 2) alterations of ventricular loading. These two may act independently or may influence each other.

Alterations of left ventricular systolic function and coronary disease

Coronary disease may affect regional systolic ventricular function by causing either infarction or ischemia. In either case, there may be failure of systolic shortening or there may be paradoxical systolic bulging, i.e., akinesia or dyskinesia. It is unlikely

118

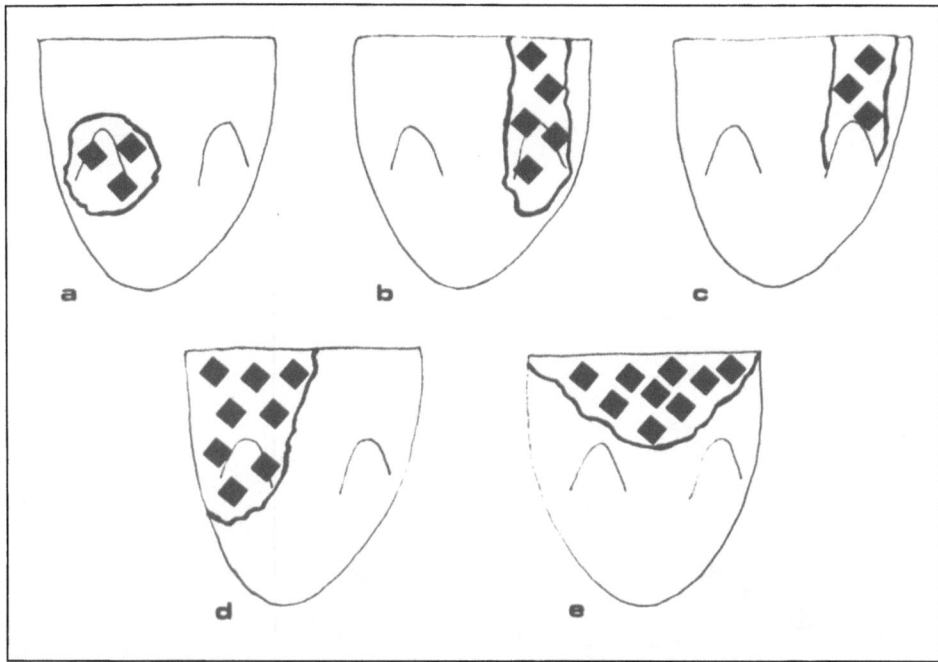

Fig. 2. Patterns of left ventricular infarctions. These generally depend on the distribution and intercorrections of the right, and circumflex coronary arteries. a) Localized infarction of a segment of posterior left ventricle to which the posteromedial papillary muscle is attached; b) Longitudinal area of ischemia: infarction from the annulus to the left ventricle beyond the papillary muscle, c) similar infarct but not involving the area of papillary muscle origin; d) Larger infarct interfering with both posterior left ventricular shortening and annular contraction; e) Circumferential basal infarct affecting annular shortening

that regional hypokinesia with normal cusps and chordae can produce mitral insufficiency. While ischemia can undoubtedly produce reversible regional dyskinesia for periods of minutes or hours, it is doubtful that it ever does so for longer periods of time. However, reversible *akinesia* due to ischemia can exist for more prolonged periods, while in the case of "stunned" myocardium it may last 2 to 3 weeks. Infarction may produce a pathological appearance of intermixed scar and muscle commonly resulting in akinesia or it may result in a thin scar that is dyskinetic. The function of ischemic myocardium may obviously be improved by pharmacologic or mechanical improvement of coronary blood flow, but may also be improved by measures which improve myocardial supply demand ratios by lowering ventricular work and wall tension and reducing cavitary pressure, i.e., measures which decrease preload and afterload and perhaps also heart rate.

Ventricular loading and mitral insufficiency

Mitral insufficiency due to fixed lesions of the mitral valve can be dramatically altered by altering the loading of the left ventricle (Fig. 4). Colloid infusions, sys-

119

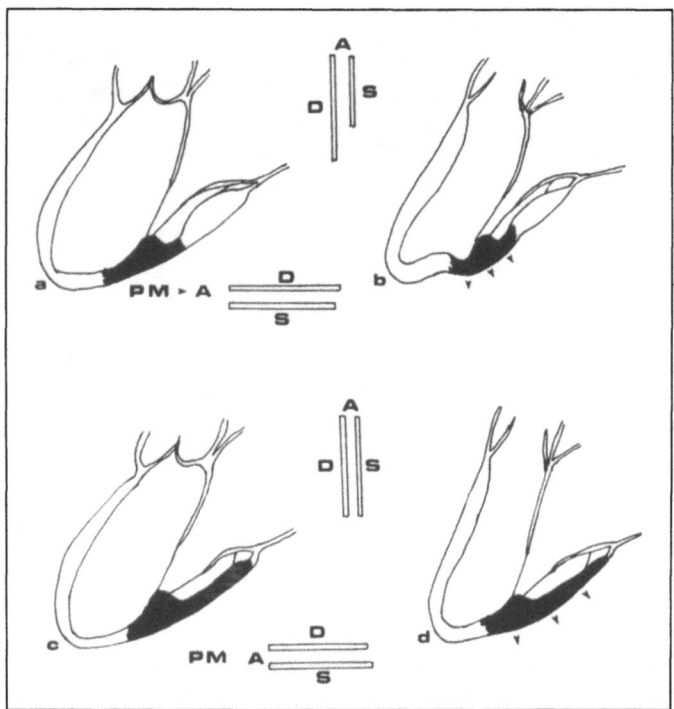

Fig. 3. a) and b) Infarction of the ventricle subjacent to and around a papillary muscle origin. Paradoxical motion in systole causes failure of PM-A systolic shortening. c) and d) More extensive infarct causing failure of annular shortening and systolic *elongation* of PM-A distance because of a combination of dyskinesia and failure of posterior ventricular shortening

temic vasoconstrictors, systemic vasodilators, and inotropic agents act more by changing the volume of the ventricle and thereby, the size of the regurgitant orifice, than by their effect on the ventriculo-atrial systolic gradient [12, 13, 14]. Inotropic agents and peripheral vasoconstrictors can be administered so as to produce equal ventriculo-atrial gradients. The inotrope will reduce insufficiency by reducing ventricular systolic dimensions thereby producing better cusp coaption and a smaller regurgitant orifice; the afterload increasing agent increases ventricular systemic dimensions thereby causing a decrease in cusp coaption and an increase in regurgitant area. This poses a problem: gross mitral insufficiency associated with coronary disease may be improved by intravenous nitroglycerine therapy either because myocardial perfusion has been improved or because the ventricle has been unloaded, or both. A change from akinetic to hypokinetic motion during pharmacologic therapy is clearly in favor of a diagnosis of recoverable myocardium, and is therefore a condition correctable by revascularization. Further evidence of recoverable ischemia is provided by a thallium test that demonstrates perfusion of the myocardial region responsible for the mitral regurgitation. Alternatively, the mitral valve with normal cusps and chordae whose proper apposition has been affected by ventricular ischemia or infarction but not to the point of incompetence may be rendered incompetent by increased ventricular loading (Fig. 5).

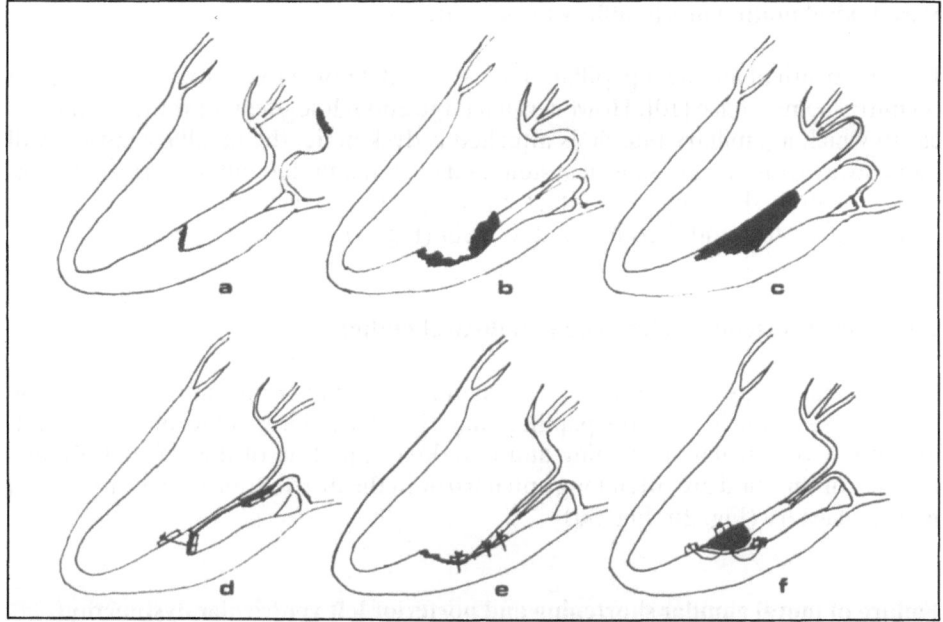

Fig. 4. a) and d) Rupture of part of a papillary muscle; flail posterior scallop; repair by chordal replacement. b) and e) Partial rupture of a papillary muscle; prolapsed anterior and posterior cusps; repair by resuture of fibrous papillary muscle tip. c) and f) Post-ischemic papillary muscle elongation; repair by shortening plasty

Ventricular mechanisms of mitral incompetence

The ventricular mechanisms of mitral insufficiency are illustrated in this article by drawings in each of which the length of the anterior and posterior cusps and anterior and posterior chordae are identical. The systolic annular diameter and posterior left ventricular papillary muscle to the annulus distance and the axis of the chordal line between cusp free edge and papillary muscle connections are altered from case to case. Thus all failures of cusp coaption and, therefore, competence, are dependent only on alterations of ventricular mechanisms.

The long axis shown is through one side or the other of the central bare areas of the mitral anterior and posterior cusps, so as to show the main anterior and posterior chordae.

Failure of posterior left ventricular shortening

Even with normal shortening of the annulus diameter, if the papillary-muscle-to-annulus distance stays at its diastolic dimension during systole, the free edges of the cusps will be held down in the ventricular cavity during systole and prevented from meeting properly (Fig. 1).

Paradoxical motion of a papillary muscle attachment

Isolated death of an intact papillary muscle is well known for its total lack of effect on mitral competence [10]. However, if a large enough segment of ventricular muscle to which a papillary muscle is attached is dyskinetic, the papillary muscle will move away from the annulus in systole and even if annular and posterior left ventricular systolic shortening are intact, the cusp edges may be pulled away from the annulus in systole and therefore fail to meet (Fig. 3).

Combined shortening failure and paradoxical motion

More extensive areas of infarction or ischemia extending from annulus towards the apex and reaching beyond the papillary muscle attachments will result in both failure of left ventricular shortening and paradoxical motion of the chordal origins. Infarcts of this kind are often long and narrow in the distribution of one circumflex marginal artery (Fig. 2b, Fig. 3d).

Failure of mural annular shortening and posterior left ventricular dysfunction

The ischemic area may have a triangular shape based on the annulus with the apex extending beyond the papillary muscle. When this happens, there is a combination of failure of mural annular systolic shortening and the posterior left ventricular akinesia or dyskinesia already described. Failure of coaptation of cusps is more likely with this combination than it is with either mechanism alone (Fig. 3d).

Pure failure of mural annular shortening due to ischemia

Occasionally the distribution of an infarct may involve the muscle adjacent to the mural annulus, but may not extend far down the left ventricular free wall. This results in more or less pure failure of mural annular shortening combined with some degree of annular dilatation. Whether insufficiency results from this depends on the degree of annular dilatation. If the dimension is such that the annular diameter exceeds the combined depths of the opposing anterior and posterior cusps, then the failure to decrease that dimension in systole will result in incompetence (Fig. 3e).

Normal and abnormal mitral valve anatomy and incompetence caused by myocardial ischemia

It is clear from clinical experience that patients with similar degrees of myocardial ischemia or infarction may or may not have mitral insufficiency. It is likely that the reason for this lies in variation in the relationship between the area of the cusps and the posterior left ventricular wall and mural annulus systolic dimensions. If the area of the cusps is relatively small, the area of coaption will be less for a given set of nor-

122

mal systolic dimensions than it would be if the area of the cusps were larger. The degree of change in systolic dimensions necessary to cause loss of coaption will be less in the patient with relatively small cusps than it would be if the cusps were larger.

This has been well demonstrated in studies by Cornelissen conducted in our laboratories. A bicuspid chordally supported valve was made of tanned xenograft pericardium. The same valve was mounted in our pulse duplicator with a fixed annular diameter of either 25 or 21 mm. The distance from the annulus to the distal chordal fixation point was varied, thus imitating changes in posterior left ventricular shortening. Regurgitant flow during systole was measured with different chordal attachment to annular plane distances. If the linear contact along the midline between the two cusps is measured, it is 7 mm with a 25 mm annulus, and 11 mm with a 21 mm annulus. With an annular to chordal attachment distance of 30 mm there is adequate apposition for both annular sizes, but an increase of annular to chordal attachment distance of only 3 mm produces deficient coaption with the 25 mm annulus while allowing still adequate coaption with the 21 mm annulus. When the cusp depths are increased by 1 mm, the annular to chordal attachment distance at which incompetence begins to occur is significantly increased.

This work illustrates the clear relationship between systolic annular size, cusp depth, and annular to chordal attachment distance. If a valve is competent at a particular annular to chordal attachment distance, incompetence may be produced by increasing the annular to chordal attachment distance or increasing the annular size or both. At a given cusp depth with a small annular diameter, there is a range of annular to chordal attachment distances over which valve closure is optimal. With deeper cusps this range is increased. At the larger systolic annular dimension there is some increase in regurgitant volume at any annular to chordal attachment distance, but more importantly, the range of annular to chordal attachment distances over which closure is optimal is much reduced.

Increased systolic annular size and increased annular to chordal attachment distance are experimentally confirmed as mechanisms of ischemic mitral insufficiency. The greater the naturally existing cusp depths and therefore cusp coaption, the greater will be the degree of disturbance of annular diameter and annular to chordal attachment distance that can be tolerated without resulting in incompetence.

These studies also confirm the possible mechanisms of surgical correction. An excessive systolic annular dimension can obviously be corrected by annuloplasty. However, it is also apparent that reducing annular size will correct insufficiency occurring because of an increased chordal attachment to annular distance. Figure 6 shows the regurgitant fraction relative to annular to chordal attachment distance for two valves mounted in 25 and 21 mm annuli. Valve B has cusps 1 mm deeper than Valve A.

Direct papillary muscle mechanisms

Papillary muscle rupture

Most clinically diagnosed cases of infarction related to papillary muscle rupture have rupture of only a part of one papillary muscle. Generally, the papillary origin

123

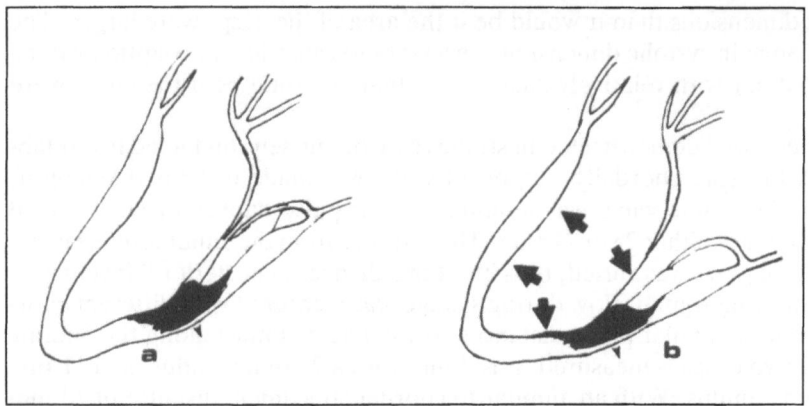

Fig. 5. a) Systole, localized infarct, mild dyskinesia, some loss of coaption, competence is maintained. b) Systole with increased ventricular loading. Increased systolic dimension is enough to increase the PM-A distance so that coaption fails; incompetence results

of only a few chordae inserted into only a part of a cusp is found to be ruptured. Quite often, however, the papillary muscle still attached to the ventricular wall looks grossly as though it too is infarcted. Rupture of only a part of one papillary muscle, even in the absence of infarction of the adjacent ventricular muscle, can result in severe congestive failure. This may occur acutely or develop over a few weeks. Complete rupture of one papillary muscle produces such gross mitral incompetence that it is far more likely to present in the autopsy room than the CCU (Fig. 4a).

Incomplete rupture and elongation

Partial rupture will allow prolapse and is liable at any time to result in complete rupture and a flail valve: it is therefore a rare clinical presentation. Carpentier has described a chronic elongation of a papillary muscle due to ischemic injury [1]. The papillary muscles do normally elongate during systole [6]. When made ischemic in animals, they have been shown to elongate enough to cause prolapse or billowing [11]. There is great variability of papillary muscles from quite sessile to finger-like [9]. A significant lengthening in response to ischemia can occur only if there is already a significant length of papillary muscles: doubling of a 1 cm muscle leads to only a 1 cm rise in systolic cusp free edge level and this may not be enough to bring it to the atrial side of the atrioventricular plane; a 2 cm change resulting from the doubling of a 2 cm muscle may be enough to produce prolapse and incompetence. If the muscle heals in an elongated state then a permanent prolapse without flail will be the consequence of the infarction (Fig. 4c).

Surgical methods of correcting ischemic mitral insufficiency

1) Failure of left ventricular systolic function

Whether annulus or posterior left ventricular wall or both are defective, annuloplasty can restore competence (Fig. 7).

124

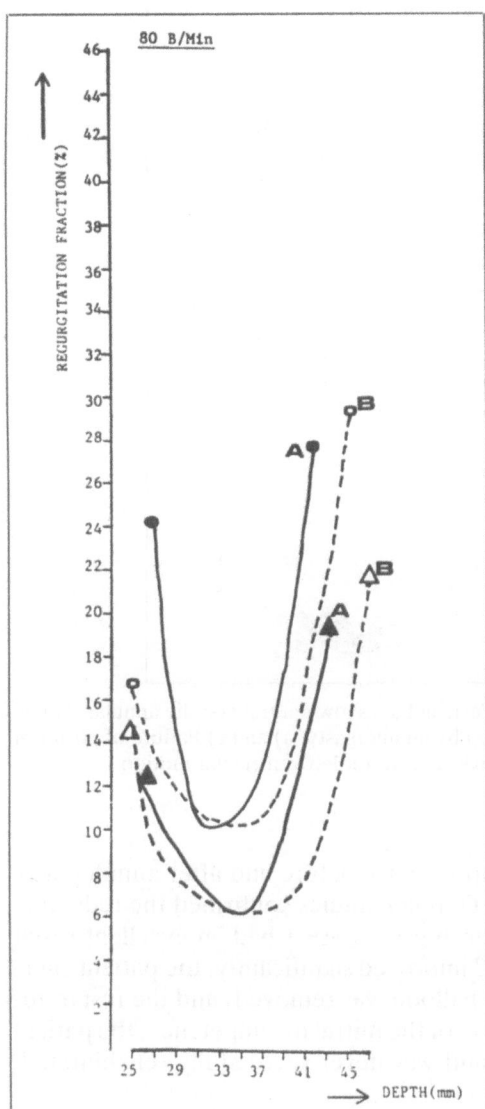

Fig. 6. Regurgitant fraction compared with chordal attachment to annular plane distance. Bicuspid, chordally supported valves mounted in a pulse duplicator. Valve B has cusp 1 mm deeper than valve A. Each valve is mounted in either a 21 mm (triangles) or a 25 mm (circles) diameter annulus. Too short a chordal attachment to annular plane distance allows prolapse. Too long a distance prevents cusp coaption. If there is regurgitation at a particular chordal attachment to annular distance with the valve mounted in the 25 mm annulus, reducing it to 21 mm will restore competence.

Two cases illustrate this:

Case 1: A 71-year-old female, 3 months post inferior myocardial infarction, class IV, intractable congestive cardiac failure, gross mitral and tricuspid insufficiency, three-vessel coronary disease, ejection fraction 45%. Surgery consisted of tricuspid and mitral annuloplasty and triple aortocoronary bypass grafts.

Case 2: A 71-year-old male, posterior myocardial infarction, cardiogenic shock, intraaortic balloon pumping, inotropes and unloading agents, echocardiography and angiography show 3+ mitral insufficiency, 35% ejection fraction, no graftable vessels. Surgery was confined to mitral annuloplasty.

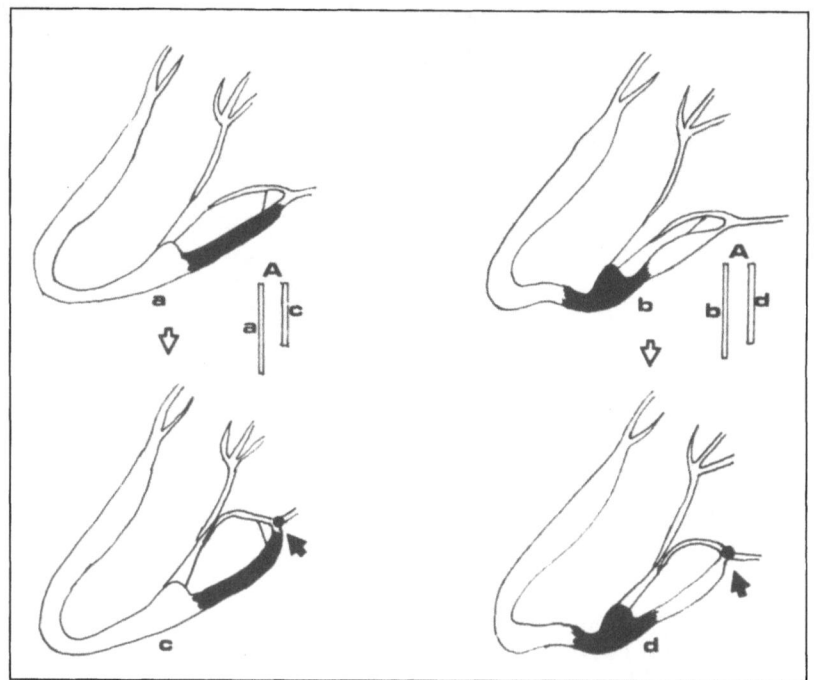

Fig. 7. Systole before and after annuloplasty. Vertical bars show natural systolic annular dimension and the systolic annular dimension produced by annuloplasty. a) and c) Failure of posterior ventricular systolic shortening. b) and d) Paradoxical posterior left ventricular motion

Systolic echocardiographic long axis appearance before and after annuloplasty are shown in Fig. 8 (case 1). Color flow Doppler studies confirmed the reduction of insufficiency from gross to trivial in each case. Case 1 had an excellent result changing from Class IV to Class I. Case 2 improved significantly: the patient came out of cardiogenic shock, the intraaortic balloon was removed, and the respirator discontinued. However, despite correction of the mitral incompetence, the patient remained in chronic congestive failure and was never successfully rehabilitated, dying 6 weeks post-operatively.

Posterior left ventricular wall including the papillary muscle origin: This may be corrected by excision of the infarct scar with reimplantation of the papillary muscle in the closure of the ventricle. While the longitudinal scar will not shorten, the papillary muscle will be closer to the annulus and will not move paradoxically in systole (Fig. 9).

2) Rupture of a papillary muscle head

Chronic cases can be treated by reimplantation or replacement by new chordae [4]. There are cases of rupture which can be managed medically during the infarct, but which soon lead to progressive critically severe heart failure. Reimplantation or chordal replacement is technically feasible in these and obviously the treatment of choice. Illustrative case: a 79-year-old patient was in terminal cardiac failure (stuporose, cardiac index 1.5, V waves 75 mm). Six weeks after a myocardial infarc-

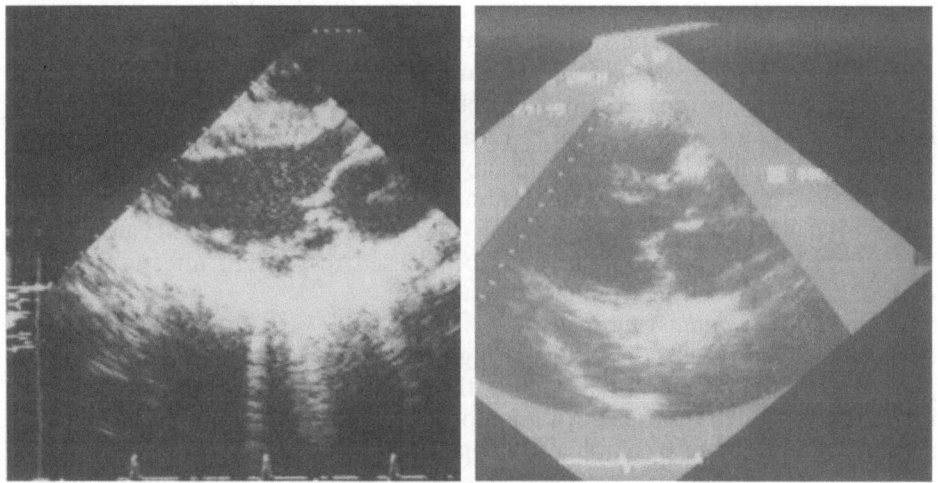

Fig. 8. Case 1: Long-axis echocardiogram; systole. a) Before annuloplasty; b) After annuloplasty

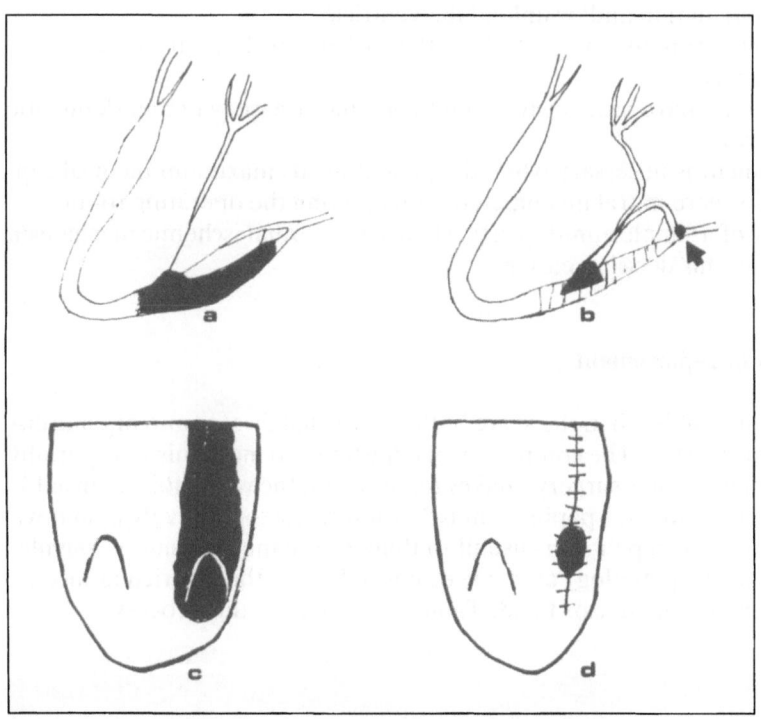

Fig. 9. Excision of scar and reimplantation of papillary muscle

127

tion, rupture of posterior chordae was treated with chordal replacement using xenograft pericardium. The valve remains competent after 8 years.

In the acute case the state of the remaining papillary muscle dictates the surgical treatment: the appearance of fresh infarction in the still attached part of the papillary muscle argues against repair. Replacement should leave as much of cusps, chordae and papillary muscles as will allow proper function of the chosen replacement device. If there is visible infarction of, as yet, unruptured papillary muscle and a mechanical valve that uses a tilting disc or discs is the proposed valve choice, the affected cusps and chordae must be excised to prevent interference with occluder motion resulting from late rupture.

3) *Elongation of papillary muscles*

A shortening plasty will correct this, bringing the free edges parallel and below the plane of the annulus but not as deep as the free edges of the cusps served by the intact other papillary muscle. An annuloplasty reducing the annulus area to the area of the anterior cusp completes the operation (Fig. 4c, f).

Indication for surgical treatment

Mitral insufficiency that may reasonably be left has the following characteristics:
a) It is no more than moderate by echocardiographic, angiographic, or hemodynamic criteria.
b) Even if gross at times, it has fluctuated and been controllable by measures that aid coronary circulation and/or unload the ventricle.
c) The muscle of the annulus and posterior left ventricular wall is still contracting or at least still perfused.
d) The valve does not have previously acquired organic disease (whether rheumatic or degenerative).

Surgical treatment is necessary when the patient needs maximum medical support and still has severe mitral incompetence on entering the operating room.

The feasibility of a simple annuloplasty when a myocardial ischemic mechanism is operative makes this decision easier.

Choice of repair or replacement

Replacement is advisable when there are both myocardial disease and organic disease of cusps and chordae. The complexity of adjusting two mechanisms especially during urgent or emergency surgery, makes replacement the wise choice. Unstable pathology with a potential for papillary muscle rupture postoperatively is an obvious contraindication to repair. It is useful to think of the mechanisms as valvular and/or ventricular, the pathology as stable or unstable, and the ventricular mechanism when present as dynamic or fixed. Table 1 summarizes this process.

Table 1. Mitral insufficiency and coronary disease

	Mitral Valve	Posterior Ventricle	Mechanisms	Surgery
1)	Normal	Ischemic (Dynamic)	Ventricular	CABG
2)	Organic	Normal	Valvular	Valve and CABG
3)	Normal	Infarcted (fixed)	Ventricular	Valve and CABG
4)	Organic	Ischemic/Infarcted	Valve and Ventricular	Valve and CABG

In 3) the valve procedure is likely to be a plasty, in 4) a replacement, and in 2) either according to the valvular pathology

The problem in perspective

In order to assess the extent of this problem the records of 275 successive cases of coronary artery disease coming to surgery during 1987 and 1988 were reviewed. This included all cases including emergencies. Twenty-five of these patients were diagnosed at cardiac catheterization to have moderate to severe mitral insufficiency (grade 3−4 on a scale of 0−4). There were six patients with rheumatic heart disease including one who presented with cardiogenic shock; all had valve replacement. Two had degenerative valve disease. One, with relatively normal ventricular function, had valve repair and the other had valve replacement. seventeen patients had myocardial ischemic mitral insufficiency. In six, the mitral insufficiency was judged to be producing serious hemodynamic compromise, and to be a critical component in the patient's acute or chronic disability. The ventricular component was fixed and severe in all six. In four of these, the patient was, or had been, in cardiogenic shock just prior to surgery. Four had annuloplasty and two, valve replacement. Two of these patients died after some time in the ICU of multiorgan failure despite correction of mitral insufficiency. All of the remaining 11 patients were, or had recently been, in unstable angina. Their mitral insufficiency had tended to fluctuate and there was thought to be opportunity for some improvement in ventricular function after revascularization. One patient died: the contribution of residual mitral insufficiency was unclear.

Discussion

The concepts presented here are based on the correlation of anatomical knowledge and clinical experience. They are backed up by a variety of observations by others. Kay has long advocated annuloplasty for ischemic mitral insufficiency [8]. Echocardiographic observations by a number of authors has confirmed that failure of cusp apposition down in the cavity of the ventricle is a major mechanism of ischemic mitral insufficiency, that the insufficiency occurs at one or the other side according to the infarct location, and that central insufficiency occurs with annular dilatation [5, 7].

Summary

The mechanisms of mitral insufficiency related to coronary occlusive disease are described. Failure of left ventricular systolic shortening is the major mechanism. Annuloplasty compensates for failure of systolic shortening of both the annulus and the posterior left ventricular wall. Other mechanisms and the choice of surgery are also discussed.

References

1. Carpentier A (1988) Personal communication
2. Frater RWM (1961) Mitral valve anatomy and prosthetic valve design. Proc staff meet. Mayo Clin Proc 36:23
3. Frater RWM (1986) Functional anatomy of the mitral valve. In: Ionescu M, Cohn L (eds) Butterworths 8:123–134
4. Frater RWM, Gabbay S, Shore S, Factor S, Strom J (1983) Reproducible replacement of elongated or ruptured mitral valve chordae. Ann Thorac Surg 35(1):14–28
5. Godley RW, Wann LS, Rogers EW, Feigenbaum H, Weyman AE (1981) Incomplete mitral leaflet closure in patients with papillary muscle dysfunction. Circulation 63:565–571
6. Hagl S, Heimisch W, Meister H, Mendler N, Sebening F (1984) In situ function of the papillary muscle in the canine left ventricle. In: Duran C, Angen WA, Johnson AD, Oury JM (eds) Recent progress in mitral valve disease. Butterworths, London, p 397–409
7. Izumi S, Miyatake K, Beppu S, Park YD, Nagata S, Kinoshita N, Sakakibara H, Nimura Y (1987) Mechanism of mitral regurgitation in patients with myocardial infarction: a study using real-time two-dimensional Doppler flow imaging and echocardiography. Circulation 76:777–785
8. Kay JM, Zubiate P, Mendez MA, Vanstrom N, Yokoyama T, Gharari MA (1980) Surgical treatment of mitral insufficiency secondary to coronary artery disease. J Thorac Cardiovasc Surg 79:12
9. McAlpine WA (1975) Heart and coronary arteries. Springer, Berlin Heidelberg New York
10. Miller GE Jr, Cohn KE, Kerth WF, Selzer A, Gerbode F (1968) Experimental papillary muscle infarction. J Thorac Cardiovasc Surg 56:611–616
11. Tei C, Sakamake T, Shah PM, Meerbaum S, Kondo S, Shimoura K, Corday E (1983) Mitral valve prolapse in short-term experimental coronary occlusion: a possible mechanism of ischemic mitral regurgitation. Circulation 68:183–189
12. Yellin EL, Yoran C, Sonnenblick EH, Gabbay S, Frater RWM (1979) Dynamic changes in the canine mitral regurgitant orifice area during ventricular ejection. Circ Res 45:667–683
13. Yoran C, Yellin EL, Becker RM, Gabbay S, Frater RWM (1979) Mechanism for reduction of mitral regurgitation with vasodilator therapy. Am J Cardiol 43:773–777
14. Yoran C, Yellin EL, Becker RM, Gabbay S, Frater RWM (1979) Dynamic aspects of mitral regurgitation: effects of ventricular volume, pressure and contractility on the effective regurgitation orifice area. Circulation 60:170–176

Author's address:
Prof. Dr. R. W. M. Frater
Division of Cardiothoracic Surgery
The Albert Einstein College of Medicine
of Yeshiva University
1825 Eastchester Rd.
Bronx, NY 10461
USA

Technical aspects and clinical experience of mitral reconstruction in ischemic mitral incompetence

C. G. Duran, J. H. Oury, W. Angell

King Faisal Specialist Hospital & Research Center, Riyadh, Kingdom of Saudi Arabia
Scripps Clinic & Research Foundation, San Diego, California, USA

Introduction

The surgery of mitral valve disease associated with coronary artery pathology is still a difficult subject. The results of mitral valve replacement with simultaneous coronary artery grafting have generally been far from satisfactory both in terms of a high hospital mortality and long-term evolution [4, 8, 13].

Extensive experience in valve reconstruction for rheumatic and degenerative mitral regurgitation has shown that these techniques are reproducible and stable [7]. It was therefore a logical consequence to attempt to apply them also in cases of ischemic regurgitation. There are, however, still many unanswered questions in this field.

Surgical problems

When dealing with mitral regurgitation in a patient who requires coronary bypass surgery, the surgeon is faced with some very specific problems:
1) The first and more general question is the lack of understanding we often have of the basic mechanism responsible for the mitral valve dysfunction. In some cases where there is a chordal or papillary muscle rupture the cause is obvious, but in the majority of patients no observable anomaly can be detected when the valve is exposed. Papillary muscle dysfunction which was claimed to be responsible for the regurgitation has been shown experimentally not to be the case [9].
2) Time constraint: Valve repair always requires a longer ischemic time than does replacement. The fact that a number of bypass grafts have to be made and the often poor left ventricular function both compound the problem.
3) Poor valve visibility: All reconstructive surgery requires an excellent exposure both to explore the whole mitral apparatus and to be able to apply the appropriate corrective surgical technique. The small size of the left atrium interferes with visibility, making any reconstructive maneuver sometimes impossible.
4) The very thin mitral valve tissue makes its surgical handling difficult and hazardous.

Surgical techniques

Mitral valve approaches

We have always favored a left atriotomy performed immediately posterior to the interatrial groove. An atrial rather than ventricular visualization of the mitral valve seems to us essential, not only because of the surgical maneuvers to be undertaken, but even more so to explore and check the result of the reconstruction. The standard atriotomy, however, is very often insufficient for a good valve visibility. In these cases the atriotomy can be effectively enlarged by extending the incision behind both venae cavae. The limiting factor is the tension on the superior vena cava which does not allow a complete retraction of the right atrium. A considerable degree of improvement is achieved by dissection of the pericardial reflection on the superior vena cava, freeing it and allowing it to be displaced anteriorly. Recently, in an attempt to further increase exposure in very small left atria the superior vena cava has been completely transected at about 1 cm from its entrance in the right atrium. This maneuver requires a right-angled metal tip cannulation 3–4 cm distal to that point. The vast majority of our mitral patients, where tricuspid surgery is not envisaged, have a single double stage right atrial cannulation, which in our opinion is not only faster, but also provides a better mitral exposure, maintaining a satisfactory venous return. Only in the presence of a very small atrium is a double cannulation performed as described in order to make possible the SVC transection and extension of the atriotomy into the atrial roof which achieves an extraordinary exposure.

Other authors favor a transeptal approach to the left atrium. This can be done either longitudinally along the fossa ovalis and upper portion of the septum [12] or transversely across the septum and lateral walls of the right and left atria [5].

Surgical maneuvers

As in any case of mitral repair the individual lesion causing regurgitation must be identified. Each component of the mitral complex must be explored: annulus, leaflets, commisures, and subvalvar apparatus. In ischemic mitral disease the appearance is of an apparently normal valve with very thin tissue and delicate subvalvar structures, a very different aspect from the thickened rheumatic or redundant degenerative valves.

Ruptured chords and papillary muscle heads are easily identified by pulling with nerve hooks along the free edge of both leaflets. The rupture is at the papillary extremity of the chord or at the tip of the muscle. The surgical maneuvers to be applied are the resection of the unsupported segment of the posterior leaflet with resuture or the transposition of the corresponding posterior leaflet chord to the anterior leaflet. This last technique can be complicated by the very thin nature of the leaflet tissue in these cases. Our "flip over" technique considerably simplifies this maneuver: a large rectangular segment of the posterior leaflet is transferred with its chordal attachments onto the actual surface of the anterior leaflet [6] (Fig. 1).

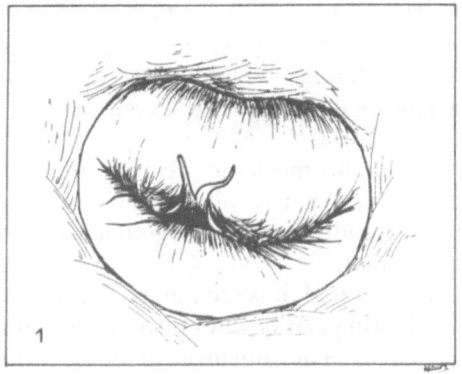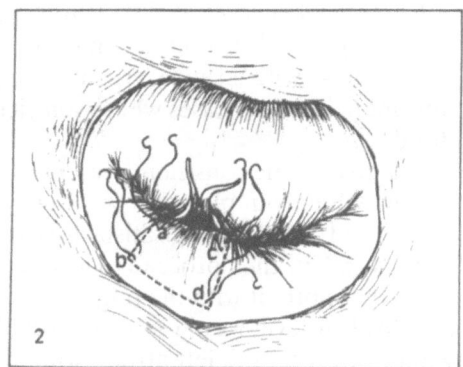
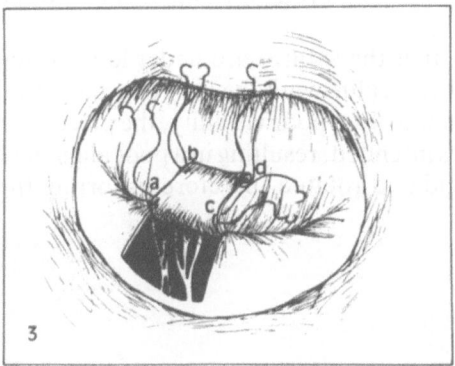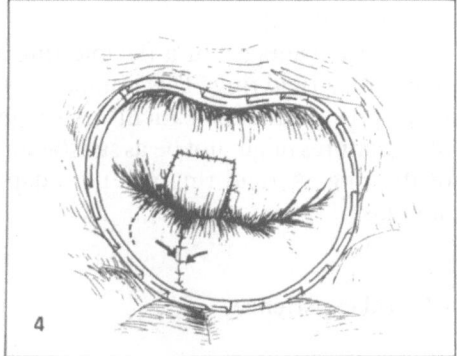

Fig. 1. The "flip-over" technique for chordal transposition. 1) Ruptured main chords to the anterior leaflet; 2) A large quadrangular area of the posterior leaflet is selected; 3) The chordal carrying segment is "flipped over" onto the anterior leaflet; 4) The segment is sutured, the posterior leaflet gap closed, and a ring annuloplasty performed

Occasionally, in chronic cases the cause of incompetence is a prolapse due to elongation of a papillary muscle head. The whitish, fibrous muscle is very easily identified. The treatment is to shorten it by suture to the ventricular wall. A pledgeted 4/0 prolene suture is used and tightened before tying so as to check that the leaflet prolapse has disappeared.

Most often the whole mitral apparatus looks normal, or at best an annulus dilatation is thought to be present. In all such cases, a ring annuloplasty is performed in the hope that either the annulus is actually dilated or due to a wall dysfunction, leaflet apposition is lost resulting in regurgitation. The reduction in the mitral orifice to its theoretical systolic dimension should achieve competence. It is surprising how often this simple maneuver solves the problem. In this context we strongly favor the use of a totally flexible ring* which has been shown to be more physiological than a rigid ring.

---

* Duran Ring, Medtronic Blood Systems, La Palma Ave., Anaheim, California, USA

Recently, David et al. [3] clearly demonstrated a significantly better left ventricular systolic function in a group of patients with a Duran flexible ring than among those with a rigid Carpentier ring. This difference might be even more significant in ischemic cases where ventricular contractility might be severely jeopardized.

Due to the time constraint present in these cases, we check the valve closure with the ring already in place but without tying it down. If the result is satisfactory the ring is tied but if it is unsatisfactory it can be rapidly removed together with its sutures and we then proceed to a valve replacement.

Furthermore, if with the ring in place but not yet tied, it is seen that a maneuver at subvalvar level would solve the problem, the ring can be cut in two halves and withdrawn from the left atrium with all its sutures. The subvalvar maneuver can then be easily done, and the two halves of the ring brought down again unto the annulus and tied.

Other advantages of a flexible ring are that the sutures are under less tension than with a rigid ring. This is important when dealing with the very delicate mitral tissue present in these patients. Also, given the often poor visibility, the placement of the sutures might not be as satisfactory as intended, resulting in a poor alignment of the ring. A rigid ring will not adapt and end rotated therefore distorting the annulus.

Clinical experience

Our total experience of mitral valve surgery combined with coronary bypass grafting amounts to 143 patients with an average age of 69 years; 80 were male and 63 female; 130 had mitral regurgitation and 32 had mitral stenosis; 25 had also aortic valve disease (16 regurgitant and nine stenotic lesions) and 16 had tricuspid involvement.

93% of the patients were in Functional Class III—IV preoperatively (II = 10, III = 80, IV = 53) and their ejection fraction was below 30 in 18 patients, 30—40 in 18 patients, 40—50 in 14 patients, and above 50 in 82 (one unknown). Forty-eight patients had a previous myocardial infarction, 15 had angina, and 31 had electrocardiographic signs of ischemia.

409 coronary bypass grafts were performed (2.8 per patient); 19 patients had simultaneous aortic valve, 16 tricuspid, and five carotid surgery.

At mitral level 79 patients had a valve replacement (55%) and 64 a conservative procedure which in six cases was a simple commissurotomy. 58 had an annuloplasty (57 with a ring) and in 25 of them a reconstructive technique was added at leaflet, chordal or papillary level.

The hospital mortality was 11% (16 patients). The perioperative complications were 16 cases of bleeding, eight thromboembolic accidents and one bacterial endocarditis on a prosthesis which was treated medically.

Seven patients were lost to follow up (4.9%) and 120 were followed for a mean of 2.2 years (total number of years 243.4).

There were 24 late deaths (one of unknown cause). Three patients (all with prosthesis) had infective endocarditis (one required prosthetic replacement), six thromboembolic accidents and two bleeding events were recorded. No thrombosis were detected. 103 patients are alive, 93 of them in functional Class I–II (92%), seven are in Class III, and three in Class IV.

Conclusion

Mitral valve surgery associated with coronary disease, although still a difficult surgical problem, can now be approached with more confidence. Recent reports in the literature indicate that a conservative attitude yields better results [1, 11, 14]. This is not surprising, not only because of avoiding the well known problems inherent to all valve prosthesis, but also due to the physiological importance of conserving the normal attachments of the papillary muscles to the mitral annulus [2, 10].

The main problems facing the surgeon are the often limited visibility of the mitral valve apparatus and the ischemic time required for complex surgery in the setting of a poor ventricular function. The question of whether to approach the reconstruction from the atrial or from the ventricular aspect is not yet solved. The last one, proposed by some authors [14], although it obviously affords a very good visibility, has the drawback of sectioning a very fragile and compromised left ventricle. Furthermore, most of the reconstructive techniques available at present have been designed to be used from the atrial level. Perhaps an individualized approach might be the correct answer.

The problem of the long ischemic time required to perform this surgery can be partially solved through a better understanding of the mechanisms responsible for the regurgitation. Once identified, an appropriately conducted preoperative study should direct the surgeon towards the correct surgical technique. Advances in myocardial protection will also improve the results of this surgery. In our experience, the use of blood cardioplegia, both in the aorta and through the saphenous grafts, together with very low, monitored, myocardial temperatures has extended very significantly the safe ischemic time.

Although a numnber or surgical maneuvers have been used and described in the literature, we strongly advocate those that have become standardized, making them reproducible, and which have shown their long-term stability. The question of the appropriate intraoperative method to check the results remains open. Although in general we favor the use of a small left apical vent to fill the left ventricle under pressure, we are reluctant to use it in ishemic cases where a transvalvular injection is preferred. Transesophageal echo-color-Doppler is an extremely useful tool but can only be used in some centers and its use requires a normally beating heart. As in most other fields further work is necessary.

References

1. Connolly MW, Gelbfish JS, Jacobowitz IJ, et al. (1986) Surgical results for mitral regurgitation from coronary artery disease. J Thorac Cardiovasc Surg 91:379–388
2. David TE, Ho WC (1986) The effect of preservation of chordae tendineae on mitral valve replacement for postinfarction mitral regurgitation. Circulation 74, Supply I:116–120

3. David T, Komeda M, Pollick Ch, Burns RJ (1988) Mitral annuloplasty: Effect of type on left ventricular function. 24th Annual Meeting Soc Thor Surg, New Orleans, September 1988
4. DiSesa VJ, Cohn LH, Collin JJ Jr, Koster JK, VanDevanter S (1982) Determinants of operative survival following combined mitral valve replacement and coronary revascularization. Ann Thorac Surg 34:484
5. Dubost C, Guilmet D, Parades B et al. (1966) Nouvelle technique d'ouverture de l'oreillette gauche en chirurgie a ceur ouvert: l'abord biauriculaire transeptal. Presse Med 74:1607–1608
6. Duran CG (1986) Repair of anterior mitral leaflet chordal rupture or elongation: The flip-over technique. J Cardiac Surg 1:161–165
7. Duran CG, Gaite L, Alonso J, Alonso L, Fleitas M, Revuelta JM (1988) Stability of mitral reconstructive surgery at 10–12 years for predominantly rheumatic valvular disease. Circulation 78, Supp I:91–96
8. Geha AS, Francis CK, Hammond GL, Laks H, Kopf GS, Hashim SW (1984) Combined valve replacement and myocardial revascularization. J Vasc Surg 1:27–31
9. Hagl S, Heimisch W, Meisner H, Mendler N, Sebening F (1984) In situ function of the papillary muscle in the canine left ventricle. In: Duran C, Angell W, Johnson AD, Oury JH (eds) Recent Progress in Mitral Valve Disease. Butterworths, London, p 397–409
10. Hansen DE, Cahill PD, Derby GC, Miller DC (1987) Relative contributions of the anterior and posterior mitral chordae tendineae to canine global left ventricular systolic function. J Thorac Cardiovasc Surg 93:45–55
11. Kay GL, Kay JH, Zubiate P, Yokoyama T, Mendez M (1986) Mitral valve repair for mitral regurgitation secondary to coronary artery disease. Circulation 74, Supp I:88–98
12. Kreitmann P, Jourdan J, Saab (1986) Abord de la valve mitrale par voie transatriale. Ann Chir 40:557–559
13. Pinson CW, Cobanoglu A, Metzdorff MT, Grunkemeier GL, Kay PH, Starr A (1984) Late surgical results for ischemic mitral regurgitation. J Thorac Cardiovasc Surg 88:663–672
14. Rankin S, Feneley MP, Hickey M StJ, Muhlbaier LH, Wechsler AS, Floyd RD, Rever JG, Skelton TN, Califf RM, Lowe JE, Sabiston DC (1988) A clinical comparison of mitral valve repair versus replacement in ischemic mitral regurgitation. J Thorac Cardiovasc Surg 95:165–177

Author's address:
Prof. Dr. C. Duran
Department of Cardiovascular Diseases
King Faisal Specialist Hospital
and Research Center
P.O. Box 33 54
Riyadh
Kingdom of Saudi Arabia

Decision-making aspects in the surgical treatment of ischemic mitral incompetence

H. Siniawski, Y. Weng, R. Hetzer

German Heart Institute, Thoracic and Cordiovascular Surgery, Berlin, FRG

Introduction

Ischemic mitral incompetence, i.e., the mitral valve dysfunction which results from the impairment of the left ventricular muscle parts that play a role in the organized valvular function cyclus − papillary muscle, papillary muscle-bearing wall segment and the ventricle on the whole − has remained to be an unclear field in cardiac surgery. This is due to the individual complexity of the underlying mechanism, the seemingly normal structures of the valve itself, and the often severely compromised ventricular function which loads surgical attempts with an increased risk.

This is most prominently true in all cases of acute mitral incompetence early after an infarct when the patient, in general, presents with cardiogenic shock and a highly vulnerable myocardium.

Results of valve replacement and repair have been reported with a high operative mortality ranging from 30% to 53% [11, 14]. Mitral incompetence either stable in the chronic postinfarction period or intermittantly occuring in transient ischemia poses the question of the prospect of coronary artery revascularization alone or the need of direct intervention on the valve. More recently, some well-documented studies have shed light on this otherwise unsolved topic [1, 3, 11].

Decision-making for surgery and procedures

In our experience, emergency surgery in acute early postinfarct mitral incompetence, in general due to rupture of an entire papillary muscle body or at least of a papillary muscletip bearing major chordae included prosthetic valve replacement in all cases. In a few instances reimplantation of a ruptured papillary muscle has been attempted, as suggested by some authors [5, 7], however, this was universally discarded in favor of replacement because of unreliable repair visible earlier during the operation.

Great attention has been paid to preserve as much of the subvalvular apparatus as possible (this has been our concept in mitral replacement during the last 10 years (9)), initially preserving the posterior leaflet and its chordal attachment and, more recently, both leaflets and the entire apparatus. In particular, in the already critical state of the ventricle in ischemic mitral incompetence, this concept (which meanwhile has been demonstrated to avoid the additional damage caused by the still widely used complete valve-resection technique), in our opinion, is of utmost importance.

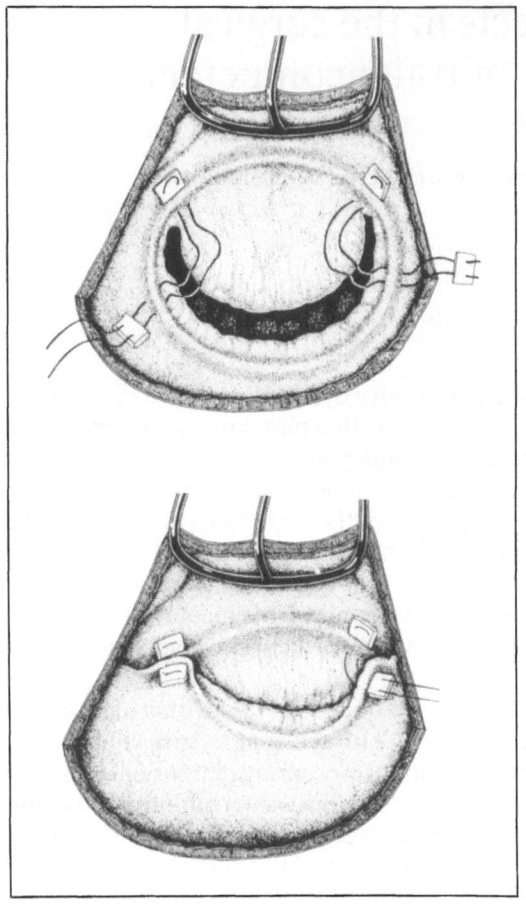

Fig. 1. Annuloplasty according to the Kay-Wooler principle in the modification of Borst and Dalichau (2).

In chronic ischemic mitral incompetence, at least in the past, most surgeons have turned towards replacement rather than repair, quite obviously since the valve leaflets and the chordae are quite normal, thus not offering a clear anatomical pathology for the usual repair procedures.

However, it has been demonstrated by long-term follow-up studies and also in more series that the simple posterior annulus shortening procedures, such as the Kay-Wooler annuloplasty, may obliviate valve incompetence in this setting [12, 14].

Thus, the underlying defects of papillary muscle and ventricular wall dysfunction may well be neutralized by increasing the leaflet coaptation area.

Following this regime, in the cases without detectable leaflet and chorda damage, we have applied the Kay-Wooler plasty [2, 12, 18] (Fig. 1) and the Paneth plasty [16] (Fig. 2), in some instances using a flexible ring (Duran) in addition or alone for annulus stabilization purpose.

138

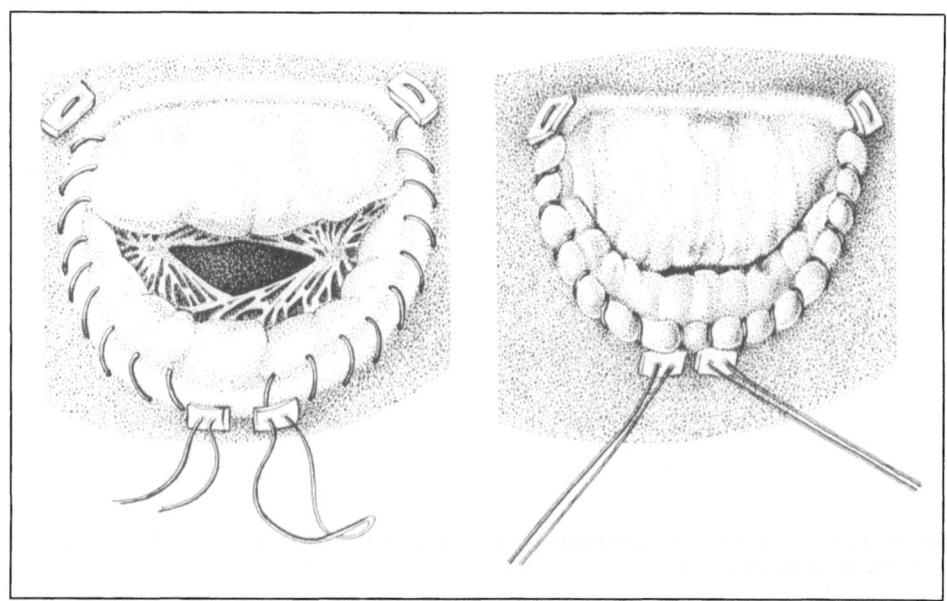

Fig. 2. Annuloplasty according to Paneth (16) (authors' modification (10)).

From our experience with valve repair in active infective mitral endocarditis (8) where we would resect all infected valve tissue and then remodel a valve which usually includes closure of a commissure, we also used this principle in cases with obvious unilateral papillary muscle fibrosis to close the coaptation line along the commissure related to the inflicted papillary muscle with interrupted sutures, a procedure we call "commissuroplasty" [10] (Fig. 3).

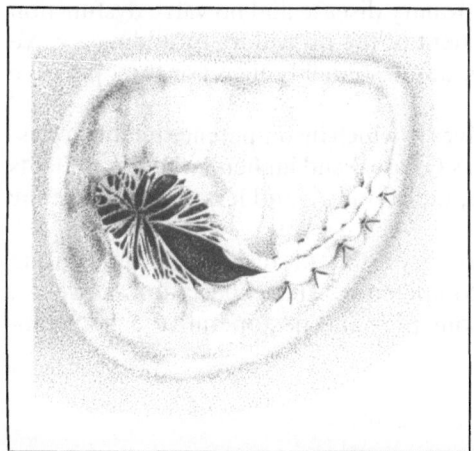

Fig. 3. "Commissuroplasty" − Unilateral closure of commissure supported by infarcted or scarred papillary muscle (10).

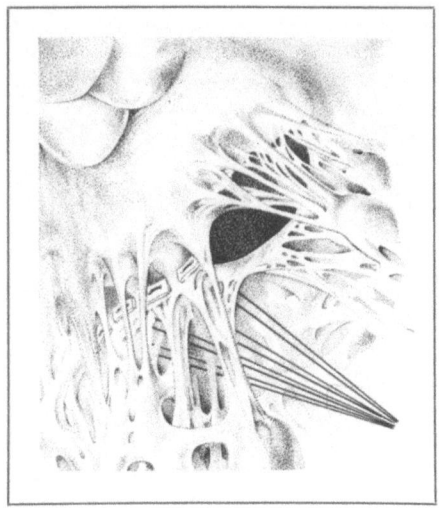

Fig. 4. Transventricular "commissuroplasty" according to Rankin (14) in cases of simultaneous ventricular aneurysm resection.

Although this plasty does not concur with the generally accepted reconstruction principles, both valve competence and sufficient residual valve opening has been achieved by this method.

In the rare case of a patient surviving with a large ventricular aneurysm and severe mitral incompetence, we have successfully used the transventricular approach to apply such a unilateral commisuroplasty, quite similar to that introduced by Rankin [14] (Fig. 4).

The decision as to when a valve repair should be added to mere coronary artery bypass operations has remained controversial and difficult. On one hand, it has been clearly demonstrated that patients with coronary artery disease and additional ischemic mitral incompetence have a poorer survival prognosis when compared to those with the same degree of coronary disease and no valve dysfunction [11, 14]. On the other hand, the enlargement of the procedure by adding a valve operation to simple bypass grafting does unquestionably increase the operative risk.

It has been our policy to attack these valves in which incompetence has been classified by preoperative echocardiography as Grade 3 and highers, whereas patients with milder forms of valve incompetence, i.e., Grade 2 and less, were treated by bypass grafting alone.

Initially, it was our hope that better coronary artery perfusion after the grafting procedure might also diminish mitral incompetence. This expectation, however, did not come true, as demonstrated by our pre- and postoperative echocardiographic studies (Fig. 9).

Methods of valve evaluation

Intraoperative valve testing after mitral repair has remained a widely-discussed subject. Reproducible good results of surgical repair depend on a reliable

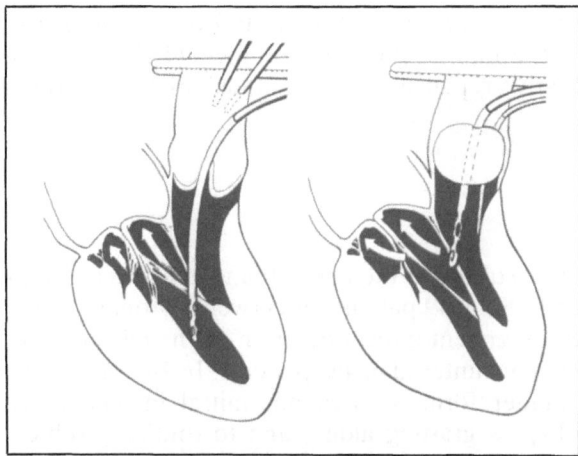

Fig. 5. Intraoperative testing method for mitral repair. In solitary mitral repair (a) a thin catheter (12 Charr) is inserted into the left ventricle via the aortic cardioplegia hole and aortic valve, and cardioplegic solution is instilled under pressure-control (< 50 mmHg). In simultaneous aortic valve replacement (b), a Folley catheter is inserted into the left ventricular outflow tract, the balloon is inflated for LVOT occlusion, and cardioplegic solution is instilled through the catheter lumen.

intraoperative testing method. While in the past pressure-controlled filling of the ventricle with cardioplegic solution and observation of the mitral valve under direct vision has been a fairly dependable method [8] (Fig. 5), this failed completely in the cases of ischemic mitral incompetence.

Intraoperative transesophageal echocardiography (TEE) has become the most reliable method to demonstrate the quality of repair [4, 6, 13, 15, 17]. This method, in contrast to intracardiac testing procedures, requires closure of the heart incisions, interruption of cardioplegic arrest, rewarming of the patient, and at least a brief period of going off bypass. However, with modern types if cardioplegic myocardial preservation and a high standard of extracorporeal circulation, one or two additional arrest periods in the case of unsatisfactory repair – be it for additional repair or for valve replacement – are well tolerated by the patient without increased risk.

The value of TEE is convincingly demonstrated by the fact that now we no longer encounter any case of unexpected early postoperative repair failure when immediate intraoperative consequences were drawn from TEE findings.

Between June 1988 and September 1990, 129 patients underwent mitral valve repair for a variety of underlying pathology. Intraoperative valve testing by ventricular filling with cardioplegic solution revealed seemingly good valve function in all. However, TEE* proved this to be true in only 108 (83.7%), whereas in the remainder mitral incompetence of a significant degree became apparent. In these cases, additional repair steps or valve replacement were added in the same session.

---

* Currently in use: Aloka 870, Transthoracic probe 3.5 MHz, Transesophageal probe 5.0 MHz.

In this series, there was only one case early postoperative TEE revealed a more significant residual valve incompetence than in the intraoperative TEE, and there were two cases of early postoperative repair breakdown after initially well-functioning reconstruction.

Patients and methods

From April 1986, when surgery was started at the newly founded German Heart Institute Berlin, until September 1990, 5849 patients underwent coronary artery bypass surgery and 1047 patients underwent direct operation on the mitral valve. Ischemic mitral incompetence was encountered in 468 patients. In June 1988, the concept was adopted to treat milder forms of ischemic mitral incompetence (Grades 1 and 2) by coronary bypass grafting alone, and to routinely subject patients with more significant mitral incompetence (Grades 3 and 4) to direct valve surgery in addition to bypass grafting.

Systematic echocardiography data were obtained pre- and postoperatively in 118 patients (Table 1): 76 patients with mild MI, treated with coronary artery bypass grafting alone, and 42 patients with MI Grades 3 and 4, who received mitral repair (n = 31) or replacement (n = 11).

In the coronary bypass grafting group, there was no significant change in the degree of MI in the majority (89.5%) of patients when comparing pre- and postoperative TEE findings (Fig. 9). In the repair group, MI went from Grades 3 and 4 to Grades 0 and 1 in 18 patients, and in 10 patients MI of Grade 2 persisted (Fig. 10).

Three patients died during the perioperative period, all of whom had left ventricular ejection fraction of below 30%.

Perioperative evaluation of mitral valve function

The following sequence of procedures (Fig. 6) has become routine in order to obtain a high degree of reliability of valve function estimation and also to allow for comparison of the various testing methods.

Table 1. Patient data of ischemic mitral incompetence echo study

	n = 118 / June '88 – Sept. '90	
Degree of MR	< 2	> 3
n	76	42
Mode of surgery	CABG alone	CABG + mitral reconstruction
Age (years)	61 ± 7.8	67 ± 8.7
Range (years)	42–76	48–87
Sex		
f	21 (27.7%)	13 (31.0%)
m	55 (72.3%)	29 (69.0%)

MR Mitral regurgitation (angio + TEE)

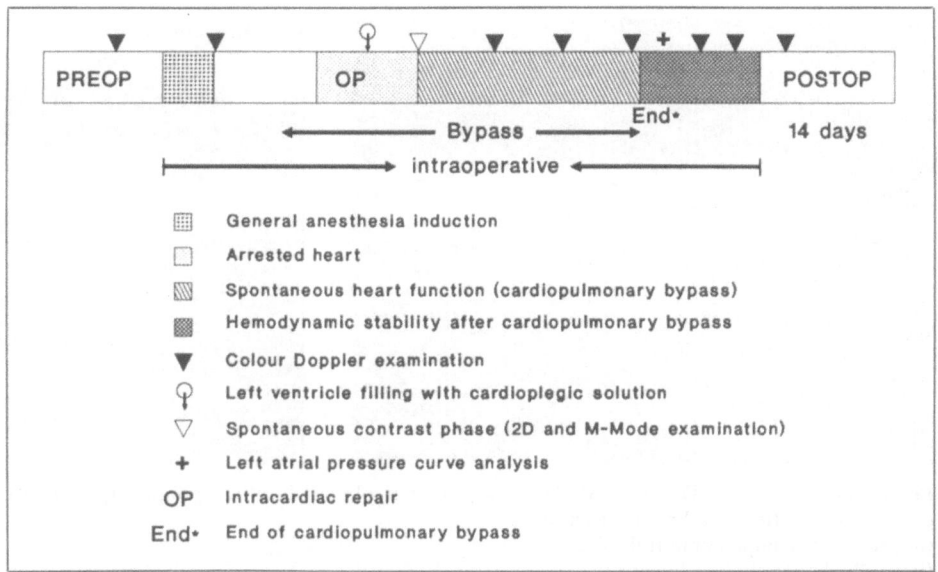

Fig. 6. Sequence of perioperative diagnostic procedures during mitral valve repair.

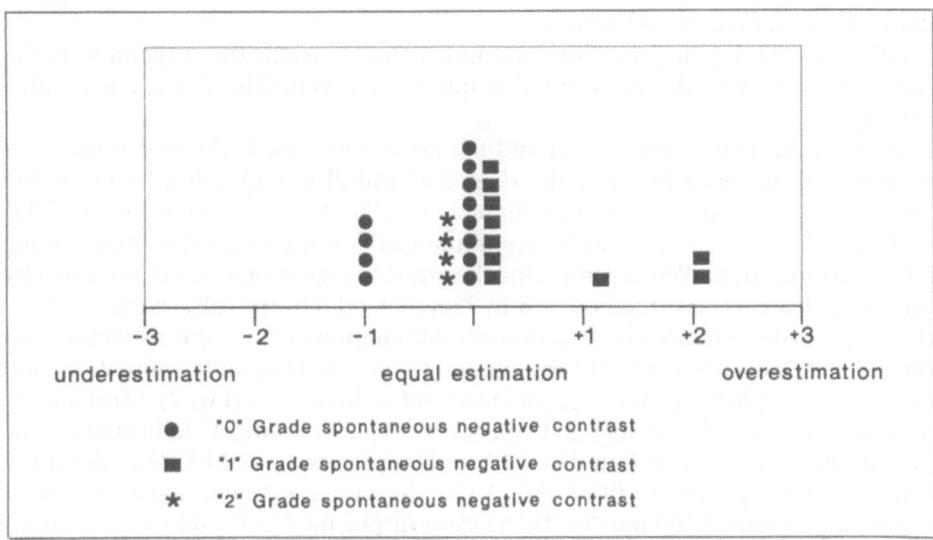

Fig. 7. Estimation of "spontaneous negative contrast" as compared to postoperative color Doppler assessment in 26 patients. Mitral regurgitation was equally graded by the two methods in most cases. It was underestimated by "negative contrast" in four cases by one grade, and overestimated in three cases by one or two grades. There was no discrepancy in any case with a competent valve.

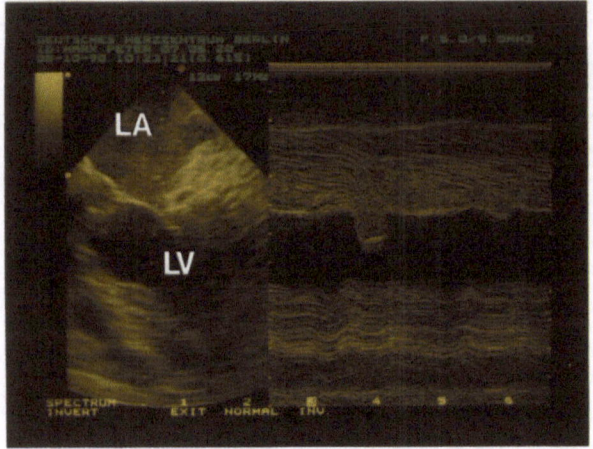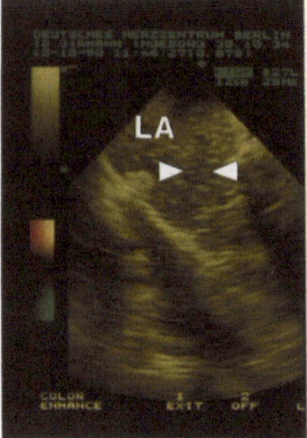

Fig. 8. Intraoperative 2-D and M-Mode echocardiogram obtained during spontaneous negative contrast phase after mitral reconstruction:
(a) presenting competent mitral valve;
(b) residual regurgitation (arrows);
LA = left atrium;
LV = left ventricle.

All patients with mitral valve disease are screened by TEE preoperative in oder to define those valves which would qualify for a repair operation. In the patients thus assigned to presumable repair after induction of anesthesia, TEE is carried out under defined hemodynamic conditions, i.e., systolic pressure of 120 mmHg and diastolic pressure of 70–80 mmHg.

Following the repair procedure and under direct vision, the surgeon tests the valve by instilling cardioplegic solution into the left ventricle via the aortic valve (Fig. 5).

With the heart incisions closed and the aorta unclamped, the first ventricular contractions are used to study the degree of mitral regurgitation by observing "spontaneous negative contrast phenomenon" (Fig. 8) in two-dimensional (2-D) TEE, which is created by the faster regurgitant jet flow within the slowly circulating left atrial blood pool. When comparing the grade of regurgitation as determined by this "negative contrast" method and by Doppler echo in the fully working heart, there was no discrepancy in estimation of regurgitation in the majority of cases and the error of "negative contrast" was limited to one grade of underestimation, and to overestimation of one or two grades in a total of three cases (Fig. 7). Most important, however, was the finding that whenever "negative contrast" indicated a competent valve, this was also found in the later Doppler study. A TEE-Doppler study is then performed during a brief period with the patient taken off bypass and with a systolic pressure of 100 mmHg. In the cases displaying significant mitral regurgitation, a second arrest period and re-cooling of the patient is now added for additional repair or mitral replacement.

In those cases with a satisfactory Doppler result at this stage, the patient is fully rewarmed, taken off bypass, and final intraoperative TEE studies are performed

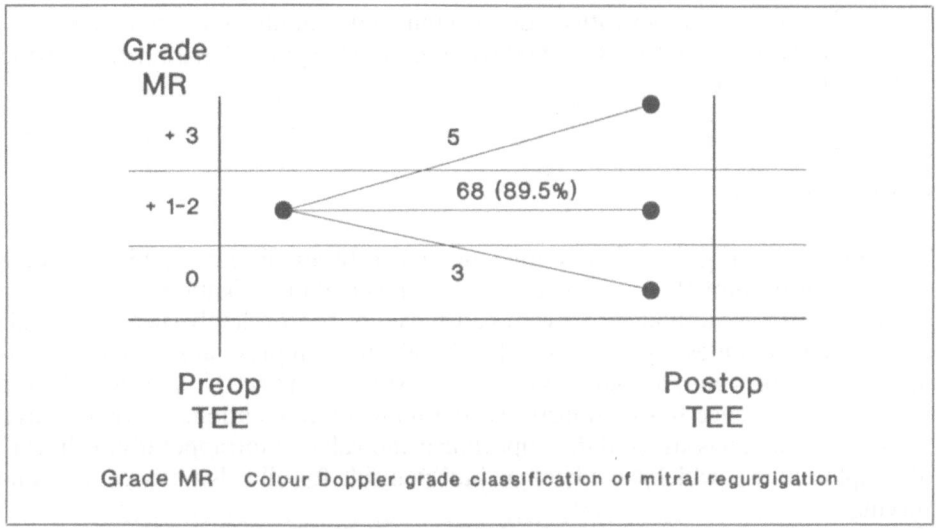

Fig. 9. Ischemic mitral incompetence Color Doppler regurgitant flow before and after coronary revascularization in 76 patients. In the majority (89.5%) there was no change in the degree of mitral regurgitation before and after operation.

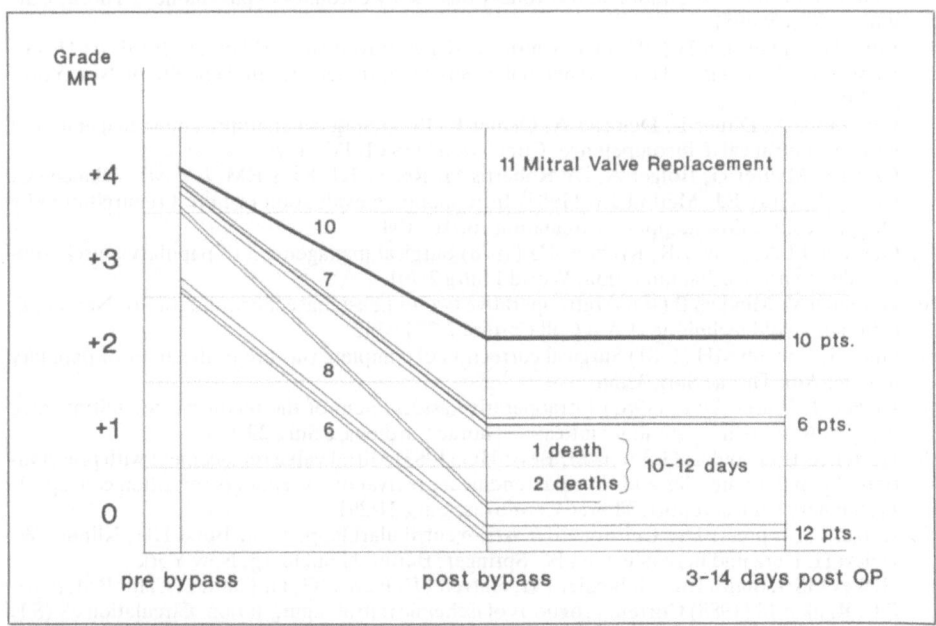

Fig. 10. Ischemic mitral incompetence regurgitant flow before and after valve repair and coronary bypass in 31 patients.
The degree of mitral regurgitation was reduced by more than two grades in all patients after operation. Valve competence was achieved in 18 patients. There were three postoperative deaths in patients with LVEF less than 30%.

145

and documented, together with cardiac rhythm and hemodynamic data, in particular left atrial pressure curve. Before discharge from hospital TEE is repeated in the fully awake patient.

Closing comment

Ischemic mitral regurgitation, until quite recently an obscure field in cardiac surgery, has become the topic of renewed interest and investigation.

Since common methods of valve repair have not been reliably successful in all cases, new techniques need to be sought whereby the complex nature of the disease needs to be taken into account. As a positive side effect, valve repair in ischemic mitral incompetence has demonstrated the limits of conventional intraoperative valve testing and has stressed the importance and value of intraoperative echocardiographic studies which have become indispensible for all valve-procedures conserving.

References

1. Arcidi JM, Hebeler RF, Craver JM, Jones EL, Hatcher CR, Guyton RA (1988) Treatment of moderate mitral regurgitation and coronary disease by coronary bypass alone. J Thorac Cardiovasc Surg 95:951
2. Borst HG, Dalichau H (1978) Die Chirurgie der Atrioventrikularklappen. In: Borst H. G., Klinner W., Senning A. Herz und herznahe Gefäße. Springer, Berlin, Heidelberg, New York, pp 495–546
3. Carpentier A, Didier L, Deloche A, Oenier P (1987) Surgical anatomy and management of ischemic mitral valve incompetence. Circulation 76:SVI, IV–1776
4. Czer LS, Maurer G, Bolger A, De Robertis M, Resser KJ, Kass RM, Lee ME, Blanche C, Chaux A, Gray RJ, Matloff JM (1987) Intraoperative evaluation of mitral regurgitation by Doppler colour flow mapping. Circulation 76:III–108
5. Gerbode FLA, Hetzer R, Krebber HJ (1978) Surgical management of papillary muscle rupture due to myocardial infarction. World J Surg 2:791
6. Goldman M, Mindich B (1986) Intraoperative two-dimensional echocardiography: New application of an old technique. J Am Coll Cardiol 7:374–382
7. Gula G, Yacoub MH (1981) Surgical correction of complete rupture of the anterior papillary muscle. Ann Thorac Surg 32:88
8. Hetzer R, Warnecke H (1981) Intraoperative assessement of the reconstructed mitral valve using a low pressure crystalloid infusion. Thorac Cardiovasc Surg 29:100
9. Hetzer R, Bougioukas G, Franz M, Borst HG (1983) Mitral valve replacement with preservation of papillary muscles and chordae tendineae: revival of a seemingly forgotten concept: I. Preliminary clinical report. Thorac Cardiovasc Surg 31:291
10. Hetzer R (in press) Die Chirurgie der Atrioventrikularklappen. In: Borst HG, Klinner W, Oelert H. Herz und herznahe Gefäße. Springer, Berlin, Heidelberg, New York
11. Hickey MStJ, Smith LR, Muhlbaier LH, Harrell FE, Reves JG, Hinihara T, Califf RM, Pryor DB, Rankin JS (1988) Current prognosis of ischemic mitral regurgitation. Circulation 78:(S I) I–51
12. Kay GL, Kay JH, Zubiate P, Yokoyama T, Mendez M (1986) Mitral valve repair for mitral regurgitation secondary to coronary artery disease. Circulation 74:SI, I–88
13. Kenny J, Cohn L, Shemin R, Collins JJ, Plappert M, Sutton MG (1987) Doppler echocardiographic evaluation of ring mitral valvuloplasty for pure mitral regurgitation. Am J Cardiol 59:341

14. Rankin JS, Hickey M, Smith LR, Debruijn NP, Clements FM, Muhlbaier LH, Lowe JE, Wechsler AS, Califf RM, Reves JG, Wolfe WG (1989) Current management of mitral valve incompetence associated with coronary artery disease. J Card Surg 4:25

15. Sheikh KH, De Bruijn NP, Rankin JS, Clements FM, Stanley T, Wolfe WG, Kisslo J (1990) The utility of transesophageal echocardiography and Doppler color flow imaging in patients undergoing cardiac valve surgery. J Am Coll Cardiol 15:363

16. Shore DF, Wong P, Paneth M (1980) Results of mitral valvuloplasty with suture plication technique. J Thorac Cardiovasc Surg 79:349

17. Stewart WJ, Salcedo EE (1989) Echocardiography in patients undergoing mitral valve surgery. J Card Surg 2:194

18. Wooler GH, Nixon PGF, Grimshaw VA, Watson DA (1962) Experience with the repair of the mitral valve in mitral incompetence. Thorax 17:49

Authors' address
Prof. Dr. R. Hetzer
Deutsches Herzzentrum Berlin
Augustenburger Platz 1
1000 Berlin 65

Results of surgical therapy in ischemic mitral regurgitation

A. W. Waibel, G. Hausdorf, H. O. Vetter, J. W. Park, W. Rutsch*, R. Hetzer M.D.
German Heart Institute and University Clinic Rudolf Virchow, Berlin, FRG

Patients and methods

The severity of mitral regurgitation and clinical symptomatology determined surgical therapy. Generally patients with moderate to severe mitral regurgitation were treated with a valve procedure. Mitral valve replacement was performed when both anterior and posterior papillary muscle fibrosis (two patients) or papillary muscle rupture (two patients, both posterior) was present.

Mitral valve repair consisted of unilateral comissuroplasty (six anterior, 12 posterior) and was combined with a coronary bypass procedure in 16 patients. Five patients had concomittant aneurysmectomy (two anterior, three posterior). Mitral valve repair was performed through a transatrial incision unless combined with aneurysm resection, in which case valve repair was carried out transventricularly. Interrupted sutures were used to coapt anterior and posterior leaflets along the line between the rough and smooth surfaces of the valve.

Mitral valve replacement was performed transatrially and combined with coronary bypass grafting in all six cases. The anterior leaflet was always resected and the posterior leaflet left in place. Three patients received mechanical valves, bioprostheses were used in the remaining three.

Catheter reports of patients who had undergone coronary bypass surgery were reviewed for mitral regurgitation. Angiograms were evaluated in a uniform manner. Patients were excluded if mitral regurgitation was limited to extrasystolic and postextrasystolic beats or if other significant valvular disease was present (i.a., MS, AS, AI, mitral valve prolapse). Mitral regurgitation was graded according to Sellers' criteria [11]. Coronary artery lesions causing 60% luminal narrowing or more were considered significant. Regional wall motion analysis of right anterior oblique ventriculograms was performed using a Cardio 200 image analyzer (Kontron) with a fixed axis reference system, calculating the percent area change in 12 segments. The first two segments near the mitral valve and the 12th segment adjacent to the aortic valve were excluded. Segments were defined as 3−5 inferior, 6−7 apical, and 8−11 anterior. Anterior wall motion was considered abnormal if the percent area change in all four segments was below normal range. Ejection fraction was calculated by the area-length method.

Follow-up data was available on all patients. The Lifetest procedure in SAS [3] was used to produce survival distribution plots and for computation of Wilcoxon rank tests of preoperative parameters for prognostic significance.

Postoperative echocardiograms were performed using an Aloka 870 ultrasound system. Color Doppler gain was increased until background noise appeared. A

149

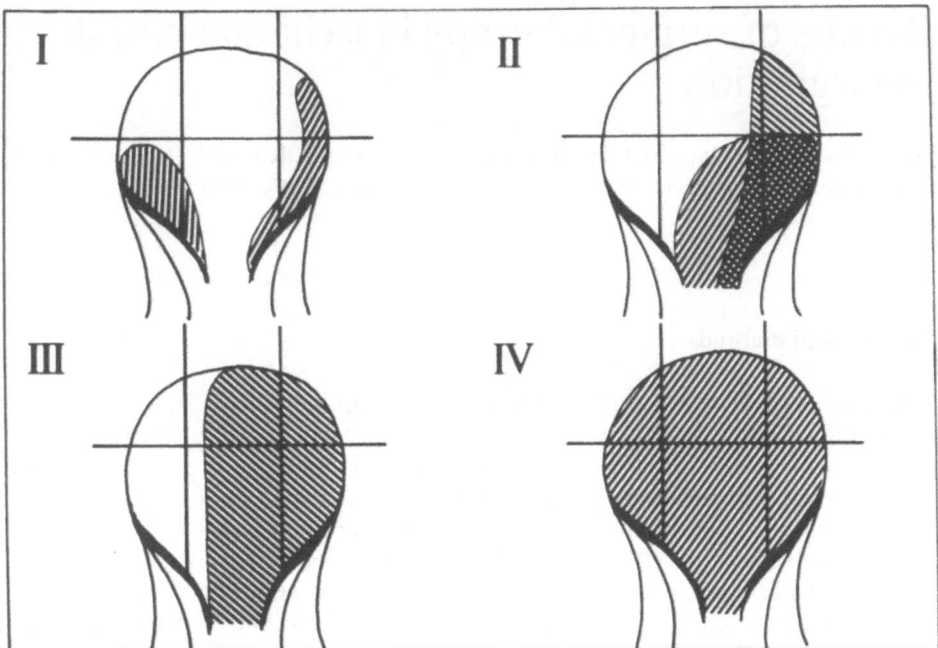

Fig. 1. Semiquantitative grading of mitral regurgitation by color flow echocardiography (sSee text for details)

3.5 MHz transducer was used for transthoracic examinations. Parasternal long axis and apical four-chamber views were recorded. Continuous wave Doppler tracings were obtained from the apical view. A 5 MHz transducer was used for transesophageal examinations. The esophageal transducer was manipulated to allow complete visualization of the left atrium. Additionally, the left atrial cavity was systematically mapped by pulsed wave Doppler to confirm the turbulent nature of observed regurgitant jets. Mitral regurgitation was graded semiquantitatively according to criteria illustrated in Fig. 1. Regurgitant jets one-third the width of the atrium confined to the anterior atrium or narrower jets extending into the posterior atrium were classified as grade 1. Jets two-thirds the width of the atrium confined to the anterior atrium or one-third wide extending further posteriorly were classified as grade 2. Regurgitation two-thirds the width of the atrium extending into the posterior atrium was classified as grade 3. Grade 4 mitral regurgitation was considered to be present if the regurgitant jet filled the entire atrium.

Results

Preoperative characteristics of the three treatment groups are summarized in Table 1. The groups were similar with respect to age, sex, ejection fraction, left ventricular end-diastolic pressure, severity of coronary disease, and history of anterior infarction. Patients treated with a valve procedure had more severe mitral regurgi-

150

Table 1. Preoperative Characteristics of Treatment Groups

	CABG only (N = 34)	Repair (N = 18)	Replacement (N = 6)
Mean Age ± SD	63 ± 7	60 ± 10	64 ± 5
Male	20 (59%)	12 (71%)	3 (50%)
Mean Ejection Fraction ± SD	49 ± 14	46 ± 13	40 ± 20
Mean LVEDP ± SD	17 ± 9	21 ± 9	20 ± 8
3 Vessel Disease	25 (73%)	10 (60%)	4 (67%)
Anterior Infarct	8 (24%)	3 (18%)	1 (17%)
Grade MR			
I	17 (50%)	–	–
II	15 (44%)	6 (33%)	2 (33%)
III	2 (6%)	8 (44%)	1 (17%)
IV	–	4 (22%)	3 (50%)

LVEDP = Left Ventricular End-Diastolic Pressure, MR = Mitral Regurgitation
SD = Standard Deviation, CABG = Coronary Artery Bypass Grafting

tation compared to those treated with bypass grafting only, reflecting the treatment strategy described above. Three-vessel coronary disease was most common in all treatment groups.

Among all patients, 48 (83%) had a history of myocardial infarction. Of these, 36 (75%) were isolated inferior infarctions and nine (19%) isolated anterior infarctions. Three patients (6%) had a history of both anterior and inferior infarction. In 41 cases (71%) the most recent infarction was dated. Four patients (7%) had had an infarct within one month prior to surgery, eight patients (14%) one to three months, eight patients (14%) three to six months and 21 patients (36%) more than six months before surgery. The prevalence of inferior infarction among patients with ischemic mitral regurgitation is reflected in the predominance of inferior wall motion abnormalities (Fig. 2). However, a substantial number of patients had anterior wall motion disturbances. Fifteen patients (26%) had abnormal wall motion in all four anterior segments.

Survival distribution curves for the three treatment groups are shown in Fig. 3. Mitral valve repair was associated with improved survival compared to mitral valve replacement, however selection biases, small patient numbers, and short follow-up time preclude statistical comparison. Among patients treated with coronary bypass grafting alone, one patient died two weeks postoperatively of multi-organ failure, another of cancer 11 months after surgery. Of the 18 patients who had mitral valve repair three died of low cardiac output one week, eight weeks, and seven months after surgery. All had a history of anterior infarction and anterior papillary muscle fibrosis, two had concomittant resection of an anterior ventricular aneurysm. All three patients who had combined mitral valve repair and posterior ventricular aneurysm resection are alive with good clinical results two, 18 and 27 months after surgery. Two of the six mitral valve replacement patients died early postoperatively of low cardiac output; one had isolated right coronary artery disease, an inferior infarction eight weeks prior to surgery and posterior papillary muscle rupture, the other had severe three-vessel disease, both anterior and inferior infarctions, anterior and posterior papillary muscle fibrosis and impaired ventricular function (EF = 24%).

151

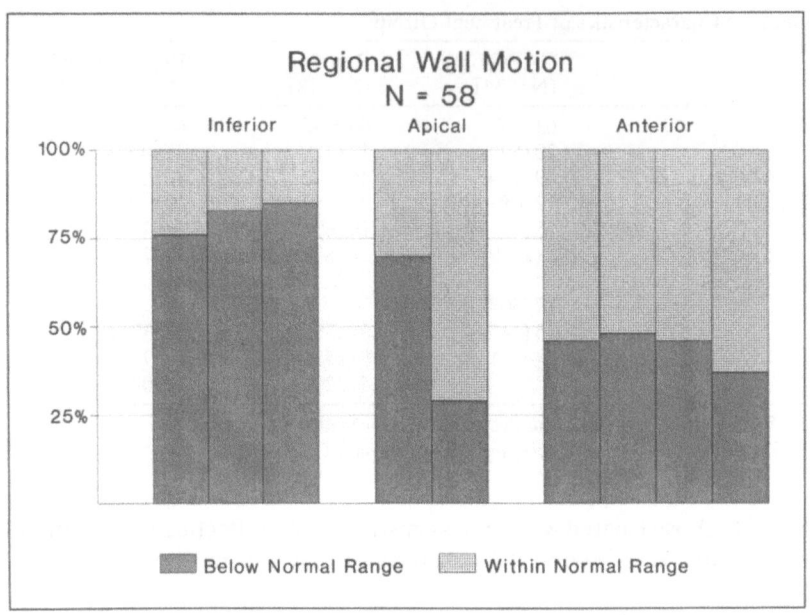

Fig. 2. Results of regional wall motion analysis of right anterior oblique ventriculograms

Among all patients, history of anterior infarction was the most significant predictor of mortality (P < 0.01). Four of 12 patients with a history of anterior infarction died within seven months after surgery. These patients uniformly had severe disease of the left anterior descending system, usually combined with circumflex disease. Three of the four patients with anterior infarction who died had three-vessel disease, one had single vessel disease limited to the LAD system. The presence of an anterior wall motion abnormality was also associated with increased mortality, though less strongly (P < 0.05).

Of all seven patients who died, four had three vessel disease, one had combined disease of the right and circumflex coronary arteries, two had one-vessel disease (one RCA, one LAD). Three-vessel disease was not associated with a higher risk of mortality. Grade of mitral regurgitation, left ventricular end-diastolic pressure, ejection fraction, recency of infarction, age and sex did not correlate with mortality in our patient group.

Eleven patients treated with revascularization only and 11 patients treated with mitral valve repair were studied postoperatively by transesophageal and transthoracic color flow echocardiography. Mean follow-up times were 13 and 17.5 months, respectively. Figure 4 compares severity of preoperative and postoperative mitral regurgitation for the two treatment groups. Six patients in the revascularized group had residual mitral regurgitation. In four patients the degree of regurgitation was equivalent to preoperative ventriculography. These patients tended to be more symptomatic with exertional dyspnea than patients in whom mitral regurgitation had resolved. There were no differences between patients with and without persistent mitral regurgitation regarding history of myocardial infarction of time between infarction and surgery. All but one patient treated with mitral

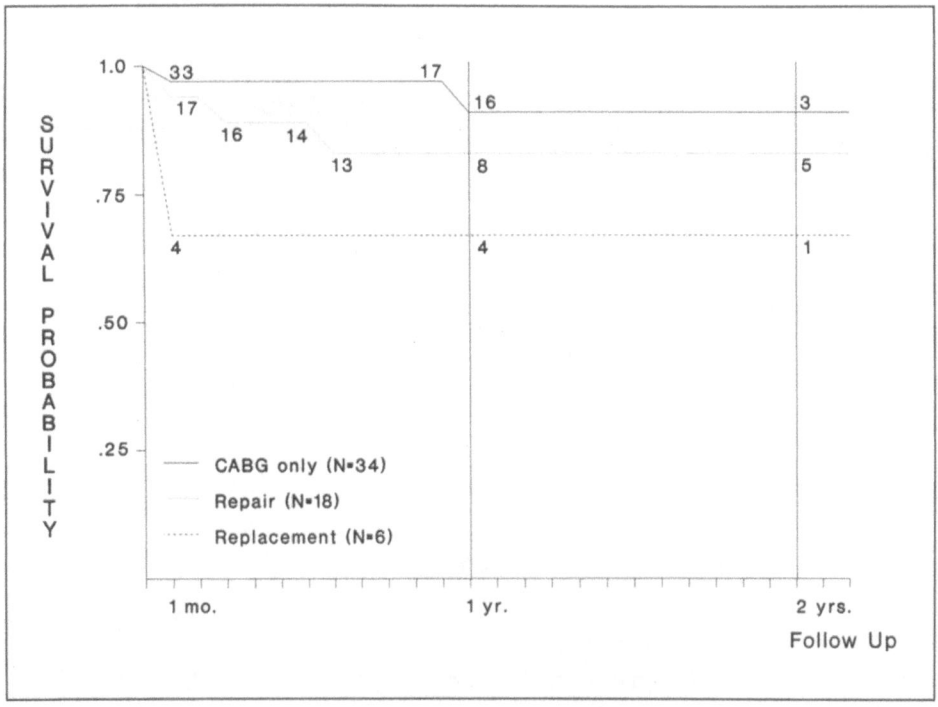

Fig. 3. Survival distribution curves stratified according to treatment modality; CAGB = coronary artery bypass grafting

valve repair had a reduction in severity of mitral regurgitation compared to preoperative ventriculography.

Transesophageal echocardiography demonstrated mitral regurgitation in 14 of 22 postoperative patients. All had characteristic continuous wave Doppler tracings with high velocity, holosystolic regurgitant flow across the mitral valve. Regurgitant flow velocity ranged from 2.6 to 5.6 m/s. Only four patients had mitral regurgitation identifiable by transthoracic color flow echocardiography. Transesophageal echo showed the degree of mitral regurgitation to be more severe than estimated by the transthoracic method in all but one case. Transesophageal echocardiography allowed more complete visualization of the left atrium and regurgitant jets. Average distance of the mitral valve anulus from the esophageal transducer was 5.4 cm compared to 10.8 cm from the apical view, with the atrium lying proximal to the mitral valve as viewed from the esophagus, distal to the mitral valve as viewed from the apex. Most regurgitant jets were eccentrically oriented, extending posteriorly and superiorly along the lateral atrial wall or interatrial septum.

Discussion

Mitral regurgitation due to coronary artery disease is associated with a poor prognosis whether treated medically or surgically. Most patients are of advanced age,

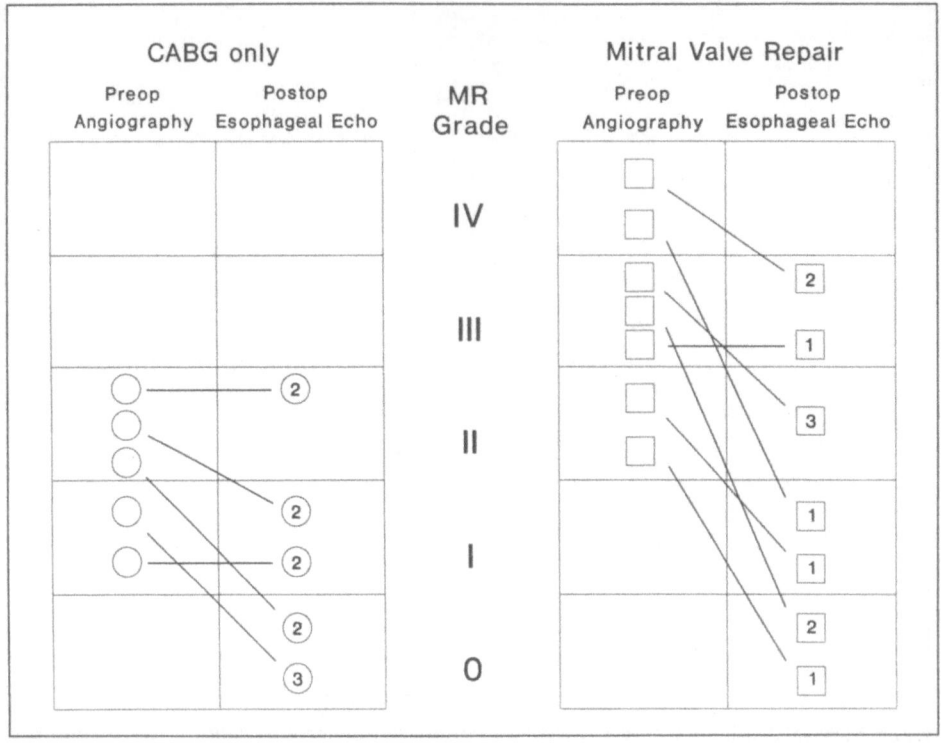

Fig. 4. Preoperative and postoperative severity of mitral regurgitation in patients treated with revascularization only (left panel) and mitral valve repair (right panel)

have severe multi-vessel coronary disease and a history of myocardial infarction. Complicating conditions such as large ventricular aneurysms are frequently present [10, 8].

Among our surgically treated patients, mitral valve repair was associated with improved survival compared to mitral valve replacement, with survival rates similar to those reported by others [8, 7]. This is probably due in part to better ventricular function after valve repair [1, 6], however selection biases such as treatment of papillary muscle rupture and concurrent anterior and posterior papillary muscle fibrosis with valve replacement or combining aneurysmectomy with mitral valve repair preclude quantitative comparison of the two groups. Other known benefits of mitral valve repair such as reduced incidence of endocarditis, thromboembolic complications and hemorrhage associated with anticoagulation [8] did not affect survival among our patients who had a relatively short follow-up time.

Anterior infarction, while less common than posterior infarction among patients with ischemic mitral regurgitation, was present in a substantial number of patients (21%) and associated with a worse prognosis (p < 0.01). Both patients who had mitral valve repair and anterior aneurysmectomy died of left ventricular failure. Dissapointing results with patients requiring anterior aneurysm resection and mitral valve repair have also been described by Rankin et al. [10], suggesting that such patients might better be treated with transplantation. Acute posterior papillary muscle rupture has previously been shown to be associated with a high operative mortality [4] and accounted for one patient death in our group.

Selection of patients with lesser degrees of mitral regurgitation for valve repair is difficult. A relatively large proportion of patients treated with revascularization alone (53%) had clinically significant residual mitral regurgitation, paralleling results of others [2]. History of infarction and time between infarction and surgery were not predictive of residual regurgitation. While intraoperative echocardiography has been shown to be accurate in detecting residual regurgitation [2, 5], it can do so only after weaning from cardiopulmonary bypass. Clearly, a preoperative method of predicting the effect of revascularization on regurgitation would be desirable.

Color flow echocardiography is increasingly used as a reliable, noninvasive means of assessing mitral regurgitation. Quantification of mitral regurgitation with transthoracic color flow echocardiography has been shown to correlate well with ventriculographic grading in preoperative patients [2, 9]. Postoperative patients, however, are more difficult to image transthoracically due to scarring. Transesophageal color flow echocardiography allows more complete visualization of the atrial cavity and more precise delineation of regurgitant jets. Reliance upon transthoracic color flow echocardiography can lead to underestimation of mitral regurgitation in postoperative patients.

Summary

Results of surgical therapy in 58 patients with ischemic mitral regurgitation operated upon during the 30-month-period through September, 1988, at the German Heart Center Berlin were analyzed in a retrospective manner. Thirty-four patients had coronary artery bypass surgery only, 18 patients had mitral valve repair, and six patients had mitral valve replacement. Preoperative parameters including age, left ventricular end-diastolic pressure, ejection fraction, degree of mitral regurgitation, localization of preceeding infarct and ventricular wall motion abnormalities were compared among treatment groups and tested for prognostic significance. Among patients who had a valve procedure, mitral valve repair was associated with less mortality than mitral valve replacement. History of preceeding anterior myocardial infarction and presence of on anterior wall motion abnormality were associated with poorer prognosis among all patients. Eleven patients treated with revascularization alone and 11 patients treated with mitral valve repair were examined postoperatively by transthoracic and transesophageal color flow echocardiography. Six patients in the revascularized group has residual mitral regurgitation. All but one patient having undergone mitral valve repair had a reduction in severity of mitral regurgitation compared to preoperative ventriculography. Transesophageal color flow echocardiography demonstrated residual mitral regurgitation in 14 of 22 postoperative patients. Of these, only four had mitral regurgitation identifiable by transthoracic color flow echocardiography. Transesophageal color flow echocardiography. Transesophageal color flow echocardiography showed the degree of mitral regurgitation to be more severe than observed by the transthoracic method in all but one case. This is due to difficulties in transthoracic imaging of postoperative patients, greater distance of the left atrium from the chest wall, more complete visualization of the left atrium by transesophageal echo and the eccentric nature of the regurgitant jet in these patients. Reliance upon transthoracic color flow echocardiography can lead to underestimation of mitral regurgitation in postoperative patients.

References

1. Bonchek LI, Olinger GN, Siegel R, Tresch DD, Keelan MH Jr. (1984) Left ventricular performance after mitral reconstruction for mitral regurgitation. J Thorac Cardiovasc Surg 88:122
2. Czer LSC, Maurer G, Bolger AF, De Robertis M, Resser KJ, Kass RM, Lee ME, Blanche C, Chaux A, Gray RJ, Matloff JM (1987) Intraoperative evaluation of mitral regurgitation by Doppler color flow mapping. Circulation 76 [Suppl III]:III-108
3. De Long DM (1985) The LIFETEST procedure. In: SAS user's guide, version 5 edition. Cary NC, SAS Institute Inc, p 529–556
4. Gerbode FLA, Hetzer R, Krebber HJ (1978) Surgical management of papillary muscle rupture due to myocardial infarction. World J Surg 2:791–796
5. Goldman ME, Mindich BP, Teichholz LE, Burgess N, Staville K, Fuster V (1984) Intraoperative contrast echocardiography to evaluate mitral valve operations. J Am Coll Cardiol 4:1035–1040
6. Goldman ME, Mora F, Guarino T, Fuster V, Mindich BP (1987) Mitral valvuloplasty is superior to valve replacement for preservation of left ventricular function: An intraoperative two-dimensional echocardiographic study. J Am Coll Cardiol 10:568–575
7. Hickey M StJ, Smith LR, Muhlbaier LH, Harrell FE Jr., Reves JG, Hinohara T, Califf RM, Pryor DB, Rankin JS (1988) Current prognosis of ischemic mitral regurgitation, implications for future management. Circulation 78 [Suppl I]:I51–59
8. Kay GL, Kay JH, Zubiate P, Yokoyama T, Mendez M (1987) Mitral valve repair for mitral regurgitation secondary to coronary artery disease. Circulation 74 [Suppl I]:I 88–98
9. Miyatake K, Izumi S, Okamoto M, Kinoshita N, Asonuma H, Nakagawa H, Yamamoto K, Takamiya M, Sakakibara H, Nimura Y (1986) Semiquantitative grading of severity of mitral regurgitation by real-time two-dimensional doppler flow imaging technique. J Am Coll Cardiol 7:82–88
10. Rankin JS, Feneley MP, Hickey M StJ, Muhlbaier LH, Wechsler AS, Floyd RD, Reves JG, Skelton TN, Califf RM, Lowe JE, Sabiston DC Jr (1988) A clinical comparison of mitral valve repair versus valve replacement in ischemic mitral regurgitation. J Thorac Cardiovasc Surg 95:165–177
11. Sellers RD, Levy MJ, Amplatz K, Lillehei CW (1964) Left retrograde cardioangiography in aquired cardiac disease: technic, indications and interpretation in 700 cases. Am J Cardiol 14:437–447

Author's address:
Dr. med. A. William Waibel
Deutsches Herzzentrum Berlin
Augustenburger Platz 1
1000 Berlin 65

Current concepts in the pathogenesis and treatment of ischemic mitral regurgitation

J. S. Rankin, M. S. J. Hickey, L. R. Smith, N. P. DeBruijn, K. H. Sheikh, and D. C. Sabiston, Jr.

Departments of Surgery, Medicine, and Anesthesiology, Duke University Medical Center, Durham, North Carolina, USA

Mitral valve anatomy and physiology

Under normal conditions, mitral valve competence is maintained by a complex interaction of the five components of mitral valve function: the ventricular wall, the fibrous annulus, the papillary muscles, the chordae tendineae, and the valve leaflets. Derangements in any single component can produce valve dysfunction, but in ischemic incompetence, the primary defect is infarction of the ventricular wall and papillary muscles. With increasing interest in valvular reconstruction in ischemic mitral regurgitation, a detailed knowledge of mitral valve anatomy has become essential.

The fibrous skeleton of the heart, to which the mitral valve attaches, is derived from the endocardial cushions [1]. The mitral annulus is a thin, incomplete ring of fibrous tissue, which is most apparent at two points, the right and left fibrous trigones (Fig. 1). The left fibrous trigone is situated at the left anterior aspect of the mitral ring and consists of fibrous tissue joining the mitral ring to the base of the aorta. The right fibrous trigone, or central fibrous body, lies in the midline of the heart and represents the confluence of fibrous tissue from the mitral valve, tricuspid valve, membranous septum, and posterior aspect of the base of the aorta.

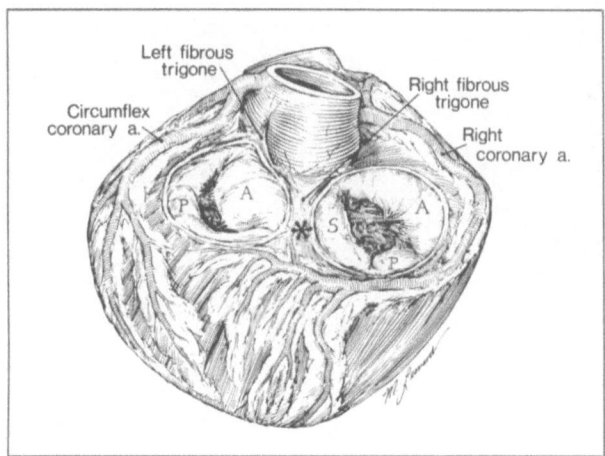

Fig. 1. Anatomic interrelationships of the atrioventricular valves. A is the anterior leaflet, P is the posterior leaflet, and S is the septal leaflet. The asterisk represents the area of the bundle of His

Supported by NIH Grants Nos. L09315, HL29536, HL17670

Embryologically, the mitral valve is initially quadracuspid, and as development continues, the accessory or commissural cusps fuse with and become part of the lateral aspects of the posterior leaflet. Persistence of these fetal commissural cusps, especially at the posterior commissure, can produce scalloping of the lateral posterior leaflet or minor posterior leaflet defects. In most adults, however, only two leaflets are evident, the broader anterior leaflet and the narrower posterior leaflet. The anterior leaflet has a much longer base-to-margin length than the posterior leaflet; however, the annular attachment of the posterior leaflet is twice as great, so that the surface area of each leaflet is almost identical [2−4]. Both leaflets have a trapezoidal shape and attach by thin fibrous chordae tendineae to *both* the anterior and posterior papillary muscles. Stated differently, the chordae from each papillary muscle fan out and attach to nearly half of both cusp margins (Fig. 2). The commissures do not divide the leaflet tissue completely to the valve annulus, and the basal aspects at the commissures are composed of continuous valvular tissue [2, 3].

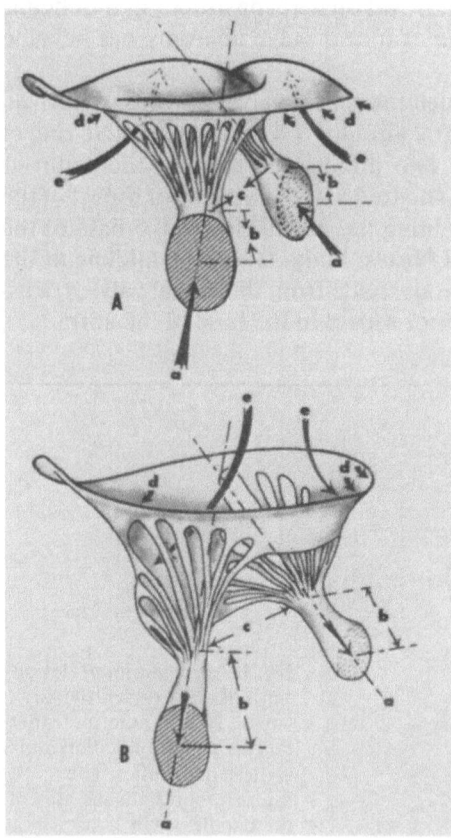

Fig. 2. Diagrammatic anatomy of the mitral apparatus. A, anatomy of the valve during leaflet closure; B, the open valve showing relationships of the papillary muscles and chordal fans to the valve axis. (Reproduced from [3])

The papillary muscles arise from the ventricular walls, at approximately two-thirds of the distance toward the apex. The anterolateral papillary muscle is single in 75% of patients, whereas its posteromedial counterpart usually has multiple heads arising directly from the ventricular wall [5]. The anterolateral muscle is supplied by branches of the proximal left anterior descending or circumflex coronary systems and is generally believed to have a more abundant blood supply. Posterolateral branches of the right coronary artery usually perfuse the posterior papillary muscle heads and are at some distance from the orifices of the coronary arteries [4, 6, 7]. In cases of left coronary dominance, posterolateral branches of the circumflex coronary artery supply the posterior papillary muscles. This more tenuous nature of posterior wall perfusion may be one explanation for the predominant involvement of the posterior coronary circulation in acute papillary-annular dysfunction.

First order chordae originate at or near the apices of the papillary muscles and insert into the free edges of the leaflets as fine strands. *Secondary chordae* also originate near the apices of the papillary muscles and insert into the ventricular surface of the leaflet 1−3 mm from the free edge. Secondary chordae usually are thicker and less numerous than primary chordae. *Tertiary chordae* originate from the ventricular walls, insert along the basal aspects of the leaflets, and are more prominent in the posterior leaflet [5]. The edge of the leaflets have a slightly serrated appearance due to the insertion of chordae tendineae on the ventricular surface; these serrations mark the line of closure of the normal valve. Thus, the point of coaptation is not the free edge but is located a short distance proximally on the leaflet; the leaflets normally coapt along a considerable area of their atrial surface [5].

The function of the mitral valve is to permit uninhibited flow of blood from the left atrium to the left ventricle during ventricular diastole and to prevent reflux of blood into the atrium during ventricular systole. The valve achieves this objective by a coordinated contraction of ventricular myocardium and the papillary muscles during the cardiac cycle. During systole, the valve is closed, and the left atrium serves as a reservoir to store blood returning from the lungs. With isovolumic relaxation, left ventricular pressure falls, and when ventricular pressure becomes lower than that of the full atrium, the valve opens and initiates rapid filling of the ventricle (Fig. 3), [8]. It is interesting to note that the highest filling velocities and the majority of diastolic ventricular filling occur during the rapid filling phase, before left ventricular pressure reaches its diastolic minimum. Early transmitral flow not only is produced by positive pressure gradients from the atrium to the ventricle, but also may be facilitated by active ventricular restorative forces related to myocardial relaxation [9].

Several factors contribute to mitral valve closure [10]. First, deceleration of mitral flow during late rapid filling and again after atrial systole is associated with partial closure of the valve leaflets. Flow deceleration produces positive pressure gradients from the ventricular to the atrial surface of the valve leaflets, and initiates closure. Second, analysis of blood velocity patterns during filling (Fig. 4) demonstrates large asymmetrical "ring vortices" produced by the incoming jet of blood striking the apex and spreading up the ventricular walls toward the base [11]. These vortices then strike the ventricular surface of the leaflets and contribute to

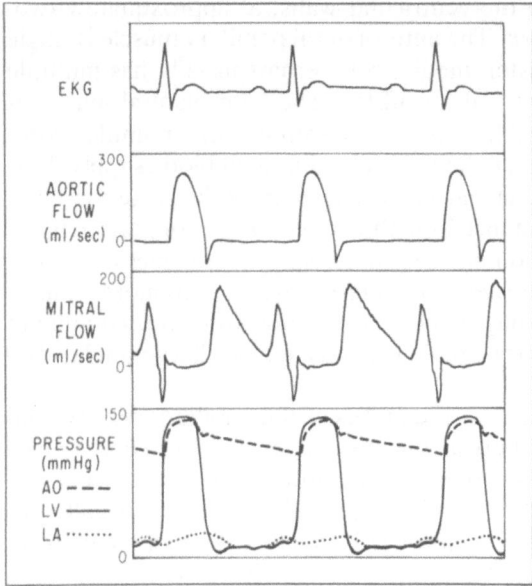

Fig. 3. Schematic of the physiology of transmitral blood flow. Note the positive atrioventricular pressure gradients during rapid filling and atrial systole, along with the associated filling velocities. Retrograde mitral flow during valve closure is minimal

closure. There tends to be an asymmetry in the size of the vortices, with the larger being located behind the anterior leaflet. Flow deceleration and vortex strength have been shown to be of nearly equal importance to valve closure, achieving almost complete leaflet apposition by the onset of ventricular contraction [10]. Finally, as ventricular systole begins, rising left ventricular pressure completely closes the valve with minimal retrograde flow (Fig. 3). If it were not for flow deceleration and vortices, the magnitude of regurgitation during normal valve closure would be substantially greater.

The active motions of the mitral annulus and papillary muscles also contribute to valve competence. Annular area, determined by echocardiography, changes dramatically during the cardiac cycle, decreasing by one-third from end-diastole to mid-systole [12]. The dynamic valve area curve appears similar to the ventricular volume curve, suggesting that active shortening of circumferential muscle bundles at the base reduces valve orifice area during systole and contributes to leaflet competence.

Since the atrioventricular valves have no intrinsic structure, intact chordae and normal papillary muscle function also are necessary for proper leaflet closure. During systole, contraction of each papillary muscle shortens the subvalvular apparatus and compensates for inward displacement of the ventricular walls. The systolic shortening characteristics of both papillary muscles are quite similar to segmental ventricular fiber shortening in the circumferential plane [13]. With posterior wall infarction, several factors, including dilatation of the mitral annulus, papillary muscle elongation, loss of papillary muscle shortening, and perhaps alterations in papillary-annular geometric relationships, all combine to reduce the surface area of mitral leaflet coaptation and predispose the valve to incompetence. Since many

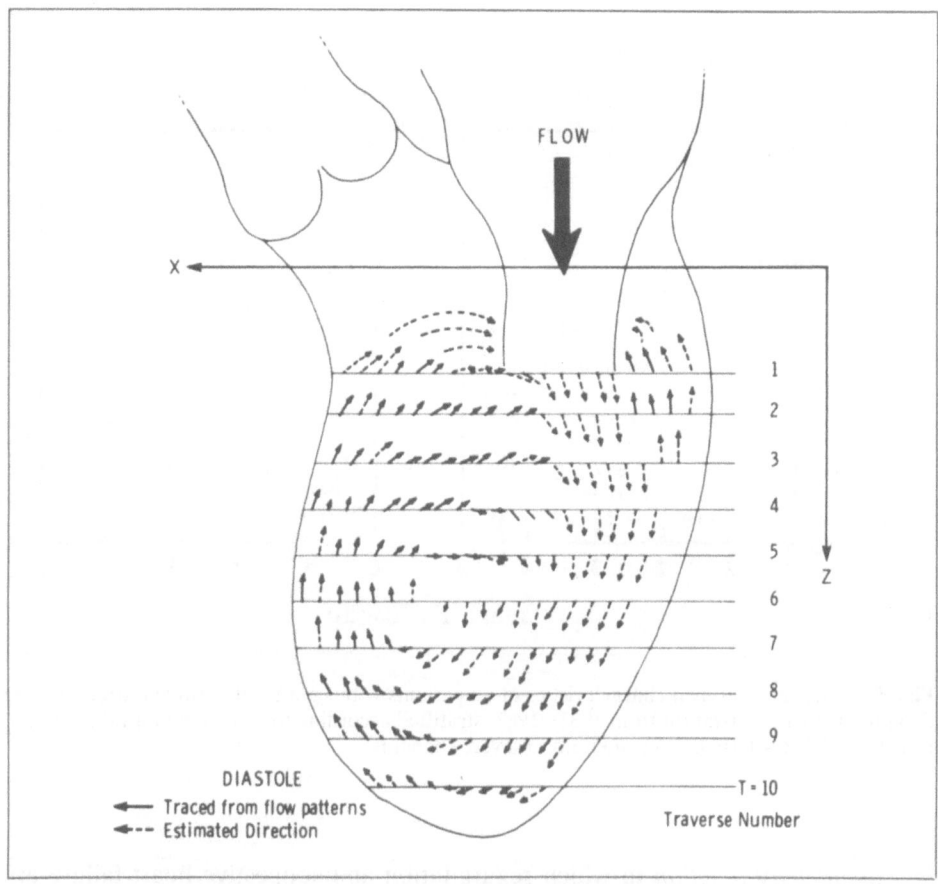

Fig. 4. Velocity profiles within the left ventricle during filling. Note the vortices spreading up the ventricular walls and localizing behind the valve to assist valve closure. (Reproduced from [11])

patients with ischemic regurgitation have peristent fetal commissural cusps or other minor anatomic defects, some degree of preexisting leaflet abnormality also may be important [14].

Clinical classification of ischemic mitral regurgitation

Ischemic mitral regurgitation is defined as valve incompetence occurring after an acute myocardial infarction with minimal leaflet or chordal pathology and is observed to a significant degree in 3% of patients with coronary artery disease undergoing catheterization [15]. The presence of moderate to servere ischemic regurgitation dramatically influences long-term prognosis (Fig. 5), being the sixth most important determinant of survival in the overall coronary artery disease population. This disorder is quite heterogeneous, both from pathophysiologic and clinical viewpoints. Physiologically, the majority of patients exhibit posterior *papil-*

161

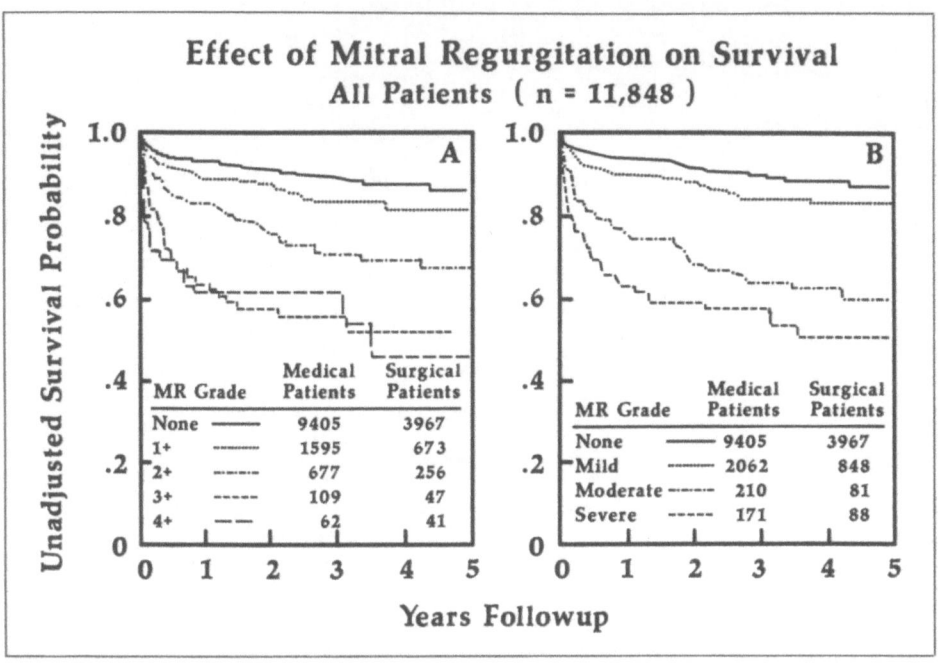

Fig. 5. Unadjusted survival characteristics of all patients with significant coronary artery disease diagnosed at catheterization from 1981–1987, stratified according to associated mitral regurgitation grade 1+ to 4+ (panel A) and mild to severe (panel B)

lary-annular dysfunction in which regurgitation and congestive heart failure are coincident with the onset of a large posterior wall infarction. As described above, combinations of posterior annular dilatation, absence of annular contraction, papillary muscle elongation, loss of papillary muscle shortening, and preexisting minor congenital leaflet defects contribute to valve incompetence in the region of the posterior mitral commissure [14]. Most patients coming to a valve procedure require surgery during the acute phase of their illness, although some present later in a more elective fashion. Fluctuating mitral regurgitation in the setting of post-infarction unstable angina is a variant of this syndrome [16].

The least common type of ischemic incompetence is *papillary muscle rupture,* occurring in only 0.1% of coronary disease patients undergoing catheterization [15]. Congestive heart failure associated with a new murmur usually develops at an interval of several days after infarction, and the majority have severe regurgitation requiring acute intervention. The infarction usually is posterior and is often small and localized; global ejection fraction frequently is maintained [14].

The third category consists of patients with diffuse left ventricular infarctions or anterior aneurysms, and the regurgitation is secondary to *generalized ventricular and annular dilatation.* A history of multiple myocardial infarctions is common, and most patients present acutely with very low ejection fractions. It is sometimes difficult to determine if the congestive heart failure is caused more by inadequate residual myocardium than by valve dysfunction. Longterm prognosis in this group is poor, independent of the therapy chosen [14].

Analysis of prognostic risk factors

Ischemic mitral regurgitation is one of the most serious disorders to be encountered in cardiac surgical practice. At a time when hospital mortality for most valve operations approximates 5% [16], mitral valve-coronary bypass procedures still carry a 10−20% mortality, partially due to the ischemic subgroup. Because ischemic cases constitute less than 10% of mitral valve operations [14], a high mortality in this category can be absorbed into the overall experience and easily overlooked. However, when examined individually, valve replacement for ischemic mitral regurgitation has been associated with a hospital mortality as high as 50% for emergency cases in most centers [17−20]. In our series [14], hospital mortality for mitral valve replacement in this setting was 53%, at a time when mortality for all other valve operations was 8.6%, and 5.6% for elective isolated valve procedures.

It is important to differentiate acute from elective circumstances, since acute clinical presentation is an overwhelming risk factor. Multivariable analysis in our series of 381 patients with moderate to severe ischemic mitral regurgitation managed between 1981 and 1987 identified several variables as influencing hospital and longterm mortality: 1) severe congestive heart failure ($p < .001$), 2) the number of comorbid disorders, such as acute renal failure, pulmonary dysfunction, and intra-aortic balloon pump requirement ($p = .001$), 3) necessity for acute CCU management ($p = .006$), 4) reduced ejection fraction ($p = .009$), 5) number of vessels diseased ($p = .016$), and 6) age ($p = .031$). In ischemic mitral regurgitation, combinations of risk factors produce a much wider spectrum of clinical results than in standard ischemic heart disease. For example, an otherwise healthy 55-year-old man with a remote infarction causing chronic mitral regurgitation with compensated congestive heart failure (currently NYHA Class II), 2-vessel coronary disease, and an ejection fraction of .55 would have an estimated hospital mortality of 4% for an elective mitral valve operation in our series (Table 1). The more common example of a 65-year-old patient in the CCU with mild pulmonary edema, 3-vessel disease, stable hemodynamics, and an ejection fraction of .40 would have a 15% mortality for a mitral valve operation. In contrast, a 75-year-old man in the CCU, intubated for pulmonary edema, on the balloon pump, in acute non-oliguric renal failure, with 3-vessel disease and having an ejection fraction of .25 would have a predicted 30-day mortality of 60% for a mitral valve procedure and only a 22% 5-year survival. Because of this wide spectrum of clinical risk, a detailed description of baseline prognostic variables is important both for data reporting and estimation of individual patient outcome.

Recent trends in therapy

Several therapeutic principles are evident from available studies. First, most would agree that patients with papillary muscle rupture should be treated with an

Table 1. The effect of preoperative risk factors on postoperative survival prognosis in ischemic mitral regurgitation*

	Low Risk Patient[a] Survival % 30 day/5 year	Medium Risk Patient[b] Survival % 30 day/5 year	High Risk Patient[c] Survival % 30 day/5 year
Medical	96/82	97/49	44/ 2
All Surgical	97/94	90/80	55/27
CAB Only	98/95	93/81	65/30
CAB + MVR	96/93	85/77	40/22

*	Survival data based on Cox model analysis of hypothetical low-, medium-, and high-risk patients derived from clinical experience of 381 patients with ischemic mitral regurgitation managed since 1981.
a	Elective operation, age = 55, EF = .55, 2 VD
b	Emergency operation, age = 65, EF = .40, CHF = mild pulmonary edema only, 3 VD, no comorbid disorders, CCU = yes
c	Emergency operation, age = 75, EF = .25, CHF = severe pulmonary edema, IV, 3 VD, 3 comorbid disorders, CCU = yes.

CAB = Coronary artery bypass
MVR = Mitral valve repair or replacement
VD = Vessels diseased
CCU = Coronary Care Unit

Note: These data are presented to illustrate the effects of baseline risk factors on prognosis in each group. Comparison between groups is inappropriate because of differences in patient composition within the model.

immediate valve operation, either prosthetic replacement or papillary muscle reimplantation [14, 21–26]. Delay of intervention can lead to multi-organ failure, whereas many patients with papillary muscle rupture have good ventricular function and an excellent prognosis after prompt restoration of valve competence. Conversely, operation currently is avoided in most patients with generalized ventricular dysfunction or anterior aneurysm associated with significant valve incompetence. Consistent with previous reports [27, 28], longterm survival in this subset has been dismal with either valve replacement or repair, even utilizing contemporary myocardial protection and supportive measures [14]. Therefore, avoiding operation, especially in cases with multiple associated risk factors, seems justified since little therapeutic benefit has been evident. This subgroup can be defined objectively as having less than 25% of normal wall motion (Fig. 6) in two of three left ventricular regions (anterior, apical, posterior) of the RAO ventriculogram [14]. The other high-risk group seems to be elderly patients requiring CCU management for severe congestive heart failure associated with multi-organ failure (as in the extreme example given above). Most of the hospital mortality in our series has occurred in these two groups [14–16], and our current policy is to avoid operation in both subsets. An intensive course of medical therapy and/or coronary reperfusion can be undertaken in elderly patients with multiorgan failure, in an attempt to convert them into better operative candidates. Basing surgical patient selection on more objective criteria and avoiding inappropriate intervention may be very important for improving therapeutic results.

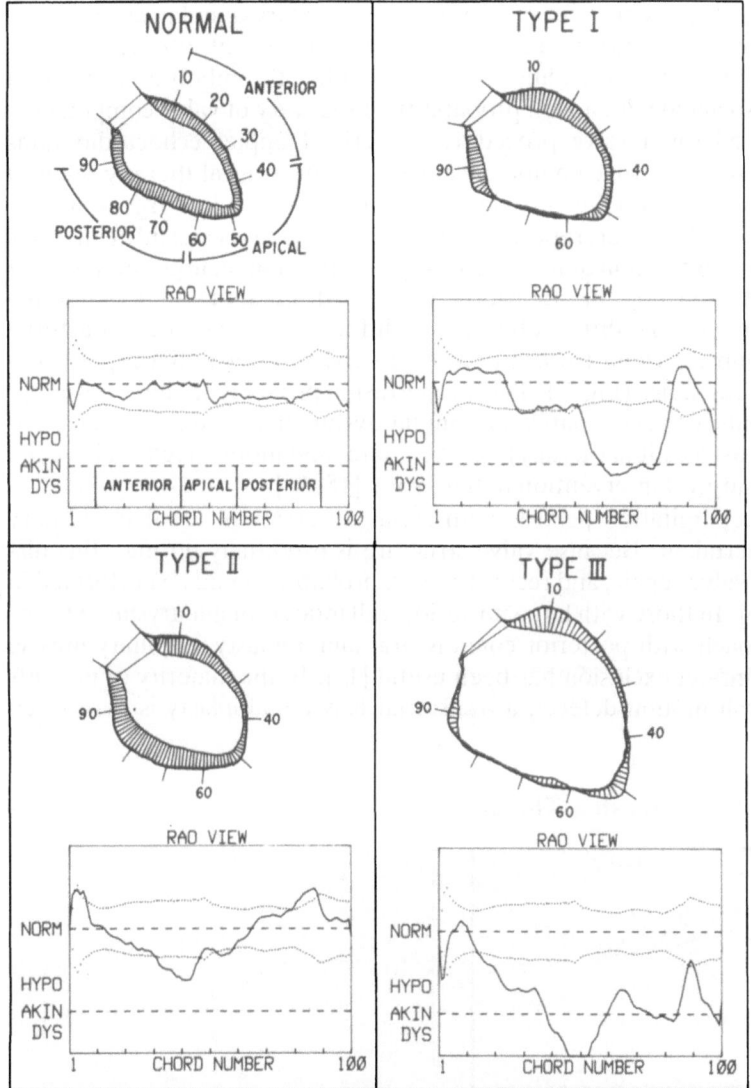

Fig. 6. Categorization into three types was performed objectively on the basis of the right anterior oblique *(RAO)* left ventriculogram. A modified center-line regional wall motion analysis was used, wherein the circumference of the right anterior oblique projection was divided into 100 equidistant chords constructed perpendicular to a center line drawn midway between the end-diastolic and end-systolic contours. The shortening fraction for each chord was normalized by defining the average shortening observed for each chord in a normal group of 50 patients as 100% wall motion, and akinesis at 0%. Average chordal shortening was computed for the *anterior wall* (chords 11 to 40), the *apical region* (chords 41 to 60), and the *posterior wall* (chords 61 to 90) Chords 1−10 and 91−100 were omitted from the analysis because of greater variability in defining normal wall motion in the paravalvular regions. *Type I,* papillary annular dysfunction; *Type II,* papillary muscle rupture; *Type III,* severe left ventricular dysfunction

In the majority of patients with *acute* posterior papillary-annular dysfunction, reperfusion therapy is the current treatment of choice [15, 16, 29, 39]. Reestablishment of blood flow in the offending artery with either thrombolysis or balloon angioplasty is associated with a high probability of recovery of valve competence, obviating the need for a valve procedure. If serial Doppler echocardiograms demonstrate recovery of valve competence, subsequent surgical therapy is based on residual coronary obstruction and can be accomplished in a less urgent fashion and at minimal risk. Moreover, reperfusion therapy has been successful at intervals of several days after infarction or in fluctuating postinfarction regurgitation, so that attempted reperfusion may be appropriate for most situations [15]. Although retrospective comparison is difficult because of differences in baseline characteristics between groups, a trend toward improved survival after initial reperfusion therapy exists in our series (Fig. 7). Thus, reperfusion probably should be attempted in most patients with acute papillary-annular dysfunction, and thrombolysis or angioplasty (at least as initial therapy) may be a safer and more effective approach than immediate surgival intervention in this group [15, 16].

If significant regurgitation persists with serial observation, a valve-coronary operation is undertaken. Because valve structure is essentially normal, this disorder is ideal for valve repair, and reconstruction probably should be performed in most patients [16]. In those with large posterior wall infarcts or aneurysms, a transventricular approach with posterior commissural annuloplasty, papillary muscle shortening, and infarct exclusion has been useful [14]. In the majority of patients without major wall motion defects, a transatrial Kay annuloplasty is performed

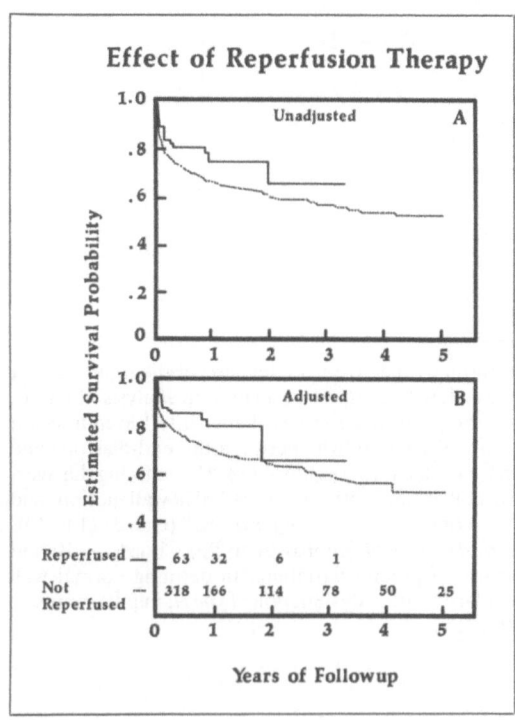

Fig. 7. Survival curves for reperfused (n = 63) vs all other patients (n = 318) with ischemic mitral regurgitation treated since 1981. Panel A represents raw unadjusted survival characteristics which were adjusted for differences in baseline characteristics (panel B) using a Cox model

[31], depending on the pathologic anatomy [16]. While retrospective comparisons are always difficult, valve repair in our experience appears to reduce operative mortality by approximately 50% [14, 15] and to significantly improve longterm survival (Fig. 8).

A difficult subgroup has been patients requiring coronary bypass for anginal symptoms with coincident moderate to severe mitral regurgitation. In recent reports, the hospital mortality for coronary bypass alone in this population has approximated 10%, which is significantly higher than for similar patients undergoing coronary revascularization without associated regurgitation [15]. Most of these patients, in general, have had moderate ventriculographic [32] regurgitation and less serious risk factors than those requiring valve procedures. The explanation for the high mortality may reflect more hemodynamically "significant" regurgitation in many patients than suspected by ventriculography. Most would agree that contrast ventriculography is not altogether accurate in defining hemodynamic regurgitant fraction [33, 34]. Although previous criteria suggested avoidance of valve procedures whenever possible, it is our current opinion that a simple Kay annuloplasty should be performed whenever a question of hemodynamic significance exists. Moreover, intraoperative valve testing, as described below, has been uniformly successful in the objective selection of patients with moderate valve dysfunction for valve procedures. Liberal application of valve repair in this subgroup based on operative valve testing with transesophageal Doppler echocardiography could reduce early complications related to residual valve dysfunction and improve longterm results [15].

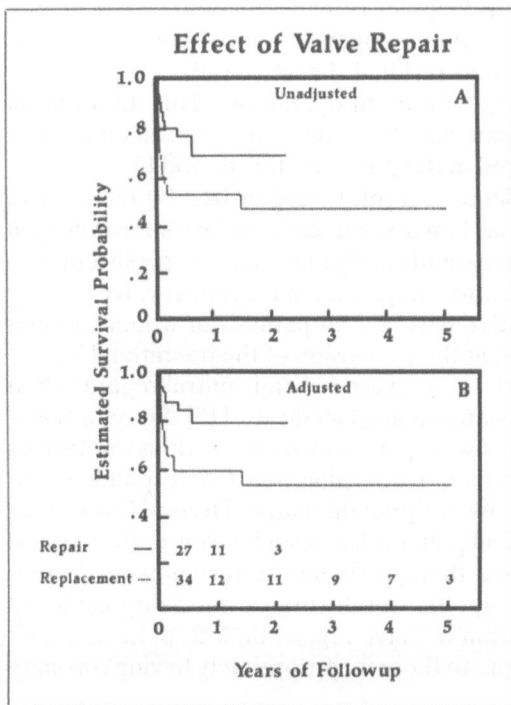

Fig. 8. Unadjusted (panel A) and adjusted (Panel B) survival curves for patients undergoing mitral valve repair (n = 27) vs valve replacement (n = 34). Adjustments for differences in baseline characteristics were accomplished with the Cox proportional hazards model

167

Information provided by transesophageal echocardiography is useful even if the patient has previously undergone both cardiac catheterization and routine chest echocardiography. In our experience, in patients undergoing mitral valve operation, findings unsuspected by preoperative evaluation, which subsequently lead to either a modification or change in the planned operation are detected in nearly 25% of all cases. Most frequently these involve an assessment of the leaflet and submitral morphology. This information is then utilized by the surgeon to decide upon the character of the repair which is most suitable. Thus, for all types of valve repair, decisions regarding the use of annuloplasty vs leaflet resection vs chordal and papillary muscle repairs can be made prior to chest incision. Furthermore, the presence of atrial thrombi or other coexistent abnormalities, such as atrial septal defects or coexistent valvular abnormalities have also been identified. A significant number of patients also have been encountered where preoperative mitral insufficiency was diagnosed by cardiac catheterization or chest echocardiography, which was then found to be insignificant when assessed by transesophageal echocardiography. In these instances, if following volume loading significant mitral insufficiency does not develop when assessed by both transesophageal echocardiography and hemodynamics, a mitral valve operation may be avoided [37].

Previous methods of assessing intraoperative competency of the repaired mitral valve have included fluid filling of the arrested ventricle, direct palpation of the left atrium for regurgitation, hemodynamic assessment using pulmonary capillary or left atrial pressures and echocardiographic assessment using agitated saline. All of these techniques have limitations in that they either create nonphysiologic conditions, are cumbersome and time consuming, or lack sensitivity. Thus, the use of transesophageal echocardiography with Doppler color flow mapping has been a significant improvement in the assessment of competency of the mitral valve following mitral repair. We have identified residual defects requiring repeat cardiopulmonary bypass in approximately 10% of all operations. This information has facilitated further immediate repair and thus, decreased the likelihood of repeat valve replacement being required in the postoperative period [37].

The importance of achieving an adequate result is emphasized by recent data indicating that patients in whom valvular function was deemed by transesophageal echocardiography to be satisfactory have significantly lower rates of persistent congestive heart failure. They also have a lower requirement for repeat valve surgery and lower mortality in the postoperative period than patients in whom valvular defects of moderate degree were noted at the conclusion of the operation [37].

Finally, 60% of patients with moderate to severe ischemic mitral regurgitation treated in our center since 1981 have been managed medically [15]. Since only 4% were rejected for operation, the majority were patients with less serious risk factors who had significant regurgitation after an acute infarction but responded well enough to initial medical therapy to allow hospital discharge. Despite less serious risk factors, longterm survival of medical patients has been inferior to the surgical group (Fig. 9), implying that operative therapy should be recommended more often in the less symptomatic subgroup. If overall surgical mortality could be reduced further by increasing application of valve repair, both to patients previously treated with valve replacement and to those inappropriately having coronary

bypass only, the difference in medical-surgical survival and the clinical utility of surgical therapy could become even more significant.

Operative approaches

As with all cardiac surgery, the quality of cardiac anesthesia is critical to patient outcome, and the current techniques employed in our center are described elsewhere [35]. The operation is performed through a median sternotomy with a transesophageal Doppler echocardiographic probe in place [36, 37]. As the incision is completed, the echocardiographer assesses the degree and location of regurgitation, as well as the functional anatomy of the mitral leaflets. In most cases, chordal or papillary muscle rupture can be identified, the exact leaflet prolapsing can be defined, and the presence of central vs lateral regurgitation can be discerned.

After aortic cannulation, a left atrial pressure line is placed, and volume loading is performed via the aortic cannula to a mean left atrial pressure of 12−15 mmHg. If hemodynamics remain stable, and minimal Doppler evidence of regurgitation exists, a conventional coronary bypass in undertaken using single venous cannulation. Conversely, if prominent V waves develop and are accompanied by significant Doppler regurgitation (Fig. 10), a mitral procedure is incorporated into the operative plan. For most mitral valve operations, individual cannulae are placed

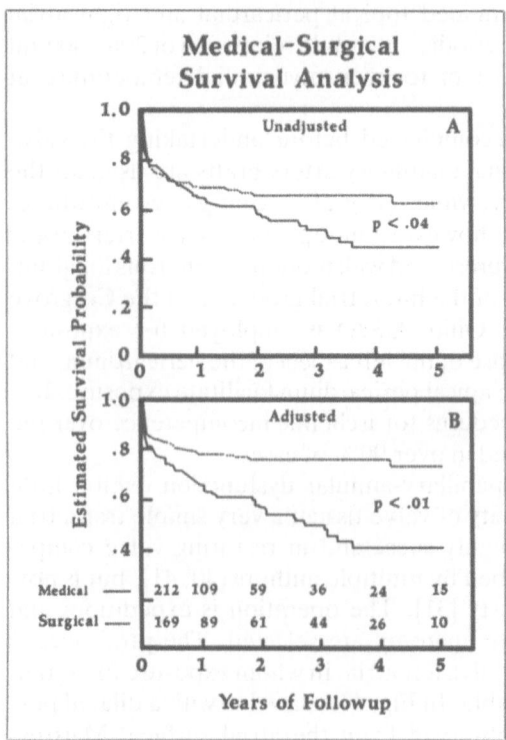

Fig. 9. Unadjusted (Panel A) and adjusted (panel B) survival characteristics for all patients receiving ultimate medical therapy (n = 212) vs surgical therapy (n = 169). Adjustments were performed with the Cox proportional hazards model

169

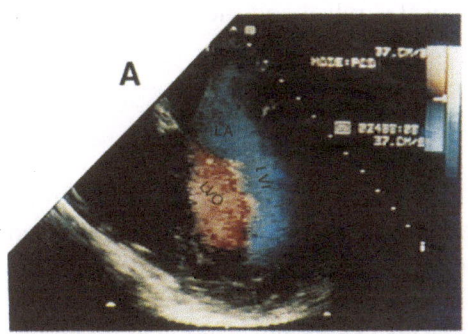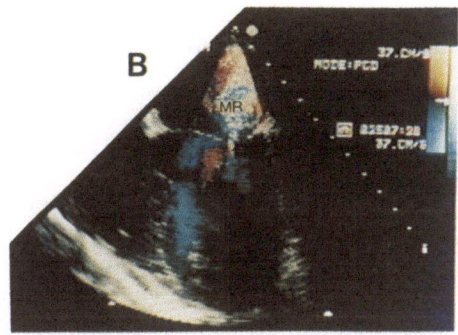

Fig. 10. Transesophageal echo/Doppler appearance of a regurgitant mitral valve in a patient with acute papillary-annular dysfunction. Panel A represents a diastolic frame and Panel B a systolic frame. Note the broad regurgitant jet in panel B.

directly into the venae cavae; however, a single right atrial cannula can be used for transventricular mitral repairs [14]. Adequacy of myocardial protection is extremely important in this subset, and this topic is reviewed elsewhere [38]. Briefly, a highly successful technique has combined 1) bicaval cannulation with occluding tapes, 2) myocardial precooling to 20°–24°C with the bypass circuit, 3) reduction in systemic flow during the arrest period to 1.0–1.5 l/min/m² with systemic hypothermia of 24°C, 4) a 1 200 ml initial antegrade crystalloid cardioplegia infusion after aortic clamping, 5) combined topical pericardial and right atrial endocardial cold saline lavage, and 6) periodic antegrade reinfusion of 200–400 ml of cardioplegia solution every 30–45 min to keep myocardial temperature at approximately 10°C.

Distal coronary anastomoses are accomplished before undertaking the valve procedure, and in most patients, internal mammary artery grafts are used for the left anterior descending coronary artery, while vein grafts are employed elsewhere. In several young patients in our series, however, multiple mammary artery grafts [39] were constructed. In patients with preserved wall motion, a generous longitudinal atriotomy is performed to the left of the interatrial groove, and the Cosgrove retractor (Kapp Surgical, Cleveland, Ohio, USA) is employed for exposure. Mobilization of both venae cavae, release of the left aspect of the pericardium, and placement of a surgical sponge into the apical pericardium facilitate exposure. In a personal series of 35 mitral valve procedures for ischemic incompetence over the past 5 years, the valve has been repaired in over 90% of cases.

Since most patients with ischemic papillary-annular dysfunction exhibit little leaflet prolapse or structural abnormality of valve tissue, a very simple transatrial lateral commissural annuloplasty is highly successful in restoring valve competence. This procedure has been described by multiple authors [40, 41], but is now commonly termed the Kay annuloplasty [31]. The operation is expeditious and effective when valves with appropriate anatomy are selected. The procedure is especially useful in patients with diminutive left atria, in whom exposure for a standard valve replacement can be formidable. In Fig. 11A, a valve with a dilated posterior annulus but little prolapse is observed from the atrial surface. Mattress

170

sutures of 3-0 polypropylens supported with Teflon felt pledgets are placed deeply into annular tissue at each commissure. The anterior bites of the annuloplasty sutures are placed into the right and left fibrous trigones, very close to the valve commissures. This maneuver leaves the anterior annulus intact as it attaches to the aortic rot and fibrous skeleton of the heart. The posterior sutures are placed at some distance from the commissures, so that the posterior annulus is selectively reduced in circumference. As with the Carpentier procedure, the posterior annulus thus is moved toward the anterior leaflet, increasing the surface area of leaflet coaptation (Fig. 11B). The echocardiographic appearance of a mitral valve after a Kay annuloplasty is shown in Fig. 12.

In the presence of a thinned-out transmural infarct or aneurysm, a transventricular approach to the mitral valve is simple and provides excellent exposure [14]. A longitudinal posterior ventriculotomy is performed to the left of the posterior descending coronary artery and toward the atrioventricular groove to avoid the bases of the papillary muscles (Fig. 13). Once the papillary muscles are identified, the incision is extended toward the apex, avoiding the papillary insertions. In most patients, a 5 cm vertical incision, placed to within 1 cm of the base, provides excellent visualization of the mitral valve and submitral apparatus. Larger incisions occasionally are necessary to resect posterior wall aneurysms.

The mitral valve leaflets and subvalvular structures are carefully inspected. In most patients, the anterior papillary muscle is single, is longer than its posterior counterpart, and has a firm consistency. In contrast, the posterior papillary apparatus usually consists of 2−3 short muscles directly arising from the posterior ventricular wall. For isolated posterior papillary-annular dysfunction, a posterior commissural annuloplasty is performed (Fig. 13, left panel), as modified from the technique of Johnson et al. [42]. A pledgetted horizontal mattress suture of 3−0

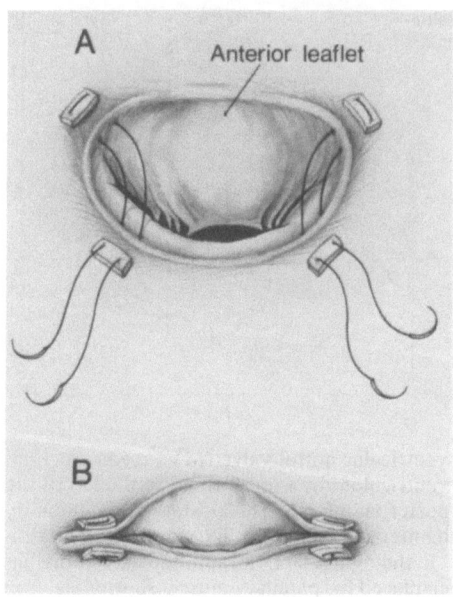

Fig. 11. Atrial view of Kay annuloplasty. See text for details

171

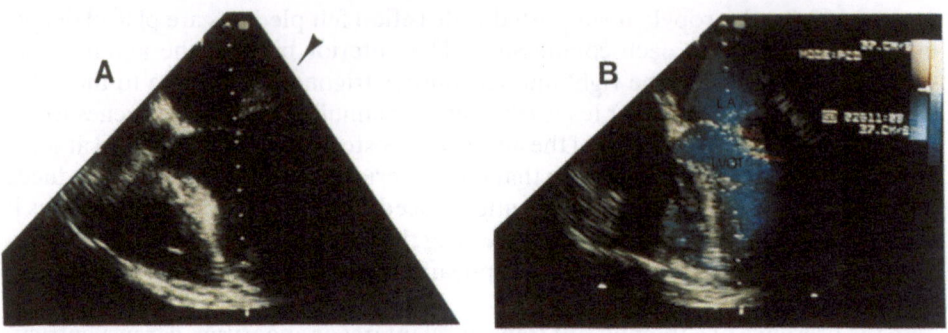

Fig. 12. Transesophageal echo/Doppler appearance of a regurgitant mitral valve after a transatrial Kay annuloplasty. Panel A is a diastolic frame and Panel B is a systolic frame. Note that regurgitation is now absent after valve repair (same patient as illustrated in Fig. 10).

polypropylene is placed deep into the valve annulus at the posterior commissure and tied firmly. It is important to obtain substantial bites of ventricular and atrial tissue with this suture, since the only failed valve repair in our series occurred when a superficially placed suture separated the valve annulus from the ventricular wall.

In most cases, the infarcted posterior papillary heads appear somewhat elongated, producing slack posterior chordae to both leaflets and a localized lateral valve prolapse. To compensate for the elongation, the papillary muscles are

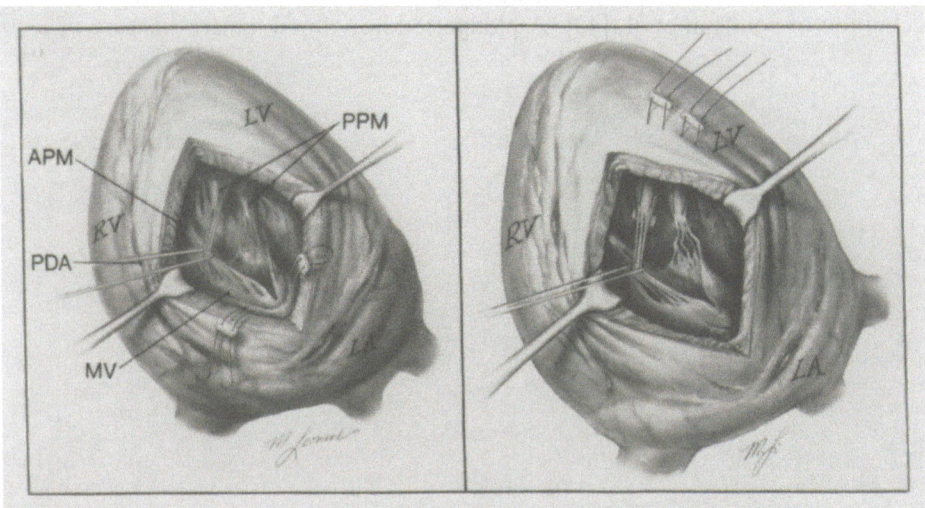

Fig. 13. Left panel represents initial steps of transventricular mitral valve (MV) reconstruction. The apex of the heart is lifted superiorly, and the ventriculotomy is performed to the left of the posterior descending artery (PDA) through the posterior infarct. The posterior annuloplasty suture is illustrated, as are the posterior (PPM) and anterior (APM) papillary muscles. The ventriculotomy is shown larger for illustrative purposes. In the right panel, the annuloplasty suture has been tied, and pledgetted mattress sutures have been placed for papillary muscle shortening

172

sutured to the ventricular wall at a slightly more apical level to prevent leaflet prolapse beyond the annular plane (Fig. 13, right panel). When pledgetted horizontal
mattress sutures are placed into a papillary muscle, the fibrous tip is utilized for at
least one of the two arms. The ventriculotomy then is closed with 4–5 large horizontal mattress sutures of No. 1 braided polyester suture buttressed with Teflon felt
strips, and over-sewn with a running No. 1 polypropylene suture for hemostasis. The
initial row of horizontal mattress sutures is placed at the margins of the infarct to
exclude the dysfunctional segment [43]. If a prominent leaflet defect is present at
the posterior commissure, the posterior valve leaflets are either closed with
pledgetted mattress sutures or the cleft is sutured directly (Fig. 14). Valve orifice
area is reduced insignificantly by this procedure, and direct leaflet closure may prevent minor residual valve leaks.

Other coincidental valve abnormalities can be corrected during transventricular
repair. If chordae to the anterior papillary muscle are elongated (Fig. 15A), a precise chordal shortening is performed by the Carpentier technique. The anterior
papillary muscle is never sutured to the ventricular wall, because of concern over
shortening the chordal apparatus too much. If a component of anterior annular
dilatation also is evident, an anterior commissural annuloplasty is performed, taking care to avoid the aortic valve by placing the cephalad sutures into the left fibrous
trigone (Fig. 15B). Coexistent rupture of minor primary chordae can be repaired
by suture transfer to adjacent secondary chordae. In patients with sustained ventricular tachycardia, electrophysiologic mapping and subendocardial resection of

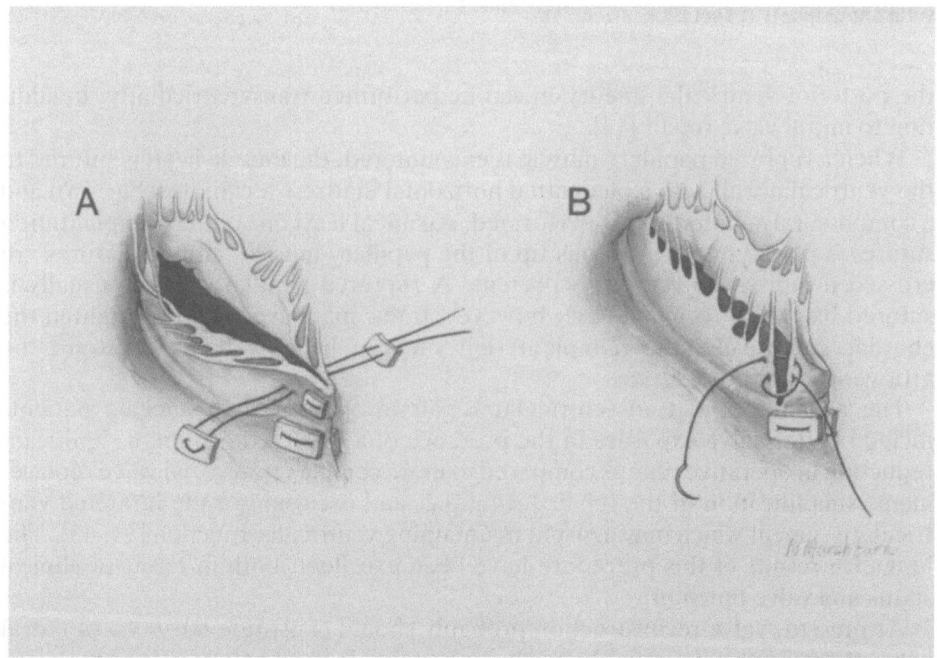

Fig. 14. Repair techniques of posterior leaflet closure when inadequate commissural leaflet tissue
is encountered. See text for detail

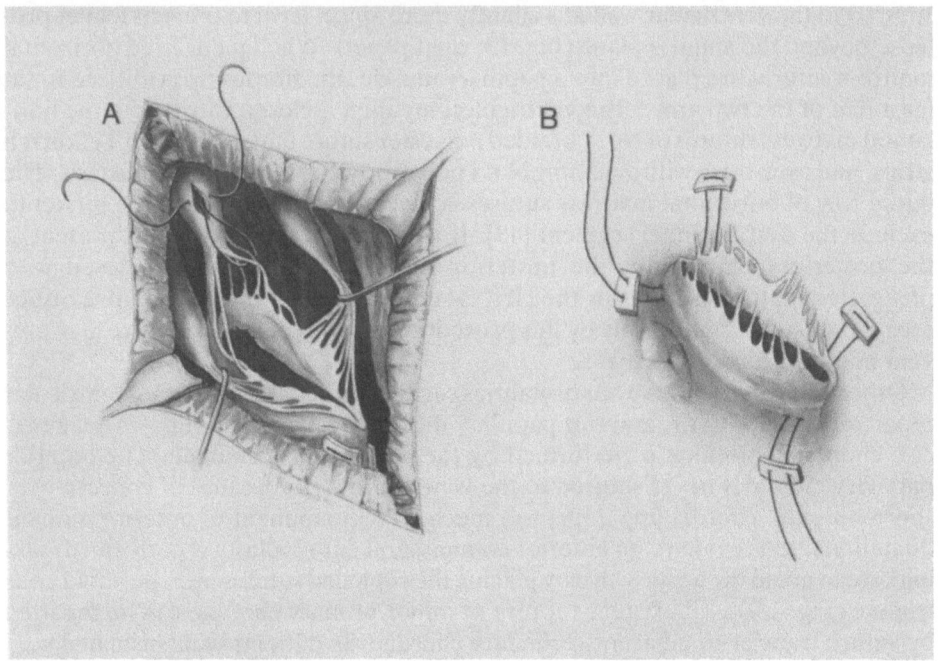

Fig. 15. A Carpentier chordal shortening procedure, as performed transventricularly for elongated anterior chordae to the central posterior leaflet (panel A), and a transventricular lateral commissural annuloplasty (panel B)

the posterior ventricular aneurysm can be performed transventricularly, in addition to mitral valve repair [14].

When a ruptured papillary muscle is encountered, the muscle head is sutured to the ventricular wall with a pledgetted horizontal mattress technique (Fig. 16), and a commissural annuloplasty is performed. Again, at least one of the reimplantation sutures is placed into the fibrous tip of the papillary muscle, and the sutures are crossed if more than one tip is present. A ruptured papillary muscle usually. is sutured back to its original base; however, if this maneuver seems to tighten the chordae excessively, the reimplantation site can be moved more toward the atrioventricular groove.

The advantages of transventricular repair in appropriately selected patients include better valve exposure in the presence of a small left atrium, a significant reduction in operative time as compared to more complex transatrial valve replacement, simplification of the repair technique, and exclusion of the infarcted ventricular segment which may assist in maintaining ventricular function [14, 43]. The longterm results of this procedure have been excellent, both in terms of clinical status and valve function.

At present, valve reconstruction probably should constitute 60–90% of mitral valve operations, but repair obviously is not possible in all patients, even with current techniques. Severely deformed valves or valves with significant primary leaflet abnormalities or associated calcification sometimes require prosthetic replacement

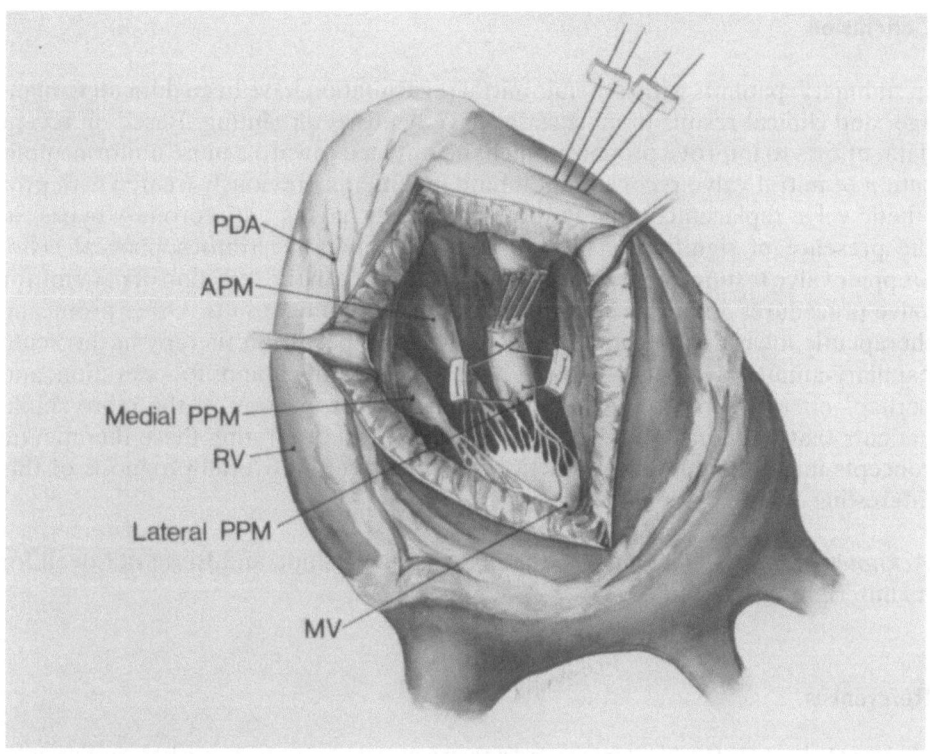

Fig. 16. Reimplantation of a ruptured lateral head of the posterior papillary muscle complex. Abbreviations are the same as for Fig. 13; see text for details

[44–46]. Several reports suggest that destruction of the mitral apparatus during valve replacement may impair left ventricular function [47–49]. This concept could account in part for suboptimal longterm results. To address this problem, techniques have been developed to preserve normal mitral-papillary continuity during prosthetic valve insertion. David described a technique in which portions of the anterior leaflet are resected but connections to the papillary muscles are maintained [50], and Cooley reported "intravalvular prosthetic insertion" of St. Jude valves. While initial results with these procedures at our center were good, one patient recently had echocardiographically demonstrated interference of St. Jude valve closure by the anterior mitral leaflet, and another had postoperative systolic anterior motion of the anterior leaflet with an asymptomatic outflow gradient. Similar findings have been reported by others [52]. For these reasons, the authors currently prefer a complete resection of the anterior mitral leaflet during most mitral valve replacements, and this procedure has been associated with minimal ventricular impairment [53]. However, the posterior mitral leaflet frequently is left intact to bolster the suture line [54, 55]. In our center, most mitral valve prostheses are inserted with interrupted pledgetted horizontal mattress techniques.

Conclusion

In summary, patients with ischemic mitral regurgitation have been difficult to manage, and clinical results in most series have been disappointing. Based on recent data, efforts to improve prognosis might be directed toward a more uniform application of mitral valve reconstruction both in patients previously treated with prosthetic valve replacement and in those previously having only coronary bypass in the presence of significant regurgitation. Intraoperative transesophageal echo/ Doppler valve testing has been an important advance in the selection of patients for valve procedures and in the assessment of hemodynamic results. Other promising therapeutic measures include the liberal use of reperfusion therapy in the acute papillary-annular dysfunction group, better selection of patients for operation, and perhaps operative recommendation to a greater proportion of the more stable patients that previously were treated medically. Incorporating these therapeutic concepts into routine clinical practice may improve the overall prognosis of this interesting disorder.

Acknowledgements: The authors thank Suzanne Yoshida and Barbara Lovell for manuscript preparation.

References

1. Van Mierop LHS (1979) Morphologic development of the heart. In: Berne RM, Sperelakis N, Geiger SR, (eds) Handbook of Physiology, Section 2: The cardiovascular system. American Physiological Society, Bethesda, Maryland
2. Roberts WC, Perloff JK (1972) Mitral valvular disease: A clinicopathologic survey of the conditions causing the mitral valve to function abnormally. Ann Int Med 77:939
3. Glover RP, Davilla JC (1961) The surgery of mitral stenosis. Grune and Stratton, New York
4. Roberts WC (1983) Morphologic features of the normal and abnormal mitral valve. Am J Cardiol 51:1005
5. Ellis FH Jr. (1967) Surgery for acquired mitral valve disease. Saunders and Company, Philadelphia
6. Perloff JK, Roberts WC (1984) The mitral apparatus: Functional anatomy of mitral regurgitation. J Thorac Cardiovasc Surg 88:663
7. Dalen JE, Alberts JS (1981) Valvular heart disease. Little, Brown, and Company, Boston
8. Yellin EL, Yoran C, Frater RWM (1984) Physiology of mitral valve flow. Chapter 4. In: Duran C, Angell WW, Johnson AD, Oury JH (eds) Recent Progress in Mitral Valve Disease. Butterworths, London
9. Yellin EL, Masatsugu H, Yoran C, Sonnenblick EH, Gabbay S, Frater RWM (1986) Left ventricular relaxation in the filling and nonfilling intact heart. Am J Physiol 250:H620
10. Bellhouse BJ (1972) The fluid mechanics of heart valves. Chapter 8. In: Bergel DH (ed) Cardiovascular fluid dynamics. Academic Press, London New York
11. Weiting DW, Stripling TE (1984) Dynamics and fluid dynamics of the mitral valve. In: Duran D, Angell WW, Johnson AD, Oury JH (eds) Recent progress in mitral valve disease. Butterworths, London
12. Shah PM, Tei C (1984) Functional anatomy of the mitral valve and annulus in man: Lessons from echocardiographic observations. Chapter 6. In: Duran C, Angell WW, Johnson AD, Oury JH (eds) Recent progress in mitral valve disease. Butterworths, London
13. Hagl S, Heimisch W, Meisner H, Mendler N, Sebening F (1984) In-situ function of the papillary muscles in the intact canine left ventricle. Chapter 32. In: Duran C, Angell WW, Johnson AD, Oury JH (eds) Recent progress in mitral valve disease. Butterworths, London

14. Rankin JS, Feneley MP, Hickey MStJ, Muhlbaier LH, et al. (1988) A clinical comparison of mitral valve repair versus valve replacement in ischemic mitral regurgitation. J Thorac Cardiovasc Surg 95:165
15. Hickey MStJ, Smith LR, Muhlbaier LH, Harrell F Jr, Reves JG, Hinohara T, Califf RM, Pryor DB, Rankin JS (1988) Current prognosis of ischemic mitral regurgitation: Implications for future management. Circulation [Suppl I] 78:I−51
16. Rankin JS, Hickey MStJ, Smith LR, deBruijn NP, Clements FM, Muhlbaier LH, Lowe JE, Wechsler AS, Califf RM, Reves JG, Wolfe WG (1988) Current management of mitral valve incompetence associated with coronary artery disease. J Cardiac Surg (in press)
17. DiSesa VJ, Cohn LH, Collins JJ Jr, Koster JK, VanDevanter S (1982) Determinants of operative survival following combined mitral valve replacement and coronary revascularization. Ann Thorac Surg 34:484
18. Tepe NA, Edmunds LH Jr (1985) Operation for acute postinfarction mitral insufficiency and cardiogenic shock. J Thorac Cardiovasc Surg 89:525
19. Gerbode FLA, Hetzer R, Krebber HJ (1978) Surgical management of papillary muscle rupture due to myocardial infarction. World J Surg 2:791
20. Merin G, Giulani ER, Pluth JR, Wallace RB, Danielson GK (1973) Surgery for mitral valve incompetence after myocardial infarction. Am J Cardiol 32:322
21. Killen DA, Reed WA, Wathanacharoen S, Beauchamp G, Rutherford B (1983) Surgical treatment of papillary muscle rupture. Ann Thorac Surg 35:243
22. Clements SD, Story WE, Hurst JW, Craver JM, Jones EL (1985) Ruptured papillary muscle, a complication of myocardial infarction: Clinical presentation, diagnosis, and treatment. Clin Cardiol 8:93
23. Nishimura RA, Schaff HV, Shub C, Gersh BJ, Edwards WD, Tajik AJ (1983) Papillary muscle rupture complicating acute myocardial infraction: Analysis of 17 patients. Am J Cardiol 51:373
24. Gula G, Yacoub MH (1981) Surgical correction of complete rupture of the anterior papillary muscle. Ann Thorac Surg 32:88
25. Carpentier A, Didier L, Deloche A, Perier P (1987) Surgical anatomy and management of ischemic mitral valve incompetence. Circulation 76 [Suppl IV]:1776
26. Cosgrove DM (1987) Valve reconstruction versus valve replacement. In: Crawford FA Jr (ed) Cardiac surgery: Current heart valve prostheses. Cardiac Surgery: State of the Art Reviews, Vol. 1, No. 2. Hanley & Belfus, Philadelphia
27. Najafi H, Hushang J, Hunter JA, Goldin MD, Serry C, Dye WS (1975): Mitral insufficiency secondary to coronary heart disease. Ann Thorac Surg 20:529
28. Radford MJ, Johnson RA, Buckley MJ, Daggett WM, Leinbach RC, Gold HK (1979) Survival following mitral valve replacement for mitral regurgitation due to coronary artery disease. Circulation 60 [Suppl I]:I−39
29. Reinfeld HB, Samet P, Hildner FJ (1985) Resolution of congestive failure, mitral regurgitation, and angina after percutaneous transluminal coronary angioplasty of triple vessel disease. Cath Cardiovasc Diagn 11:273
30. Heuser RR, Maddoux GL, Goss JE, Ramo BW, Raff GL, Shadoff N (1987) Coronary angioplasty for acute mitral regurgitation due to myocardial infarction. Ann Int Med 107:852
31. Kay GL, Kay JH, Zubiate P, Yokoyama T, Mendez M (1986) Mitral valve repair for mitral regurgitation secondary to coronary artery disease. Circulation 74 [Suppl I]:I−88
32. Connolly MW, Gelbfish JS, Jacobwitz IJ, Rose DM, Mendelsohn A, Cappabianca PM, Acinapura AJ, Cunningham JN Jr (1986) Surgical results for mitral regurgitation from coronary artery disease. J Thorac Cardiovasc Surg 91:379
33. Rokey R, Sterling LL, Zoghbi WA, Sartori MP, Limacher MC, Kuo LC, Quinones MA (1986) Determination of regurgitant fraction in isolated mitral or aortic regurgitation by pulsed Doppler two-dimensional echocardiography. J Am Coll Cardiol 7:1273
34. Lopez JF, Hanson S, Orchard RC, Tan L (1985) Quantification of mitral valvular incompetence. Cath Cardiovasc Diag 11:39
35. Lell WA, Reves JG, Samuelson PN (1986) Anesthesia for cardiac surgery. In: Kirklin JW (ed) Cardiac surgery. Wiley Medical Publishers, New York, pp 109−138
36. DeBruijn NP, Clements FM, Kisslo JA (1987) Applications of color flow imaging. Echocardiography 4:557
37. Sheikh KH, deBruijn N, Rankin JS, Stanley T, Clements F, Wolfe W, Kisslo J (1989) Utility

of transesophageal echocardiography in patients undergoing cardiac valve surgery. J Am Coll Cardiol (in press)

38. Rankin JS, Sabiston DC Jr (1989) Physiology of the coronary circulation, myocardial function, and intraoperative myocardial protection. In: Sabiston DC Jr, Spencer FC (eds) Gibbon's surgery of the chest. Saunders, Philadelphia
39. Rankin JS, Newman GE, Bashore TN, Muhlbaier LH, Tyson GS, Ferguson TB Jr, Sabiston DC Jr (1986) Clinical and angiographic assessment of complex mammary artery bypass grafting. J Thorac Cardiovasc Surg 92:832
40. Wooler GH, Nixon PG, Grimshaw VA, Watson DA (1962) Experience with the repair of the mitral valve in mitral incompetence. Thorax 17:49
41. Reed GE, Pooley RW, Moggio RA (1980) Durability of measured mitral annuloplasty — seventeen year study. J Thorac Cardiovasc Surg 79:321
42. Johnson WD, Pedraza PM, Kayser KL (1984) Preservation and restoration of the mitral mechanism during inferior wall aneurysmectomy. In: Duran CMG, Angell WW, Johnson AD, Oury JH (eds) Recent progress in mitral valve disease, Butterworths, London
43. Rankin JS, Newman GE, Muhlbaier LH, Behar VS, Fedor JM, Sabiston DC Jr (1985) The effects of coronary revascularization on left ventricular function in ischemic heart disease. J Thorac Cardiovasc Surg 90:818
44. Carpentier A (1983) Cardiac valve surgery — the "French correction." J Thorac Cardiovasc Surg 86:323
45. Lessana A, Escorsin M, Romano M, Andes F, Vergoni W, Lorenzoni D, Menozzi C, Monducci I (1985) Transposition of posterior leaflet for treatment of ruptured main chordae of the anterior mitral leaflet. J Thorac Cardiovasc Surg 89:804
46. Dawkins K, Paneth M (1986) Mitral repair versus replacement [letter]. J Thorac Cardiovasc Surg 91:150
47. Bonchek LI, Olinger GN, Siegel R, Trensch DD, Keelan MH Jr (1984) Left ventricular performance after mitral reconstruction for mitral regurgitation. J Thorac Cardiovasc Surg 88:122
48. Hansen DE, Cahill PD, Derby GC, Miller DC (1987) Relative contributions of the anterior and posterior mitral chordae tendineae to canine global left ventricular systolic function. J Thorac Cardiovasc Surg 93:45
49. David TE, Ho WC (1986) The effect of preservation of chordae tendineae on mitral valve replacement for postinfarction mitral regurgitation. Circulation 74 [Suppl I]:I−116
50. David TE (1986) Mitral valve replacement with preservation of chordae tendineae: rationale and technical considerations. Ann Thorac Surg 41:680
51. Cooley DA, Ingram MT (1987) Intravalvular implantation of mitral valve prostheses. Tex Heart Inst J 14:188
52. Come PC, Riley MF, Weintraub RM, Wei JY, Markis JE, Lorell BH (1987) Dynamic left ventricular outflow tract obstruction when the anterior leaflet is retained at prosthetic mitral valve replacement. Ann Thorac Surg 43:561
53. Harpole DH, Rankin JS, Wolfe WG, Smith LR, Young WR, Clements FM, Jones RH: Assessment of left ventricular functional preservation during isolated cardiac valvular operations. Circulation 80 (Suppl III): (In press)
54. Cohn LH: The surgical treatment of valvular heart disease. In: Gay WA Jr (ed), Cardiovascular surgery, Chapter 18 Harper & Row, Philadelphia
55. Spencer FC, Galloway AC, Colvin SB (1985) A clinical evaluation of the hypothesis that rupture of the left ventricle following mitral valve replacement can be prevented by preservation of the chordae of the mural leaflet. Ann Surg 202:673

Author's address:
J. Scott Rankin, M.D.
Department of Surgery
Box 38 51
Duke University Medical Center
Durham, North Carolina 27710
USA

Surgical treatment of ischemic mitral regurgitation by repair and replacement

L. H. Cohn

Division of Cardiac Surgery, Harvard Medical School, Brigham and Women's Hospital, Boston, Massachusetts, USA

Introduction

The combination of mitral regurgitation and coronary artery disease presents a most significant challenge to the cardiac surgeon. Over the years this entity has the highest operative risk of any of the commonplace, acquired cardiac lesions treated surgically. Previous results from our clinic and others have documented relatively high operative mortality rates due to the urgency of the presentation, the extremely precarious myocardial function, severe triple-vessel coronary disease and prolonged operative insult, or a combination of all four of these factors [3, 7, 8, 10, 14, 16, 18]. Superimposed on a scenario of congestive failure due to severe valvular regurgitation is an often compromised ventricle derived from factors normally related to mitral regurgitation. In addition, the lack of deliverance of appropriate blood supply to these areas may be further complicated by a previous myocardial infarction and scarring. Many reported series have indicated an operative risk of 12−20% using valve replacement alone.

Never concepts in the surgical treatment of mitral valve disease have stimulated the critical evaluation of reparative methods as opposed to replacement methods for the oblation of mitral regurgitation in patients with ischemic mitral regurgitation. Presented here are some of the pathophysiologic features of the ventricle in ischemic mitral regurgitation, suggesting that reparative procedures preserving the papillary muscles' occular continuity are more important than originally believed. We have briefly reviewed some patients who had mitral valve replacement and repair for coronary artery disease and have summarized some of the current thinking in the approach to this challenging problem.

Pathophysiology

The mechanisms in patients with coronary heart disease or ischemic heart disease of mitral regurgitation are several. Mitral regurgitation may be transitory, occurring primarily with episodes of myocardial ischemia which clinically may be represented by angina and shortness of breath. It is clear that when acute ischemia occurs, there is initially left ventricular dysfunction, increase in left ventricular size, and often times transitory mitral regurgitation due to dilatation of the annulus. Patients with this syndrome may have a systolic murmur only during these periods of ischemia. These phenomena will usually subside when ischemia abates. Coro-

179

nary revascularization, either by coronary bypass graft or angioplasty, should relieve this permanently without any mitral valve operation [2].

A second variety is papillary muscle dysfunction where there may have been scarring and chronic changes in the papillary muscles so that the papillary muscle does not perform normally during valve opening and closing. In these patients there is persistent mitral regurgitation which progresses because of significant secondary valvular changes as well, i.e., rolled edges with leaflet contraction, thickening, etc.

A third type is the ruptured chordae tendenae which may often be a result of the ischemic process, although in our experiences it seems to be more commonly associated with myxomatous degeneration of the valve. In fact in our 139 cases of mitral valve repair that we have done in the past 4 years, mitral valve prolapse and myxomatous degeneration is, by far, the most common diagnosis, representing about 60% of all patients undergoing mitral valve repair at our center. This may theoretically be due to an ischemic process, i.e., a very small micro-vascular problem associated with this, or it may simple be a "wearing out" of the valve. In those with an ischemic etiology, the ruptured chord would be in association with one or more coronary artery lesions; most commonly seen in the posterior leaflet, this may also be seen in any portion of the mitral valve. These patients have a loud systolic murmur and present with longstanding mitral regurgitation with an increasing ventricular volume size both systole and diastole requiring surgery, often times in the absence of symptoms. Acute chordal rupture may rarely present with severe congestive symptoms but to a much less marked degree than if a whole papillary muscle is infarcted.

The most flagrant pathophysiologic manifestation of ischemic heart disease and mitral regurgitation is that of the ruptured papillary muscle. In this situation there has been frank infraction of the papillary muscle with usually severance of one or both heads of a muscle from actual necrosis from an occluded coronary artery. The papillary muscle controls chordae tendenea to both anterior and posterior leaflet. A removal of the stabilization of these two leaflets by one head of the papillary muscles is a profound insult resulting in an immediate flooding of the pulmonary system retrograde because of this enormous regurgitant flow. When this occurs in a setting of a normal pulmonary vasculature it promotes immediate profound pulmonary edema, cardiogenic shock, and it requires balloon counterpulsation insertion for hemodynamic stabilization and immediate mitral valve surgery. A rare combined cause of ischemic mitral regurgitation occurs in patients who have suffered a severe myocardial infarction in the past of the inferior left ventricle causing left ventricle aneurysm, ventricular septal defect, and a papillary muscle dysfunction.

Finally, there is an association, of course, of patients who have other etiologies of mitral regurgitation such as endocarditis or myxomatous degeneration or even congenital abnormalities where co-existant coronary artery disease may arise independently and be a part of this patient's pathophysiology requiring concommitant coronary bypass surgery. It is the policy at our center to evaluate the coronary arteries angiographically in every patient over the age of 40 who is to undergo valve surgery. There is often a significant number of coronary lesions detected angiographically that require concommitant bypass grafting at the time of surgery. The incidence of concommitant coronary bypass and other etiology varies considerably but in a recent review of our total experience with myxomatous degeneration of the mitral valve and reparative procedures, approximately 10% of those patients require concommitant coronary bypass.

It is of interest to note that a predominant pathology in mitral valve regurgitation varies considerably with the geographic location. As stated, prolapse and myxomatous degeneration, particularly in the aging population, is the most common diagnosis in our series of mitral valve repairs [6]. In other areas of the U.S.A., ischemic mitral regurgitation is the most commonly found etiology of mitral regurgitation and in other countries, particularly developing ones, rheumatic activity is by far the most common diagnosis. There is overlap of these pathologic entities so that sometimes classification may be somewhat difficult in terms of a pure singular valvular etiology.

Clinical materials and methods

Since 1972, over 1500 mitral valve operations have been carried out at our center for a variety of etiologies and with a variety of different operative procedures. Porcine valve replacement has been a mainstay of our valve replacement therapy since 1972 [4]. For mechanical valves we first used the standard Bjork-Shiley valve for prosthetic mitral valve replacement (1972–1983) [4] and most recently (1983–1988) our prosthetic valve of choice has been the St. Jude bileaflet valve.

For mitral stenosis our treatment of choice in the appropriate valve which was not extensively calcified has been open mitral valvuloplasty [5] which has been accomplished in about 200 patients so far. As more aggressive decalcification techniques were attempted, there has been a higher rate of reoperation in this mitral stenosis group. Currently, with the advent of successful balloon mitral valvuloplasty for compliant non-calcified valves, there have been fewer patients with this diagnosis coming to surgical correction.

Since March, 1984, a concerted effort to perform mitral valve repair rather than replacement has been carried out for patients with primary mitral regurgitation. From March, 1984 to November, 1988, 524 consecutive mitral valve operations have been performed; 274 replacements; 247 repairs. Since November, 1988, 139 repairs have been carried out for primary mitral regurgitation. The etiology of these cases is noted in Table 1. The highest percentage of cases were myxomatous degeneration. In Table 2 is a summary of data in ischemic mitral regurgitation

Table 1.

Etiology	Number of operations	Number of reoperations
Prolapse	78	8
Ischemia	34	5
Rheumatic	19	–
Endocarditis	8	–
	139	13 (10%)

Table 2. Surgical Results

	Ischemic MR
Total:	34
M/F:	25/9
Age:	47−79, 64
CABG:	100%
	1−5, 2.8
Op death:	2/34
late death:	5
reoperation:	5
LTFU:	0
FU time:	30 months

patients. 34 patients have had chronic mitral regurgitation on an ischemic basis who have undergone repair; mean age is 64 years with a range of 47−79 years. All patients in this group were functional Class III or IV and all received at least one coronary artery bypass graft [2, 8].

The indications for mitral valve surgery were volume overload, as detected by two-dimensional echocardiography studies with serial changes, indicating diastolic and systolic volume overload and annular dilatation, acute presentation with congestive failure secondary to papillary muscle infarction, mitral regurgitation from papillary muscle dysfunction, or a combination of the above with ruptured chordae. No patient with ruptured papillary muscle has been repaired − only replaced.

Operative techniques

The operative techniques for mitral valve repair or replacement vary with pathology. As indicated, there are multiple etiologies of mitral regurgitation and each must deal with a specific anatomic technique. For mitral valve replacement, we believe that the preservation of the papillary muscle structure, where possible, is very important. Work from the experimental laboratory and from the clinic worldwide [9, 12, 21] has suggested that the original concepts by Lillehei [15] were correct: Preservation of the eliptical shape of the ventricle is important particularly in patients with mitral regurgitation in order to sustain the normal cardiac output through longterm results. Thus in mitral valve replacement, we may often insert a bioprosthetic valve into a valve which is left completely in place in terms of its anterior or posterior attachments to both the anterior and posterior leaflets. This can be done safely with a porcine bioprosthetic valve since the leaflets are protected by the stent and stent post. There are techniques to do this with prosthetic valves, such as the St. Jude valve, but extreme care must be taken so that subvalvular tissue does not interfere with the motion of the leaflets. This is even more important in patients in whom a single tilting leaflet valve such as the monostrut Bjork-Shiley or Medtronic-Hall valve is inserted. Orientation of the prostheses and careful suturing techniques must be meticulously performed.

182

For bioprosthetic valves we generally use a ventricular to atrial non-everting stitch. This is quite easily done with the bioprosthetic valve because of the stent in post flow is essential and thus no interference with valve leaflet function would be anticipated. This can also be done with a Starr-Edwards ball valve which is the only other valve that has central flow and where the poppit mechanism is protected by a cage.

The re-suturing of a ruptured papillary muscle head recently has been advocated by Rankin et al. [19]. This technique requires a good bit of fortitude since the papillary muscle itself may be necrotic. But innovative techniques either by suturing the papillary muscle to the free wall of the left ventricle or re-approximating it to the papillary muscle from which it was transected is possible, given that much work with the papillary muscle is now being done with the reconstructive procedures and mitral valve surgery in general. In our clinic, ruptured papillary muscle has been an indication for a mitral valve replacement. Few patients are sicker than these people who have immediate flooding of their lungs from massive pulmonary edema. Again, trying to preserve as much valve papillary muscle continuity as possible, we believe that valve replacement, at least at this time until the long-term results of these very bold reparative techniques of ruptured papillary muscles are known is the treatment of choice.

For other types of ischemic mitral valve regurgitation, reparative procedures are utilized whenever possible. The common technique includes a resection of a leaflet area when chordal rupture has occurred and suture repair of the leaflet. We have begun using a running suture for this technique and feel that it has significant advantages. In several patients with only annular dilatation we have simply placed the rigid Carpentier-Edwards annuloplasty ring. In patients who have a fixed dilated annulus as a result of chronic ventricular dilatation producing mitral regurgitation on an ischemic basis simply stabilizing the annulus with CABG ablates the MR. In many of our other repairs, however, particularly in the mitral valve prolapse where there is a hugely dilated annulus, we have generally preferred the Duran completely flexible annuloplasty ring. In some instances where the valve is extremely fragile and the pathology is very localized, simple resection and suture of the valve leaflet may be possible with no implantation of the annulo-plasty ring as originally suggested by McGoon et al. [17]. Residual MR is checked by filling the LV via the trans-aortic vent site. Echo-Doppler is the "gold" standard, but the patient is unclamped and off bypass when evaluated [11].

All patients are operated upon with cardiopulmonary bypass with cold potassium cardioplegia with an increasing number utilizing blood cardioplegia for this very high-risk group of patients, particularly in emergency situations and re-operations. Post-operative monitoring includes pulmonary artery catheter for measurement of cardiac output by thermo dilution, left atrial and right atrial catheters and right atrial and right ventricular pacing wires. Careful monitoring is needed in these patients for maximum flexibility of maintenance and manipulation of cardiac output in the postoperative period. Prosthetic valve replacements are maintained on long-term anticoagulation at 50% above normal as is any patient with a valve ring who has undergone repair who is in atrial fibrillation. Patients with bioprosthetic valves are weaned off coumandin if the patients are in sinus rhythm at 6 weeks, and patients who have a prosthetic annuloplasty ring who are in normal sinus rhythm are maintained on one aspirin per day. All patients undergo 2D-color-Doppler echo prior to discharge from hospital. All patients are seen annually for follow-up with echocardiology.

Clinical results

Overall results of both MV repair and replacement for MR and ischemic MR have improved. In a recent report of our results at the Society of Thoracic Surgery [6], four of 64 patients (6.2%) undergoing concommitant bypass grafting and mitral valve operation died, whereas only one of 76 patients (1.3%) not undergoing coronary bypass grafting with either valve replacement or repair died in the perioperative period.

In Table 2 are summarized clinical data in 34 patients operated upon for ischemic mitral regurgitation with CABG and mitral valve repair. The late postoperative mortality was 5/34 in the ischemic MR group. It was apparent in evaluation of all patients with mitral regurgitation and, particularly, in the individuals undergoing repair or replacement for ischemic disease that patients with a valve replacement, regardless of whether some element of the valve is preserved for maintenance of papillary muscle and annular continuity, did not do as well in long-term survival. Patients with valve replacements tend to die more commonly of congestive failure and cardiac related events than do patients undergoing mitral valve repair although this tends to be masked in patients requiring concomitant CABG. Thromboembolism has not been seen in valve repair patients but has been noted in varying degrees in patients who had either a St. Jude or porcine valve series. While thromboembolism rates are considerably better with the hemodynamically superior valves such as the St. Jude and the porcine valve, the rates are still higher than for patients who have had a valve ring or other reparative procedure. And anticoagulant levels are much lower because of the better hemodynamics of the prosthetic valves and the rings, and the incidence of anticoagulant hemorrhage has decreased substantially. Comadin levels have been maintained no higher than 50% above control in those in chronic atrial fibrillation. Reoperations have not occurred in the valve replacement group, but in the valve repair group there were five reoperations in the ischemic group due to either residual or new MR. There have been 13/139 (10%) reoperations in our overall mitral repair group. These usually occur within the first 6 months and may not be related to the repair procedure but to a developed new pathology. Therefore, a learning curve is the rule rather than the exception.

Discussion

Reparative surgery for ischemic mitral valve disease is in a state of flux at the present time. We still do not have enough evidence of long-term results of the varied operations that are performed, but present results are encouraging. There is the perception that ventricular function is much better following reparative procedures because of the papillary muscles annular continuity. In addition, any valve replacement device has some morbidity associated with it whether it be bileaflet, tilting

184

Table 3.

Author	Patients		Graft/ot.		Op mort		Reoperation	
	rep	repl	rep	repl	rep	repl	rep	repl
Angell[1]	112	72	1.4	1.9	6(5%)	13(18%)	9(8%)	0
Cohn[6]	75	65	2.7	2.0	3(4%)	2(3%)	6(8%)	0
Rankin[19]	23	32	3.0	2.2	6(26%)	17(53%)	–	–
(all acute)								
Sand[20]	101	389	–	–	5(5%)	32(8%)	7(7%)	25(6%)

rep = repair
repl = replacement

disc, or bioprosthetic [4]. With a competent mitral valve repair the elipsoid character of the left ventricle is maintained and improved cardiac output is usually achieved post-operatively. With improved cardiac output comes improved functional class, decreased thromboembolism, and improved quality of life.

Table 3 shows results of mitral valve replacement and mitral valve repair for ischemic and non-ischemic mitral regurgitation in a variety of series worldwide. The results are striking for decreased long-term morbidity and mortality in patients undergoing reparative procedures.

As we understand more about the pathophysiologic mechansims of the papillary muscle and the mitral valve and the left ventricular performance before and after various mitral valve procedures, we will develop a better understanding of the technical requirements for mitral valve repair and replacement and the results in this very high risk group will be consistently improved.

References

1. Angell WW, Oury JH, Shah P (1987) A comparison of replacement and reconstruction in patients with mitral regurgitation. J Thorac Cardiovasc Surg 93:665–674
2. Arcidi JM, Hebeler RF, Craver JM, Jones EL, Hatcher CR, Guyton RA (1988) Treatment of moderate mitral regurgitation and coronary disease by coronary bypass alone. J Thorac Cardiovasc 95:951–959
3. Cohn LH (1985) Mitral valve surgery: reconstruction versus replacement. Z Kardiol [Suppl 6] 74:1–5
4. Cohn LH, Allred EN, Cohn LA, Austin JC, Sabik J, DiSesa VJ, Shemin RJ, Collins JJ (1985) Early and late risk of mitral valve replacement. J Thorac Cardiovasc 90:872–881
5. Cohn LH, Allred EN, Cohn LA, DiSesa VJ, Shemin RJ, Collins JJ Jr (1985) Long term results of open mitral valve reconstruction for mitral stenosis. Am J Cardiol 55:371–374
6. Cohn LH, Kowalker W, Bhatia S, DiSesa VJ, Shemin RJ, Collins JJ (1988) Comparative morbidity of mitral valve repair versus replacement for mitral regurgitation with and without coronary artery disease. Ann Thorac Surg 45:284–290
7. Connolly MW, Gelbfish MW, Jacobowitz IJ, Rose DM, Mendelsohn A, Cappabianca PM, Acinapura AJ, Cunningham JN (1986) Surgical results for mitral regurgitation from coronary artery disease. J Thorac Cardiovasc Surg 91:379–388
8. Czer LS, Gray RJ, DeRobertis MA, Bateman TM, Steward ME, Chaux A, Matloff JM (1984) Mitral valve replacement: impact of coronary artery disease and determinants of prognosis after revascularization. Circulation [Suppl I] 70:I-198
9. Davis TE, Uden PE, Straus HS (1983) The importance of the mitral apparatus in left ventricular function after correction of mitral regurgitation. Circulation 68(III):71–82

10. DiSesa VJ, Cohn LH, Collins JJ Jr, Koster JK Jr, Van Devater SH (1982) Determinants of operative survival following combined mitral valve replacement and coronary revascularization. Ann Thorac Surg 34:482−489
11. Goldman ME, Mora F, Guarino T, Fuster V, Mindich BP (1987) Mitral valvuloplasty is superior to valve replacement for preservation of left ventricular function: an intraoperative two-dimensional echocardiographic study. JACC 10:568−575
12. Goor AD, Mohr R, Lavee J, Serraf A, Smolinsky A (1988) Preservation of the posterior leaflet during mechanical valve replacement for ischemic mitral regurgitation and complete myocardial revascularization. J Thorac Cardiovasc Surg 96:253−260
13. Harold JG, Bateman TM, Czer LSC, Chaux A, Matloff JM, Gray RJ (1987) Mitral valve replacement early after myocardial infarction: attendant high risk of left ventricular rupture. JACC 9:277−282
14. Kay PH, Nunley DL, Grunkemeier GL, Pinson CW, Starr A (1985) Late results of combined mitral valve replacement and coronary bypass surgery. J Am Coll Cardiol 5:29−33
15. Lillehei CW, Levy MJ, Bonnabeau RC (1964) Mitral valve replacement with preservation of papillary muscles and chordae tendineae. J Thorac Cardiovasc Surg 47:532
16. Lytle BW, Cosgrove DM, Gill CC, Stewart RW, Golding LAR, Goormastic M, Taylor PC, Loop FD (1985) Mitral valve replacement combined with myocardial revascularization: early and late results for 300 patients, 1970 to 1983. Circulation 71:1179−1190
17. McGoon DC (1960) Repair of mitral insufficiency due to ruptured chordae tendinae. JTCVS 39:357−361
18. Magovern JA, Pennock JL, Campbell DB, Pierce WS, Waldhausen JA (1985) Risks of mitral valve replacement and mitral valve replacement with coronary artery bypass. Ann Thorac Surg 39:346−352
19. Rankin JS, Feneley MP, Hickey M St.J, Muhlbaier LH, Weschsler AS, Floyd RD, Reves JG, Skelton TN, Califf RM, Lowe JE, Sabiston DC (1988) A clinical comparison of mitral valve repair versus valve replacement in ischemic mitral regurgitation. J Thorac Cardiovasc Surg 95:165−177
20. Sand ME, Naftel DC, Blackstone EH, Kirklin JW, Karp RB (1987) A comparison of repair and replacement for mitral valve incompetence. J Thorac Cardiovasc Surg 94:208−219
21. Sarris GE, Cahill PD, Hansen DE, Derby GC, Miller DC, Handen CE, McConnel MV, Niczyporuk M, Williams CA (1988) Restoration of left ventricular systolic performance after reattachment of the mitral chordae tendineae. J Thorac Cardiovasc Surg 95:969−979

Author's address:
Lawrence H. Cohn, M.D.
Chief, Division of Cardiac Surgery
Brigham and Women's Hospital
75 Francis Street
Boston, MA 02115
USA

Surgical results with severe ischemic mitral regurgitation

J. S. Swanson, A. Starr

Division of Cardiopulmonary Surgery, The Oregon Health Sciences University, Heart Institute at St. Vincent Hospital and Medical Center, Portland, Oregon, USA

Introduction

In a previous paper [16] we reviewed our operative experience with ischemic mitral regurgitation (IMR) and compared the entire group of regurgitant ischemic patients with a control population who underwent coronary artery bypass and had no mitral regurgitation (MR). Significant differences in these two populations were noted. Mean age was older for those with IMR (63 years vs 58 years for the non-regurgitant group). Similarly, the IMR group had a higher incidence of prior myocardial infarction (MI) (56% vs 43%), more patients with acute MI (17% vs 6%), more cardiomegaly (31% vs 5%) and more left heart failure (42% vs 6%) than the control population. Arteriographic evaluation also indicated more severe disease in the patients with IMR than those without mitral incompetence. The mean number of diseased vessels was 3.3 as compared to 2.6 and the percentage of occluded vessels and presence of wall motion abnormalities was all greater in those patients with IMR.

Furthermore, when wall motion score was evaluated by the CASS method [12], fully 40% of the patients with IMR were noted to have moderate to severe ventricular dysfunction as indicated by a wall motion score of greater than 10.

The patients in the IMR group were stratified according to the degree of regurgitation: mild, moderate, and severe. In this earlier study, coronary bypass alone was performed in all patients with mild IMR and two-thirds of those with moderate IMR. In contrast, nearly all patients with severe IMR underwent mitral valve surgery in addition to coronary artery bypass.

When operative mortality was evaluated it was noted to be strongly related to the severity of regurgitation. Those patients in the control group who had no MR had an operative mortality of only 2%. Among the population with IMR however, the mortality was 4%, 10%, and 38% in the groups with mild, moderate, and severe regurgitation, respectively. The prognostic significance of the degree of regurgitation has been confirmed elsewhere [3]. Other significant predictors of operative mortality were: cardiogenic shock, cardiomegaly, left heart failure, and acute MI.

Similarly, long-term survival was seen to be significantly decreased in the group with IMR as compared to the non-regurgitant coronary population. Once again, severity of mitral regurgitation was the strongest negative influence on long-term survival. As with operative mortality, cardiogenic shock, cardiomegaly, heart failure, and acute MI were all seen to prejudice long-term survival. Additionally, a high wall motion score and antecedent MI were both noted to be significant negative influences on overall survival.

187

When isolated as a group, those patients with severe IMR who underwent coronary artery bypass plus a mitral valve procedure had an operative mortality of 38% and a five-year survival of only 44%. This corresponds to similar dismal numbers in the literature [1, 4, 11, 14–17]. Thus, with this background on the whole spectrum of patients with IMR we decided to more closely scrutinize this frustrating subset of patients with *severe* IMR.

Clinical material

This study concerns a retrospective review of 29 consecutive patients with severe ischemic MR operated upon at the St. Vincent Heart Institute and The Oregon Health Sciences University between 1984 and 1987. Of these 29 patients, 17 underwent coronary artery bypass and mitral valve replacement and 12 had coronary artery bypass and mitral repair. There were 15 males and 14 females and the mean age for all patients was 69 years. In 10 of these patients, operation was precipitated by an acute myocardial infarction within 30 days prior to surgery (Table 1).

From an angiographic point of view there were three patients with single-vessel disease, four patients with two-vessel disease and 22 (76%) had three or more diseased vessels. All but two patients had significant stenosis of the right coronary system and 17 (59%) had right coronary occlusion.

Left ventriculography was evaluated and the mean LV ejection fraction was 0.42. Wall motion abnormalities of some degree were seen in all patients. The distribution of these abnormalities is exemplified by Table 2 which shows the percentage of patients with "severe dysfunction" present in each of the five segments of the RAO ventriculogram. Severe dysfunction refers to a segmental score of 3 or more using the CASS method.

Hemodynamic characterization of this group also pointed to significant myocardial compromise. The mean LVEDP was 22 torr and only 20% of the patients had

Table 1. Clinical Material

Number of patients	29
CABG + replacement	17
CABG + repair	12
Male sex	15
Mean age (years)	69
Acute MI	10

Table 2. Distribution of wall motion abnormalities

Segment	Severe Dysfunction
1. Anterobasal	12%
2. Anterolateral	27%
3. Apical	35%
4. Diaphragmatic	58%
5. Posterobasal	73%

a LVEDP less than 16. The mean PCWP was 24 and the mean PA systolic and dias-tolic pressures were 51 and 20, respectively. The mean RA pressure was 10. Eleven of the 29 patients required intra-aortic balloon counterpulsation.

Results

Seventeen of the 29 Patients in this series underwent coronary artery bypass plus mitral valve replacement (CAB-MVR). The remaining 12 patients were treated with coronary artery bypass and mitral valve repair (CAB-repair). Comparison of those patients having valve replacement with those having reconstruction showed the two groups to be comparable in most respects. The mean wall motion score for those with CAB-MVR was 10.7 and was 11.3 for the CAB-repair group. Seventy-one percent of the CAB-MVR patients had three or more diseased vessels as com-pared to 75% of the CAB-repair patients. The mean ejection fraction for patients with valve replacement was 0.45 and was 0.40 for those with valve repair. Similarly the mean pulmonary capillary wedge pressure was 25 torr in the CAB-MVR patients and 24 torr in the CAB-repair group. However, 41% of those patients undergoing CAB-MVR had suffered an acute MI within 30 days prior to surgery, whereas only 25% of those in the CAB-repair group faced this prejudice (Table 3).

Evaluation of the type of surgical procedure as a function of year of operation showed a trend toward increasing use of mitral reconstructive techniques. In 1984, 83% of patients with severe IMR underwent CABG with prosthetic replacement of the mitral valve. By 1987 this figure had dropped to 43% and CAB-repair accounted for 57%.

The overall operative mortality for this group with severe IMR was 24%. Those patients who underwent CAB-MVR had an operative mortality of 29% as com-pared to 17% for those in the CAB-repair group. When operative mortality was examined by year of operation there was again a trend toward improving results. Fifty percent of patients with severe IMR died in 1984 but only 14% died in 1987 (Fig. 1).

Analysis of risk factors revealed a strong correlation between operation in the acute phase of myocardial infarction and operative death. Those patients operated upon within one month of this acute event suffered a 40% mortality as compared

Table 3. Distribution of risk factors by surgical procedure

	CABG + replacement	CABG repair
Number of patients	17	12
Acute MI	41%	25%
Wall motion abnormality score	10.7	11.3
3 or more diseased vessels	71%	75%
Pulmonary artery wedge (mmHg)	25	24
Ejection fraction	.45	.40
Total		

189

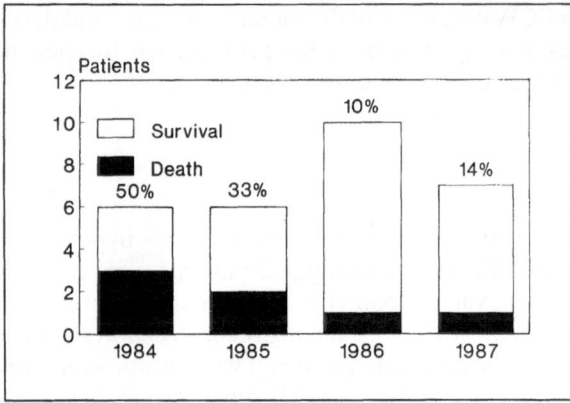

Fig. 1. Operative mortality by year of operation

Table 4. Operative mortality

Variable	Value	Mortality
Acute MI	yes	40%
	no	16%
Diseased vessels	1–2	14%
	3–6	30%
Ejection fraction	<.30	25%
	>.30	27%
LVEDP	<15	25%
	>15	25%

with only 16% for patients undergoing operation at a greater time interval from infarction.

Likewise, a negative outcome was more strongly associated with a greater number of diseased vessels. Those patients with severe IMR who had only one or two diseased vessels had an operative mortality of only 14% while this figure rose to 30% for those with three or more diseased vessels (Table 4).

Ejection fraction was not predicitve of an increased operative risk. Patients with an EF less than 0.30 had an operative mortality of 25% and this number was 27% for those with an EF greater than 0.30. Similarly the mortality was 25% for those patients with an LVEDP less than 15 torr and remained at 25% for all those whose LVEDP was greater than 15 torr.

The average age of patients surviving surgery was 69 years and it was 71 years for the operative deaths. The mean wall motion score was 11 for both the survivors and those who died. The mean PCWP was 23 torr for patients who survived and 29 torr for patients who died. Thus, within this select group of physiologically compromised patients, commonly accepted risk factors such as age, ejection fraction, wall motion score and filling pressures did not further stratify operative risk.

190

Conclusion

Our previous experience with IMR led us to envision this diagnosis as representing a broad spectrum of patients with varying degrees of pathology who suffered greatly different levels of physiologic consequence. Both operative outcome and long-term survival had been seen to be most strongly correlated with the severity of mitral regurgitation as judged angiographically.

This study of that subpopulation with severe IMR confirms the predominance of wall motion abnormalities in the posterobasal segment. A correspondingly high incidence of right coronary disease was seen in these subjects. We feel the reason for this distribution to be twofold. First, the anterobasal ventricular wall, including the anterolateral papillary muscle, is a watershed area benefitting from circulation derived from both the anterior descending and circumflex coronary arteries, whereas the posterobasal segment is more frequently an end-circulation derived predominantly from the right coronary artery. Secondly, the anterior portion of the mitral annulus, between the two trigones, is a fixed fibrous structure which participates less dynamically in mitral closure and is affected less by ischemic dilatation than the more muscular annulus posteriorly. These facts highlight the importance of serious consideration of right coronary disease in view of prevention of IMR.

The current study population was at high risk by several parameters. The mean age for these patients was 69 years. By contrast, during the same period the mean age for patients undergoing isolated coronary artery bypass was 64 years and for patients undergoing isolated mitral valve replacement it was 62 years. Furthermore, 75% of these patients had three-vessel disease and one-third were in the acute phase of myocardial infarction.

The overall operative mortality for this group (24%) compares favorably with the 38% mortality for the same category of patient noted in our earlier series and this decreasing trend in operative mortality seemed to continue throughout the four-year span of this review. During the same four years our experience with the use of reconstructive techniques in patients with IMR increased. A number of authors have recently reported an improvement in operative survival related to the use of mitral valve repair rather than replacement in the management of IMR [2, 8−10, 18].

Closer scrutiny, however, demonstrated a strong correlation between acute MI and operative death. It was noted that a larger percentage of patients treated during the acute phase of MI underwent valve replacement rather than repair and this factor alone could explain the disparity between results with the two techniques.

From a pathologic point of view, IMR is best thought of as a kind of wall motion abnormality. In this conceptualization, the entire mitral mechanism is an extension of the ventricular wall and its function is intimately related to ventricular dynamics. Ischemic compromise of myocardial contractility in the basilar segments leads to impairment of the coordinated, synchronous shortening of the annular and basilar ventricular radii during systole. Different degrees of impaired leaflet coaptation result and, when the margin of error of apposition is surpassed, mitral regurgitation occurs. It is obvious that akinetic or dyskinetic ventricular segments will impact this function more extensively than will hypokinesis. Similarly, it is evident that complete disruption of ventriculo-mitral continuity, such as with papillary muscle rupture, will yield profound incompetence.

We feel that the unifying principle common to both mitral valve replacement and repair which contributes most strongly to a successful outcome in these severely compromised patients is the recognition of the mitral apparatus as an integral part of the left ventricle. Preservation of ventriculo-mitral continuity is implicit in all mitral reparative techniques. The conservation of the mural leaflet with its chordae intact during mitral valve replacement was originally described by Lillehei [13] and the salutary effects of this technique with regard to ventricular function and operative outcome have recently been underlined [5, 6]. Goor [7] has shown a dramatic improvement in operative results for mitral valve replacement in patients with IMR when the posterior leaflet is preserved.

In conclusion, patients with severe mitral regurgitation due to coronary artery disease continue to represent a subset of more physiologically compromised individuals with a markedly increased operative mortality. The ischemic etiology must be addressed with expeditious coronary revascularization and mitral competence must be restored with maintenance of ventriculo-mitral continuity. The decision to repair the valve under these circumstances must be made after consideration of the extent and nature of the structural defects as well as the experience of the surgeon. If the valve is replaced, the mural leaflet should be preserved with its chordae to lessen the impact on ventricular function. We feel it is paramount to recognize the central etiologic importance of the right coronary artery and to use aggressive interventional management of stenotic disease in this vessel to prevent the syndrome of IMR.

References

1. Christakis GT, Kormos RL, Weisel RD, Fremes SE, Tong CP, Horst JA, Schwartz L, Mickelborough LL, Scully HE, Goldman BS, Baird RJ (1985) Morbidity and mortality in mitral valve surgery. Circulation 72 [Suppl II]:II120–128
2. Cohn LH, Kowalker W, Bhatia S, Di Sesa VJ, St. John-Sutton M, Sherwin RJ, Collins JJ (1988) Comparative morbidity of mitral valve repair versus replacement for mitral regurgitation with and without coronary artery disease. Ann Thorac Surg 45:284–290
3. Connolly MN, Gelbfish JS, Jacobowitz IJ, Rose DM, Mendelsohn A, Cappabianca AM, Acinapura AJ, Cunningham JN (1986) Surgical results for mitral regurgitation from coronary artery disease. J Thorac Cardiovasc Surg 91:379–388
4. Czer LSC, Gray RJ, DeRobertis MA, Bateman RM, Stewart ME, Charux A, Matloff AM (1984) Mitral valve replacement: impact of coronary artery disease and determinants of prognosis after revascularization. Circulation 70 [Suppl I]:I198–207
5. David TE, Ho WC (1986) The effect of preservation of chordae tendinae on mitral valve replacement for postinfarction mitral regurgitation. Circulation 74 [Suppl I]:I116–120
6. David TE, Uden DE, Strauss HD (1983) The importance of the mitral valve apparatus in left ventricular function after correction of mitral regurgitation. Circulation 68 [Suppl II]:II76–82
7. Goor DA, Mohr R, Lavee J, Serraf A, Smolinsky A (1988) Preservation of the posterior leaflet during mechanical valve replacement for ischemic mitral regurgitation and complete myocardial revascularization. J Thorac Cardiovasc Surg 96:253–260
8. Hickey MS, Smith LR, Muhlbaier LH, Harrell FE, Reves JG, Hinohara T, Califf RM, Pryor DB, Rankin JS (1988) Current prognosis of ischemic mitral regurgitation: Implications for future management. Circulation 78 (3 pt 2):I51–59

9. Kay GL, Kay JH, Zubiate P, Yokoyama T, Mendez M (1986) Mitral valve repair for mitral regurgitation secondary to coronary artery disease. Circulation 74 [Suppl I]:I88–98

10. Kay JH, Zubiate P, Mendez MA, Vanstrom N, Yokoyama T, Gharavu MA (1980) Surgical treatment of mitral insufficiency secondary to coronary artery disease. J Thorac Cardiovasc Surg 79:12–18

11. Kay PH, Nunley DL, Grunkemeier GL, Pinson CW, Starr A (1985) Late results of combined mitral valve replacement and coronary bypass surgery. J Am Coll Cardiol 5:29–33

12. Kennedy JW, Kaiser GC, Fisher LD, Maynard C, Fritz JK, Myers W, Mudd JG, Ryan TJ, Coggin J (1980) Multivariate discriminant analysis of the clinical and angiographic predictors of operative mortality from the Collaborative Study in Coronary Artery Surgery (CASS). J Thorac Cardiovasc Surg 80:876–887

13. Lillehei CW; Levy MJ, Bonnabeau RC (1964) Mitral valve replacement with preservation of papillary muscles and chordae tendinae. J Thorac Cardiovasc Surg 47:532–543

14. Merin G, Ginliano ER, Pluth JR, Wallace RB, Danielson RK (1973) Surgery for mitral valve incompetence after myocardial infarction. Am J Cardiol 32:322–324

15. Miller DC, Stinson EB, Rossiter SJ, Oyer PE, Reitz BA, Shumway NE (1978) Impact of simultaneous myocardial revascularization on operative risk, functional result and survival following mitral valve replacement. Surgery 84:848–857

16. Pinson CW, Cobanoglu A, Metzdorff MT, Grunkemeier GL, Kay PH, Starr A (1984) Late surgical results for ischemic mitral regurgitation. J Thoracic Cardiovasc Surg 88:663–672

17. Radford MJ, Johnson RA, Buckley MJ, Dagett WM, Leinbach RC, Gold HK (1979) Survival following mitral valve replacement for mitral regurgitation due to coronary artery disease. Circulation 60 [Suppl I]:I39–47

18. Rankin JS, Fenely MP, Hickey MS, Muhlbaier LH, Wechsler AS, Floyd RD, Reves JG, Skelton TN, Califf RM, Lowe JE, Sabiston DC (1988) A clinical comparison of mitral valve repair versus valve replacement in ischemic mitral regurgitation. J Thorac Cardiovasc Surg 95:165–177

19. Scott WC, Miller DC, Haverich A, Mitchell RS, Oyer PE, Stinson EB, Jamieson SW, Baldwin JC, Shumway NE (1985) Operative risk of mitral valve replacement: discriminant analysis of 1329 prodecures. Circulation 72 [Suppl II]:II108–119.

Author's address:
Jeffrey S. Swanson, MD
Assistant Professor
Division of Cardiopulmonary Surgery
The Oregon Health Sciences University
3181 SW Sam Jackson Park Road
Portland, Oregon 97201
USA

Surgery for acute ischemic mitral incompetence

A. Piwnica, Ph. Menasche, C. Kucharski, I. Abdelmeguid, J. B. Subayi

Service de Chirurgie Cardio-Vasculaire, Hôpital Lariboisière, Paris, France

Introduction

Emergency surgical correction of severe mitral incompetence complicating acute myocardial infarction still remains a therapeutic challenge for various reasons including the poor hemodynamic condition of these patients preoperatively, the potentially limited amount of residual viable myocardium, and the technical difficulties associated with the surgical procedure. On the basis of a clinical experience that encompasses 25 patients who underwent emergency surgery for acute ischemic mitral incompetence, we address the main surgical issues that continue to be raised by this life-threatening clinical entity.

Patient population

From 1972 through 1988, 25 patients required an acute operation for early postinfarction mitral incompetence. There were 23 men and two women who ranged in age from 46 to 83 years (mean: 60 years). Twenty-three patients had inferior and two had anterolateral wall infarctions. The interval between acute myocardial infarction and the appearance of the murmur of mitral insufficiency ranged from 1 to 14 days. At the time of admission, all patients were in cardiogenic shock or in intractable left ventricular failure with pulmonary edema. Six of them were supported by the intraaortic balloon pump prior to surgery.

The clinical diagnosis of mitral regurgitation was confirmed by echocardiograms and cardiac catheterization. Coronary angiograms were performed in only seven patients; three of them were found to have a tight stenosis of the left anterior descending coronary artery in addition to occlusive disease of the artery supplying the infarcted myocardium.

At operation, 15 patients had a complete rupture of the posterior papillary muscle; six had partial rupture involving the posterior papillary muscle in five cases and the anterior papillary muscle in one case. The remaining four patients had papillary muscle dysfunction involving the posterior papillary muscle in three cases and the anterior one in one case.

The 25 patients underwent prosthetic valve replacement. All of these were performed through a left atrial approach. Of the 25 prosthetic valves, 15 were mechanical valves and 10 were bioprostheses. Three patients had additional single bypass grafts to the left anterior descending coronary artery.

Results

Six patients died intra-, or postoperatively. Two patients could not be weaned from cardiopulmonary bypass. Two additional patients died in the Intensive Care Unit of persistently low cardiac output. Two other patients died 6 and 19 days after operation, respectively, one of pulmonary sepsis and the second, suddenly.

There were 19 hospital survivors, 11 of whom had required intra-aortic balloon pump support postoperatively.

Discussion

Patients with postinfarction mitral incompetence can fit into three categories: 1) those with an early and transient murmur, without hemodynamic consequences; 2) those with a mitral insufficiency of delayed onset, and which can be treated electively; and 3) those with a life-threatening left ventricular failure in the early post-infarction period (i.e., within 1 month of infarct). The present report only deals with this last subgroup, the management of which still raises several concerns which will now be discussed.

Timing of surgery

Analysis of our observations as well as those of the litterature [6] suggests that patients with acute, poorly tolerated ischemic mitral incompetence should undergo emergency surgery, regardless of whether the predominant clinical presentation is that of a true cardiogenic shock or that of an intractable left ventricular failure with pulmonary edema. Attempts at "stabilizing" the patient with the intraaortic balloon pump for a few days prior to operation are usually useless and harmful, in that they increase the likelihood of postoperative multiple organ failure resulting from a prolonged preoperative period of peripheral hypoperfusion. This concept is well illustrated by the results reported by Tepe and Edmunds [6]: The interval between mitral murmur and operation was 1.8 day in hospital survivors and 10.5 days in hospital nonsurvivors while the interval between cardiogenic shock and operation was 1.7 day and 9.3 days, respectively.

Mitral valve exposure

The small size of the left atrium is a well known difficulty of operations on acutely incompetent mitral valves. In our series, we have consistently used a left atriotomy which is made parallel to the interatrial sulcus. By dissecting the left atrial far behind the venae cavae, it is possible to extend the left atrium incision line both anteriorly and posteriorly, thereby improving exposure of the mitral valve apparatus without excessive tractions on the retractor. It is probably safer, in these patients, not to divide the superior vena cava, as it has been proposed to deal with small left atria. Alternatively, some authors have advocated a transseptal approach but this technique seems to be associated with an increased probability of postoperative supraventricular arrhythmias. A last option is to approach the mitral valve through a left ventriculotomy, but this technique remains limited to patients in whom a transmural infarct results in a significant wall motion defect and, as such, is deemed amenable to resection [5].

196

Perioperative management

Preoperatively, the intra-aortic balloon should be inserted whenever indicated [1], provided it does not result in delayed surgery. We tend to be more liberal in its use postoperatively, in particular if there is any difficulty in weaning the patient from cardiopulmonary bypass. In case of left ventricular failure refractory to conventional pharmacological therapy and to balloon pumping, the implementation of more aggressive systems of circulatory assistance should now be considered with the hope that temporary support of the left ventricle may allow for recovery of reversibly injured myocardium.

In these patients, intraoperative myocardial protection is of utmost importance. While emphasis is generally put on measures implemented during ischemic arrest, i.e., hypothermia and cardioplegia, it is our belief that equal attention should be paid to the limitation of reperfusion injury. There is now good evidence that this objective can be achieved with an appropriate control of the physico-chemical environment during the early phase of reflow, and that the use of these specifically designed reperfusion solutions may help in enhancing postoperative recovery.

Selection of procedure: In patients with papillary muscle rupture or dysfunction, there is no question about the indication of valve procedures. Up to now, the more common form of operation has been mitral valve replacement, usually with a low-profile artificial valve, as in the present series. The fragility of the anulus is a frequent finding in these patients with freshly infarcted tissues. This problem however, can usually be circumvented by the use of pledget-supported figure-of-eight horizontal sutures. A more secure fixation of the prosthesis can also be achieved by incorporating into the suture line the preserved posterior leaflet, which may have the additional advantage of reducing the deleterious consequences of mitral valve replacement upon left ventricular function [3].

More recently, some authors [2, 5] have advocated the use of repair techniques, in particular in patient subgroups with papillary muscle dysfunction. Depending on the operative findings, the repair may consist of an annuloplasty or of the re-suturing of the papillary muscle to the left ventricular wall at a more apical level in order to compensate for chordal elongation. Regardless of the technique, conservative procedures seem to be associated with a better hospital survival than mitral valve replacement. Although the number of documented cases still remains scarce, a similar trend seems to exist in the patient subgroup of papillary muscle rupture. Potential explanations for this finding may relate to preservation of the mitral valve apparatus and shortened operative time. In turn, the shorter time required for valve repair might allow for more liberal indications of associated coronary artery bypass grafting. It is therefore conceivable that, in the future, expanded application of valve repair may improve the outcome of these critically ill patients.

A last surgical issue is that of the management of patients with generalized annular dilatation associated with diffuse left ventricular dysfunction. In these cases, the hemodynamic deterioration is more predominantly related to myocardial than to valvular factors. It is therefore not unexpected that mitral valve replacement has consistently yielded poor results due to the limited amount of residual viable myocardium [4, 5]. Consequently, it may be that, in this setting, cardiac transplantation rather than valve procedure (with or without bypass) may be the operation of choice.

References

1. Buckley MJ, Mundth ED, Daggett WM, Gold HK, Leinbach RC, Austen WG (1973) Surgical management of ventricular septal defects and mitral regurgitation complicating acute myocardial infarction. Ann Thorac Surg 16:598−609
2. Carpentier A, Loulmet D, Deloche A, Perier P (1987) Surgical anatomy and management of ischemic mitral valve incompetence. Circulation [Suppl] 76:IV-446
3. David TE, Ho WC (1986) The effect of preservation of chordae tendinae on mitral valve replacement for postinfarction mitral regurgitation. Circulation [Suppl] 74:I-116−120
4. Najafi H, Javid H, Hunter JA, Golding MD, Serry C, Dye WS (1975) Mitral insufficiency secondary to coronary heart disease. Ann Thorac Surg 20:529−537
5. Rankin JS, Feneley MP, StJ Hickey M, Muhlbaier LH, Wechsler AS, Flyod RD, Reves JG, Skelton TN, Califf RM, Lowe JE, Sabiston DC (1988) A clinical comparison of mitral valve repair versus valve replacement in ischemic mitral regurgitation. J Thorac Cardiovasc Surg 95:165−177
6. Tepe NA, Edmunds LH (1985) Operation for acute postinfarction mitral insufficiency and cardiogenic shock. J Thorac Cardiovasc Surg 89:525−530

Author's address:
Prof. Dr. A. H. Piwnica
Service de Chirurgie Cardio-Vasculaire
Hôpital Lariboisière
2 Rue Ambroise Paré
75475 Paris
France

Discussion

HETZER:

We now have had a large spectrum of surgical presentations. I think Dr. Rankin's paper has really set a present state of the art of decision making and discussion. He also pointed to some of the important facts that we have to discuss and to decide in terms of going further with indication and applying those techniques to the more milder forms of ischemic mitral incompetence, which we have ignored up to now. I think we should organize the discussion somehow and we should probably start with the indications for surgery. It has been also our impression that ischemic mitral incompetence, grade II, for instance, persists after bypass only and as Dr. Rankin's follow-up data in the large catheter series has shown, those patients are definitely at a higher risk in the long run as compared to patients where we have no mitral incompetence. Now, whether the mitral incompetence adds itself as much or whether the ventricular condition, which results in mitral incompetence, is the factor that determines survival. There are probably controversial opinions about that. But I would like to open the discussion in that aspect and also go to indications for surgery or no surgery.

GAMS:

I think the problems we have with patients suffering from ischemic mitral incompetence might be due to the inadequacy of the assessment of the mitral regurgitation, preoperatively, intraoperatively, and postoperatively. Referring to this I have two questions to Dr. Cohn and Dr. Frater: Is the mitral ring dilatation transient or acute, is it chronic or permanent? I mean, how can we judge it, how can we assess it? Are we sure it remains transient and does not change to permanent or chronic? The other question is: Is the ejection fraction a reliable parameter to judge mitral incompetence as well as ventricular function in ischemic mitral incompetence?

FRATER:

I think this is very difficult, because as I pointed out, the measures that you can use to correct insufficiency by unloading the ventricle are the same measures you use to improve myocardial perfusion. So it is extremely difficult to decide, if you can, for example, treat a patient, see a benefit from that, whether you are in fact unloading the ventricle or improving the ischemia. The critical issue is: if you can see hypokinetic and, therefore, *alive* myocardium, served by an obstructed coronary artery, which has a good run-off, then you can have some hope of improving the insufficiency by grafting, but I think if you see *akinetic* myocardium, which, although it could still be alive, is more likely infarcted in the area that seems to be affecting the mitral valve competence (usually the posterior left ventricular wall), then I think you have to assume that this is going to be permanent. With regard to the annulus: if you see an infarct at the base clearly that will produce a permanent dilation of the annulus or permanent failure of contraction, and it must be measured surgically if it is to be corrected. If you enter the operating room with gross mitral insufficiency you should do something about it. I think the very difficult case is the one who had gross mitral insufficiency last week and now seems much better because he is in the ICU, he is on a balloon pump, he is getting nitroglycerin and so on. Should you be reassured by the fact that the mitral insufficiency is less now than it was before? Probably not, because all the evidence we have had in this conference is that bypass alone does not change the degree of insufficiency when you look at it a month or more later. So I think probably we should stop trying to be too clever about that and do the repair if either there is or recently has been significant mitral insufficiency. As we have pointed out, the repair is generally easy, i.e., an annuloplasty for the ventricular mechanisms of mitral insufficiency.

COHN:

Well, there are several different kinds of regurgitation, as you have seen today. I think we have to look sometimes at the patient not necessarily just the echocardiogram. The patient history is also of interest, which I think is a very important factor. If the patient gets ischemic mitral incompetence transiently – and that has been documented in a number of instances – the appearance of a mitral regurgitation murmur occurs and then it goes away. We do not do anything except a coronary bypass grafting in those patients. Now, it is a clinical decision and I do not think anybody who does this kind of surgery can go into an operation on a patient like this with a fixed plan. You have an idea what you think is usually the case. But, for example, when you come off bypass and you find there was an excellent cardiac output, there is low left atrial pressures, there is no evidence of a thrill and the color Doppler, whatever else you use, is fine, that patient is fine. However, even though you thought this was a transient phenomenon prior to surgery, if you come off bypass with a low cardiac output and these other kinds of signs, then obviously your original game plan was wrong. You go back and you do an annuloplasty. So, I think, there is a lot of judgement involved. It would be nice to be able to quantitate every judgemental aspect of the surgery. But I know of no other kind of surgery where your actual clinical judgement, observations, and putting together all the information is as important as it is in this situation. With the case that Dr. Frater describes, the acute onset, which gets better with a mass of afterload reductions such as the balloon pump. I think that is a different story, that patients in our clinic would have a mitral valve operation. I am talking about the chronic or subacute transient kind of regurgitation. To our experience a coronary bypass grafting works very well in that particular situation.

HETZER:

Have you seen patients where you have only done a bypass grafting in patients with a transient ring dilatation where you had to reoperate, let's say, a few months later and correct the mitral valve? Was there worsening of the mitral regurgitation?

COHN:

I would say essentially if I had to do that it has been more like years that this patient has done well, but to the ravages of coronary disease the patients come back and at that point, there has been a few that have had chronic severe fixed mitral regurgitation, that is true, but I do not recall that we had any in the category that you described. Unless there has been new pathology, we have that occasional case that has done well and then 6 months later they have new pathology and now have the ruptured chordae.

DURAN:

Can we try to simplify the subject because you are getting walled in and as a surgeon I want to have as clear an explanation as possible, which is not always easy. I think this morning it became quite obvious, to me at least, with the data presented by Dr. Rankin and the Berlin Heart Institute that those cases that had mild to moderate mitral regurgitation with ischemic disease and you were going to do bypasses and your question in your mind was, shall I do something to the mitral valve or not? That is a very frequent or fairly frequent case and the tendency was, leave the mitral valve as it is because I have been told that if you get a good reperfusion that mitral regurgitation is going to disappear. To me the evidence this morning is, it just does not disappear. Therefore, I am more inclined to operate at the mitral valve, that is number 1. Number 2: it seems that a lot of this dysfunction, of the papillary muscles and the left ventricular wall, you get away with if you just do an annuloplsty. So this is a fairly simple procedure to correct this type of mitral regurgitation, not the minimal one, but those that are in between mild and moderate. If I know mitral regurgitation ist not going to disappear with my bypasses so I go ahead and do just a straight annuloplasty. I do not look at the valve, do not test anything, do an annuloplasty and finish the operation. Well, I do not know whether that is universally accepted.

HETZER:

I think we should ask Dr. Hugenholtz the one question whether he thinks that he can differentiate transient ischemia from stable fibrosis in those patients. I think this is the same question that we have in all acute forms of coronary insufficiency, not only with the mitral incompetence. We have no methods available that would tell us if the myocardium is ischemic and thus not working well but reversibly — let's say — paralyzed and can recover?

HUGENHOLTZ:
With current techniques I would say no. We do not know how to separate the stunt myocardium, which can be stunt for hours and days from what is on biopsy later a fibrotic piece of tissue. Of course, everybody is working with various methods trying to use radionuclide methods to try to prove some kind of a viability to a tissue. And I think Dr. Gams' comments were very good, I mean that is the issue and Dr. Frater's answer was very clar, you study the whole case and you take your chances. I would tend to believe that the reperfusion is the key in a sense that you cannot do a repair without having looked at a vessel that supplies the piece that you are going to repair, so definitely you must know that. And then if you want to add a ring quickly as Dr. Duran says or not is exactly why we have thoracic surgeons.

VINCENT:
I was very pleased to hear from Dr. Rankin to bring back the Kay plasty. It is not only coincidence, I remember a discussion about 15 years ago between Charles Dubost and Charles Hahn concerning concomitant tricuspid insufficiency with the mitral insufficiency. The consensus became important between these two men concluding that all we need is a simple gesture to put some two or three stitches to have little repair of the tricuspid valve. It is not a coincidence the name of Kay is coming back on this mitral level. I think that is very important. We need something which takes little time because the patient is at risk being on extracorporeal circulation. Let me ask a question because there is one point concering these very bad patients with a low ejection fraction where we finally are obliged to put a valve prosthesis in. Last year Dr. Cooley emphasized replacement of the valve in the intact valvular apparatus and this is something I did not hear yesterday, even today. But I think it might be quite important in a case where we need a valve replacement it is reasonable to keep all the mitral apparatus in situ and the implant in this case may be only the St. Jude valve which fits in this procedure. Can you comment on that?

RANKIN:
After Dr. Cooley's presentation on intravalvular prosthetic insertion at the American Thoracic Meeting two years ago, we performed the operation in half a dozen patients. In general, it worked pretty well, but in two patients we had trouble. In one patient, the anterior leaflet of the native mitral valve closed with systolic contraction, limited St. Jude leaflet closure, and caused prosthetic regurgitation. We identified this problem on transesophageal Doppler echo, went back in and excised the anterior leaflet through the prosthetic valve, and then the patient did fine. We also had another patient who underwent double valve replacement, and then had a peculiar systolic murmur postoperatively. She did okay with the murmur, but on echo exam, she had systolic anterior motion of the retained anterior leaflet with left ventricular outflow tract obstruction and a 30 mmHg systolic gradient. The patient has been asymptomatic and has done well, but I think that experience along with the paper recently published from Beth Israel Hospital on left ventricular outflow tract obstruction from a retained anterior leaflet has caused us to revert to resect on of the anterior leaflet in all cases. In regard to Dr. Duran's statement, I very much appreciate simple, clear ideas, and if there are two we have derived from our experience with ischemic mitral regurgitation, the first would be that, in the past, the philosophy of leaving the mitral valve alone in patients undergoing coronary bypass with concommitant significant mitral regurgitation produced an inordinately high operative risk. Thus, our current philosophy is to repair the valve whenever there is a question. Second, we have been very impressed with transesophageal echocardiography as the primary guide to intervening in these patients, and we now base the decision for valve repair on intraoperative Doppler echo. There would not have been many things in the last couple of years that I could say have been uniformly successful, but transesophageal Doppler has been perfect so far in defining the patients who need mitral valve procedures, and in avoiding unnecessary interventions in those who do not. These are the two ideas that I would like to emphasize from our experience.

FRATER:
Just a brief word on leaving the valve in. Ignacio Gallo when he was with us about 6 years ago did a series of animals in which he put bioprotheses in without excising the valve at all and at 1 year

there was no dysfunction of those bioprothetic valves as result of this technique. I have certainly done it clinically. If you are going to use a bioprothesis for young patient in this circumstance then it is extremely easy and extremely safe and probably also helps to prevent perivalvular leaks because there is valve tissue under the suture line, I think it is a very good thing to do. Granted you have to be much more careful if you are going to use a tilting disc valve with natural valve left in place.

BRAIMBRIDGE:
I was particularly interested in what Dr. Rankin said about the advantages of reperfusion prior to accepting a case for surgery. I was not clear what he meant exactly by that. Is that streptokinase and PTCA or are you talking about surgical reperfusion. It seemed to me that for many of us who see relatively few cases we could say to our cardiologist "you reperfuse a lot of them first and see if you can make that mitral regurgitation better, because the overall operative mortality is going to be much lower", could you be a little bit more precise about that?

RANKIN:
As we get more follow-up time, we may write a specific paper on the reperfusion group; it is a very interesting subset. Of the 63 patients that had early reperfusion, approximately two-thirds had thrombolysis acutely and then went on to have definitive therapy of the residual lesions electively; one-third had an angioplasty as the method of reperfusion. Recently, we have avoided surgical reperfusion, and with improved techniques of catheter reperfusion, we very rarely operate on acute involving infarction. In my opinion, the mortality and morbidity is too high in these really sick patients, and I would agree that taking a patient with acute papillary muscle dysfunction directly to the operating room is not indicated in my practice at this time. We believe it is probably better to obtain initial catheter reperfusion. In fact, we had nine patients out of that group that were over 2 days beyond infarct onset, and the reperfusion was successful in reducing the regurgitation in five of those nine. So even in patients who are beyond the initial phase of acute infarction, or if they have influctuating postinfarction angina and influctuating regurgitation, we believe thrombolysis and/or angioplasty is the initial procedure of choice. This may be the one area where angioplasty produces better results than surgical therapy at this time.

COHN:
I just wanted to underscore a little bit what Dr. Frater said about putting a valve replacement with totally intact papillary muscles. In my opinion, I think, to put a prothetic valve device, it is difficult, then you can get into the kind of problems that Dr. Rankin was talking about. The bioprothetic valve — and we had such a case last week, a 75 year old woman with a ruptured papillary muscle — one can put that valve in entirely, I think it is a much safer thing to do than leaving the entire valve structure intact. I have a question to Dr. Rankin referrable to the group that did the valve replacement concomitant with the valve repair. I would suggest that they resected all the papillary muscles in those valves and I think that immediately, if not chronically, this makes a very major difference in postoperative cardiac output in that critical group, is that true?

HETZER:
May I add a little point from our experience. I have been routinely using this technique of preserving both papillary muscles and the posterior leaflets since 1980 for all mitral valve replacements, also in calcified leaflets, where you can decalcify the leaflet and still have the mitral apparatus left. We also use it in mechanical protheses, St. Judes, and I have never encountered a case where the leaflets got stuck with the mitral apparatus. I think especially for the ischemic mitrals that have already compromised left ventricular function it is extremely important to have this preservation.

RANKIN:
Most of the replacement patients in that early 1980 series would have had total resection of the valve tissue, and I think now, for the last several years virtually all of our surgeons whenever possible leave the posterior leaflet in, that may be important. What we are seeing here, both in the patients requiring prothetic replacement, repairs, and the ones undergoing coronary bypass, is a general improvement in our knowledge based on the fact that when we looked at our early 1980 data, they were terrible. By small advances in multiple different areas I think we have seen the

202

same thing that you showed in the Berlin data that the overall mortality now is coming down gradually, and hopefully by the turn of the next decade we can get it down to very acceptable levels.

ZIEMER:
I would like to ask Dr. Cohn and Dr. Rankin about the comparability of their patient groups which got mitral valve replacement or repair. The indications for valve replacement relate to a more seriously ill patient group. The question to Dr. Rankin is: Would those patients where you just do the Kay annuloplasty be the same patients in which Dr. Wexler would implant a mechanical valve?

RANKIN:
As I have become more involved with biostatistics in the last few years, I have become more familiar with the problems of retrospective analysis, and questions always exist with observational studies. Were the groups comparable? Were there, in fact, undefined selection or treatment biases? However, it turns out that when two surgeons or two surgical groups working within the same practice are working over time with different treatment philosophies, a pretty good pseudo-randomization is obtained based on random referral practices within a hospital. This type of procedure probably comes as close as possible to a good randomization, and most of us would agree that a true randomization is likely impossible within a busy clinical practice. During this period, the patients undergoing valve repair were sicker on average than the ones receiving replacement, because the surgeons who were interested in repair where operating on most of the CCU patients. Because we are now expanding annuloplasty into less critically ill cases undergoing coronary bypass, there would be a problem doing the study now. But over the period in question, we came out with extremely comparable groups, and at least in my practice, I feel confident that the surgical results are much better with valve repair. I would like to make a comment about the Berlin data. The difference in operative mortality rate and long-term survival between repair and replacement did not turn out to be statistically significant, but the comparison had a small sample size. One might propose that the difference is quite significant clinically, and as the sample size increases a very important improvement in survival may be evident with valve repair in this series too.

COHN:
You bring up a very good question. In our particular group we looked at relatively the same time period as Dr. Rankin mentioned. We made a conscious effort in 1984 to do those sick patients with ischemic mitral regurgitation and in fact if you look at our groups, the total group of repair and replacement for mitral valve disease of all kinds, the mitral valve repair had a higher incidence of coronary bypass surgery, higher incidence of ischemic disease. I do not think you can ever get a truly prospective randomized study. In our particular series with the same surgeons doing both repair and replacement, depending upon what the valve looked like or what the situation was, these groups are biostatistically difficult to be put in a neat package. I would say from my observations that the acute phase is significantly improved because the cardiac outputs and the cardiac function, if you measure these immediately postoperatively, they are much better in these patients than in those that have had valve replacement with resection of papillary muscles. And I am impressed that the long-term survival in our study and many others that you have heard here is better because I think the cardiac output is maintained in a much better way if the papillary muscle annular continuity is maintained and as cardiac output remains up the survival remains up.

DURAN:
Well, I am sorry to say, but we try to show, not just in ischemic, that valve repair was better than valve replacement and except for operative mortality we have not managed to demonstrate it; I hope somebody else does it. For up to 10 years we looked at the figures and there is a big difference in operative mortality, very significant whatever you look at: ejection fraction, age, functional classe, etc.

We have heard conflicting reports about what to do with a ruptured papillary muscle. So I would like to have some light on that, if I have to operate on a ruptured papillary muscle tomorrow do I suture it or do I take the valve away? Dr. Rankin, any opinion about it? Are you doing a repair every time you see a ruptured papillary muscle whether it is acute, chronic, very acute, not so acute?

RANKIN:

It is interesting, as many have said here, that papillary muscle rupture has become a rare entity now, perhaps, because of widespread use of early reperfusion or better coronary care. It is difficult to say that reimplantation of a ruptured papillary muscle is an accepted procedure based on three patients; however, the procedure has worked well in my experience. I plan to continue to develop this technique, and I think it is worthwhile, again, to point out that the valve itself is totally normal in this disorder. If one can restructure the submitral geometry properly, the valve should function entirely physiologically. However, I would put this procedure in the category of clinical investigation right now, and I cannot say that reimplantation is the right thing to do. The majority of these patients have good ventricular function, and the valve should be approached transatrially most of the time. I really cannot argue with the policy of routine valve replacement if a surgeon choses to do so.

FRATER:

Dr. Rankin, I think it depends very much on when you see the patient, for example, 3 days ago I saw an acute papillary muscle rupture, it was one-half of the postero-medio papillary muscle, that portion to which were attached the chordae to the medial half of the posterior cusp and that clearly had infarcted, causing acute insufficiency. When you looked inside the ventricle, however, the adjacent papillary muscle to which the anterior cusp chordae were still attached and which was not ruptured had a yellow kind of buttery looking appearance; to reattach that papillary muscle to that area of infarct would, I think, be dangerous. Therefore, under those circumstances the appropriate thing to do was to replace the valve. You may well say, why not do a quadrangular excision? But how do you know that the anterior cusp attached to a yellow papillary muscle is not going to rupture next week. So in the acute circumstance, 24 h after an infarct when the papillary muscle is ruptured acutely you are going to replace, but give us 10 days or 2 weeks and the patient is in severe congestive cardiac failure and needing ICU or CCU treatment and at surgery you find a papillary muscle already somewhat fibrotic then you can change your plan and do a repair.

PIWNICA:

I think you should work with clear ideas and not complicate things. The main idea if you want to do proper clinical evaluation should be if you have a very small infarct and if you can tell by all the reasons, clinically, echocardiogram, and everything, but it is a very localized infarct on the papillary muscle you can try to do a repair. If it is a big posterior infarct, where the rupture is just part of a complicated lesion you should do a replacement, because the patient is not going to survive, nobody says that it is good to have a valve inside your heart.

Closing remarks

P. G. Hugenholtz

It seems to me that this conference was an effort, well organized and well intentioned, to bring different disciplines together and that, I think, is one of the excellent basic principles on which the meeting was organized. Obviously, we have listened to experts. Yet, if a meeting is critically looked at and there are statistica on this in terms of what information was transferred to the audience, some critics and cynics say that, at best, 25% actually ended up in your brains. So s'll try to refresh your memory. The meeting here had three clear sections. We had a very good session on the basic principles and I would like to review that as a whole. We then talked about the functional analysis and the weaknesses therein and the excitement of the Transeuropean Express – and I will come back to that in a minute – and this morning we talked about the therapy as the surgeons see it and I heard many exciting things. So I will review these three blocks separately.

Before I do that, I will try to echo the cry for help from Dr. Duran yesterday afternoon: "please give me a simple definition". I want to also echo what Dr. Yellin said: "if it has to be a definition, give it a sexy name so we all know what we are talking about", and finally I have been most impressed with the reasonings that Dr. Frater has given us. So I have coined a new title, abbreviated MIMI, for myocardial ischemic mitral insufficiency and that is, according to my friend, the pathologist Dr. Becker, exactly what we ought to call it, because he attaches three conditions to MIMI. We must accept that it is based on some form of dilatation, the normal geometry, as we have heard, has been disturbed. This is a conditio sine qua non. Second, there must be – and there probably is – in 90-odd percent of the cases, obstructive coronary artery disease underlying it, afterall; otherwise you would not put the bypasses on. There must be a cause for this dilatation for it to be called ischemic. And thirdly the ischemic part is terribly important because that connotes its potential reversibility. So, I propose to this audience that we call the syndrome Myocardial Ischemic Mitral Insufficiency, and that we accept that it must have these three conditions.

Now the first set of data which back up MIMI as a concept came from Dr. Puff, who with his hight-speed camera clearly showed, that the AV ring is relating to the rest of the valve structure; apparently it is a very tensile and, shall we say, mobile element, and not at all the stilt skeleton of the heart as we have been taught to see it in the past. He also pointed out to us the helical fiber arrangement, which together with the twisting that he showed clearly in the papillary muscles appears to me to make sense. That goes back to the Streeter model from many years ago where we conceded the heart has a lot more dynamism to it than we are giving it credit for. He mentioned the significance of the posterior wall cusp, the mural cusp, for the inflow function, the anterior cusp for its outflow function and he ended up with the concept (and used the word only once; I wish he had used it a bit more), of a trellis, like you grow flowers against. I think that mobile kind of structure that is disturbed by ischemic heart disease is the concept that he wanted us to take from his talk. Becker in a perhaps more classical fashion looked with his excellent techniques, that he has in Amsterdam, at the coronary blood supply in a set of autopsy cases pointing out that he, against his original thinking, saw the right artery to be dominant in something like 75%, circumflex 8%, while 16% had an intermediate kind of supply. So that when he looked at his autopsies of the acute 23 myocardial infarctions of the anterior wall the antero-lateral papillary muscle was involved in something like 12 cases, never in the posterior, whereas in the posterior infarctions the posterior papillary muscle was always involved. He pointed out there was only one exception to the rule, namely the syndrome of the subendocardial circumferential type of infarction, which involves the whole inner layer of the heart. So he set up together with what we have heard from Dr. Puff the concept that it is the extent of involvement of the coronary artery system and its supplied area that sets up the syndrome called MIMI. Dr. Yellin pointed to the importance of the flows; particularly the interrelations are pointed in a number of very elegant slides to the interactions between pressure differences and how they actually determine how the valve apparatus works. He sald at the end that sum of left ventricular dysfunction and the reduced diastolic compliance actually dominate and determine the changes in the mitral valve apparatus. No saw this later in some of the slides, Dr. Frater showed, where temporary interactions clearly changing afterload or preload can make the mitral valve apparatus change in a major fashion. This was also very elegantly and thoroughly backed up by Dr. Gams with the series of dog experiments he had been carrying out taking out various pieces of the complex system that together then make the syndrome of MIMI and he "mimicked", if you wish, coronary artery disease by either taking out pupillary muscle, a piece of the free wall, or other manipulations. They showed how minor manipulations by themselves, such as cutting the chordae, could elicit major diameter changes to the left ventricle in a range of some 10% and enddiastolic volume by up to 18%. So the factor and the significance of the left ventricular geometry enters into our thinking. This is of interest in the sense that we now have compounds such as the ACE inhibitors, but there may well be others also, which have been shown in some early clinical data to actually intcract with the recovery process after an acute ischemic episode such that the geometrical disturbance after acute myocardial infarction may well be reduced. I refer to the data of Sharp in the New England Journal and the data of Pfeffer's group from Boston, who have clearly shown a much better ejection fraction over time, lower endsystolic volumes and diastolic volumes if you very early-on treat with ACE inhibitors. If you combine that with my final topic, namely reperfusion, it may well be that we will see quite a different set of mitral regurgitation syndromes in the next decade. Dr. Rankin had a nice intervention in the discussion, basically backing up from a surgical point of view what the pathologists are predicting, that the posterior wall is nearly always involved. That is the moment, I think, that Dr. Frater got to the microphone and said "let's stop using the term papillary muscle dysfunction", and, again, I refer to my answer. "Sir, to your plea for stopping what was basically meant to be good definition of a syndrome, it does not fit with what we were talking about."

In the second session we had the cardiologists who tried to help us. Fleck went through a large number of patients; he had something like 1605 patients with coronary artery disease of sufficient severity that the stenosis was 70% or more, and he found only 12% of patients with mitral regurgitations. He tried to quantitate and find out by either univaried or multivaried analysis what might be predictors; he came to the conclusion that there really was not anyone strikingly better than the others, although endsystolic volume index appeared to be most often to come out of the formulae for example, in terms of specificity and sensitivities. If there was three-vessel disease he gave these interesting figures, at least to me, that for a specifity of 87% but a poor sensitivity of 58% there was just age and systolic and enddiastolic volume. If you had just the circumflex and the RCA then the specificity would rise to 96% but you kept a poor sensitivity of 57% for endsystolic volume, enddiastolic volume, and ejection fraction. So he set the stage, which was then echoed by the subsequent speaker, that actually the incidence in the kind of population you and I see is relatively low in the cath labs, I am not talking about CCUs now; they are definitely dependent on the vessels affected and that the endsystolic volume and wall motion abnormalities appear to contain the best information. This was backed up by Dr. Berghöfer's analysis of 550 catheterization films, which he had obtained before and after revascularization. He actually ended up with 463 patients and found, for example, that mitral regurgitation, in the group that had acute PTCA, occurred in 64%. Now this goes back to the acute papillary muscle dysfunction or acute infarction. In the 420 patients with elective PTCA – there, again, the figure of 8% for mitral regurgitation occurred. These are incidence figures, if you wish, from two sides bearing in the same direction and demonstrating that the incidence is not really so high. He concluded that mitral regurgitation in coronary artery disease – and that is what we are talking about – is slight and that it is rather common while the severe forms are uncommon. This was the first and only time I have heard that figure during this conference, that revascularization in his experience reducced the degree of mitral regurgitation in some 50% of the patients and that occurred most often if the preoperative ejection fraction and the ventricular function was good. We then went into the never-neverland of the echo Doppler world and we got very clear warnings from Dr. Bolger about how we ought to handle this new signal very carefully. She explained the fundamentals and warned us about the many factors that may confound its interpretation. The same story came in a way from Dr. Erbel who gave us a rapid-fire of beautiful examples of transesophageal echocardiography, which, as you know, is abbreviated TEE. Here enters the Trans European Express. In Mainz, just recently, there was a 2-day conference on the use of TEE in diagnostics. There were well over 650 people in the hall. I was absolutely astounded; there was an awful lot of work beeing presented and, again, the warning came out "be careful how you interpret the signal". Yet, it may well be the Pizazz factor and the Jazzy technique that is going to be used by anesthesists as well as by neurologists now. We saw pictures of the TEE being turned around and looking backwards and finding observations of the spine and of the spinal cord, just to fire your imagination a little bit further but they too pointed out the difficulties. Actually, there was a vital and vivacious discussion between the surgeons and the cardiologists in the room and one of the cardiologists was heard to say that this tool, including that of the perloperative intracardiac assessment, should never be given in the hands of the surgeons, because they would certainly not have the time to interpret it correctly — it will be too difficult fot them, etc. The old traditional kind of battle for a new tool is on again. What Dr. Erbel also mentioned were the data from the Mayo Clinic and his own 307 cases with mitral regurgitation and finding that prolapse appeared to be occurring in 32 out of these 307, valve thickening in 19%, and normal valves with mitral regurgitation in about 30, I think now is a bit early to make echo the replacement of other techniques, but clearly it is moving up very rapidly as a major diagnostic tool.

In the surgical session Dr. Cohn gave us an elegant talk from the Harvard group, stating first the dismal results of the past and pointing for the need for improvement and then holding out to us that the Carpentier-induced valve reconstruction methodology, the better myocardial protection, all sorts of other factors and certainly the ambitious use of revascularization reperfusion were the keys. I think the helped me in my coding of MIMI by specitying a number of sub-causes that could lead to it, such as the now obvious chordne rupture and so forth. I also notet that he was the first in a series of speakers, who indicated that repair was now more often practiced than replacement. And as we just heard in the discussion, replacement seems to be pushed in a specific corner. The list that he ended with for his 1980–1987 experience of actual procedures led to a recommendation to replace the valve when we have acute papillary muscular rupture, whereas we heard again in the discussion just now that if it is papillary muscle dysfunction with some more time element to it, it would be repair and only occassionally, replacement. If there would be ruptured chordac he would prefer repair and, of course, if there is dilatation of the annulus, this certainly would be the indication for the ring mentioned by each of the surgeons, apart, of course, from the need for bypass. Repair then has become the dominant theme, together with revascularization, and, Dr. Frater echoed these plus once more elegantly pointing out how he sees the valve to move and how it is so important for the muscle underlying the papillary muscle, that is the posterior wall, to move properly for the apparatus to work accurately and again, this reiterated what we now, I think, must take as dogma, experimentally proven by the work of Dr. Hagl's group. Mitral insufficiency is an extremely dynamic process. It is something that even if you think you understand it either on an echocardiogram or on the Doppler or by direct inspection can be altered the very next moment by different loading conditions. I want to come back to someone who said, that simple technique of filling the valve is not really necessary. I think that, to me, if I were a surgeon, it would be the test I want to see, although I will know that the loading upon closing the chest and upon leaving the operating room may well be different. Still I would make a modeatly strong recommendation that even in the operating room loading conditions could be changed and that you might get much more information about how the operative ultimately would come out. Dr. Piwnica gave us then an excellent example of the cuisine nouvelle Francaise with a number of specific recommendations of how to improve our lot. I had the feeling that each papilla of my tongue was addressed with the finer points of care for the total system. I disagreed with him openly about the rupture, but I will come back to it when I show two more transparencles at the end. We then had Dr. Duran who talked about the four T's, which I have paraphrased slightly, I call it your expression of the total lack of understanding to time constraint, too limited visbility and the thin tissues that bother you when you had to repair the valve. Nevertheless, you showed us some very good tricks and we are, of course, in eternal debt to you for pushing on with your concepts of how to repair the valve. Dr. Swanson then talked about a large series of patients with low mortality. He talked a bit about the clinical classification and wall motion and eventually ended up with a relatively small series of 29 patients which they had done between 1984 and 1987, of which 17 were replacements, 12 repairs, and all got bypass surgery. He talked about wall motion abnormalities, which (and that fits wis all the series we heard,) mainly affect the postcrobasal wall, 73%, and the diaphragmatic region 58%. We then had the three papers from the German Heart Institute Drs. Vetter, Waibel and Siniawski. They too had a wonderful statistic of 2541 patients operated since April 1986. I was pleased to see a number of points, all be it small, pointing consistently in the direction that you would like them to go, namely repairs, good technique in the operating room, and I wish you a lot of luck in collecting more cases. Dr. Rankin has the advantage of having had a computer generaliet data base, which I helped to be born many years ago in the mid 1960s, when we talked about data base systems when I used to visit a few people at Duke, some of them known to both of us. He gave this historical perspective and then proceeded to give us some very solid hits of data from the ret when aspective analyses, again pointing out that in the survival curves the most important predictors were ejection fraction, age, presence or absence of congestive heart failure, and the number of vessels affected in coronary artery disease and only afterwards mitral regurgitation is a predictor. He had 55 patients in his more recent experience with MIMI and of those 31 were posterior muscle dysfunction kind, nine had anterior or posterior and 15 were diffuse dilatations. He ended with much technical detail which I listened to but could not really do justice to. I apologize at this time for anyone whom I may not have done justice to by abbreviating their presentation so drastically. Nevertheless, his methods of using the two surgeons versus the rest in terms of having different habits to me appeals, because this is, of course, the way critical practice evolves and I think the statisticians, and I like to make that point here strongly, ought to follow what we are doing in practice in oder to get significant interpretation.

Then we finally come to what I think in Dr. Rankin's presentation was the most important thing, namely the word reperfusion, and fortunately Dr. Baimbridge came to the rescue and mentioned it also. So I would like to end with why I think that some data, which now are in the literature, perhaps can in the future change our attitude in terms of what we should expect to be going on in the operating room. I refer to a study which has been published from the Netherlands but of which not all the details are in print, and I would like to give you some that are not in print. This is a study that was set up in 1981, by the Interuniversity Cardiology Institute in the Netherlands, (ICIN). The five hospitals, Rotterdam and Amsterdam, Maastricht and Leiden and another hospital in Rotterdam a collected 533 patients from 1981 to 1983 and these patients have been randomized to either streptokinase or control therapy. These days that would be impossible to do. The patients have been followed until recently and we have a 4-year follow-up. Now, the significance of this is that this is one of the few series on streptokinase or thrombolytic agents which there are now many in which we very carefully lokked at the clinical course of the patient over a full year after initial therapy. This is not a study in which you

209

do body-counting, as some of the large scale studies do, and they simply refer to statistic of so many less deaths and you are left in a quandary; a) what were the patients that were included, b) how did they behave under the therapy, and c) what happened to them? All you know is whether they did or not early on. The series here contains the 533 randomized patients who were all treated within 4 h with an avcrage of 2,9 h. So it comes very close to the ideal of what the animal experimentalists have told us all along, that if you go for reperfusion in avoidance of congestive heart failure, mitral regurgitation, MIMI, and whatever you have, you must be there early. Now, the Dutch patients were all treated with intracoronary streptokinase and roughly half of them even got an intravenous dose as they entered the hospital door, so in them the interval was even shorter. Of course, this is not practical and I am not advocating this study as being the model, it simply is the closest to an experimental kind of study in humans I would like to address what I think we might have wanted study, had we known more about the whole problem of MIMI. Then we probably would have designed the study differently but I can only give you indirect data at this point. Now the data were randomized to 264 controls and 269 for lysis and it was an intention to treat analysis. We see here the hospitalmortality: 26 in the control group and 14 in the lysis group, that is a highly significant difference, this is 14-day mortality. The three-year survival, and I now have the 5 year survival and you have to subtract a few percent, by the three-year there were 80% alive in the control group and 89% in the lytic group. Congestive heart failure and the occurrence of a murmur indicating mitral regurgitation are the important factors in the table I have shown. In those, who had severe ischemic conditions or shock the figures are considerably lower after lysis. This is a bit confusing. We defined shock as being hypotensive below 100, so it is not really classic cardiogenic shock and there was always a murmur. Now, if you were to take this as the condition we are talking about it would seem as if lysis early on drastically reduces that complication. An indirect bit of evidence comes from the need for Dopamine or Dobutamine, 42 in the control group, 26 in the lysis group. The need for balloon pumping was somewhat greater and I explain that by the fact that more people were kept alive in that group and then got to the pump. Congestive heart failure in the reconvalescence period, i.e., after the second week for the full follow-up, 53 vs 37, a very significant reduction. Interestingly, ventricular fibrillation showed roughly halving of the rates, despite the so-called reperfusion arrhythmlas. Very interesting is the low incidence of pericarditis and the absence of rupture. There were no ruptures in this group despite giving streptokinase. Of course, the neee for PTCA was much higher, in this group because they have returning symptoms of ischemia. Now, why do I show this? Because I think that there is some encouragement from these data to tell to the surgeons of tomorrow that if the doctors of today, Dr. Piwnica, try to avoid rupture, try to avoid an necessary myocardial tissue loss by treating much earlier, getting our system in order "on time" we may well have much less of a problem of MIMI in terms of an ischemia-induced dilatation leading to eventual destruction of the mitral valve function. That is really what I would like to end up with, and I have only one more comment and that is to you, Dr. Hetzer and Dr. Vetter thank you very much for organizing a very good conference.

Subject index